A WALK ALONG THE RIVER

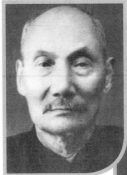

CHEN
DING-SAN

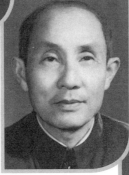

JIANG
ER-XUN

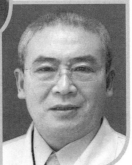

YU GUO-JUN

A WALK ALONG THE RIVER

Transmitting a Medical Lineage
through Case Records
and Discussions

YU GUO-JUN

TRANSLATED BY

Andrew Ellis / Craig Mitchell / Michael FitzGerald

EASTLAND PRESS ▶ SEATTLE

Originally published in 2006 by China Press
of Traditional Chinese Medicine as part of a larger
work entitled *Zhongyi shicheng shilu* (中医师承实录).
This English translation is authorized by the publisher.

English language edition © 2017 by Yu Guo-Jun,
Andrew Ellis, Craig Mitchell, and Michael FitzGerald
Cover photo © Jun Wei Fan

Published by Eastland Press, Inc.
P.O. Box 99749 Seattle, WA 98139, USA
www.eastlandpress.com

ISBN: 978-0-939616-85-5
Library of Congress Control Number: 2017934177

Printed in the United States of America
2   4   6   8   10   9   7   5   3   1

Cover design by Gary Niemeier and Patricia O'Connor
Book design by Gary Niemeier

Table of Contents

Translators' Foreword

Why this book?

Bookstores in China have shelves and shelves of books on Chinese medicine. A great many of these books chronicle a practitioner's experience with and thoughts about the practice of the art. What drew us to select this book and to choose, through our translation, to offer it to Western readers is its unique depth, nature, and tangible clinical utility.

The uniqueness of this work lies in Dr. Yu's decision to base the format and content of the text on records of discussions from a study group that he led. The aim of the group was to systematically study the lineage of Chinese medicine of which Dr. Yu and his teacher, Jiang Er-Xun, were a part.

The text is structured as a case study book with each case first presented in standard fashion followed by a section entitled "Differentiation of Patterns and Discussion of Treatment." It is in this section that the book begins to show its unique character, as Dr. Yu discusses the case emphasizing the following points:

1. Differentiation of disease and differentiation of pattern
2. Careful consideration of the case history, including previous treatment
3. Clear understanding of the pathodynamic
4. Consideration of both the disorder and the patient's constitution
5. Possible pitfalls in determining the pattern or disease and prescribing treatment

The physicians in the study group ask questions that lead to in-depth discussions of important aspects of the case. In concluding this section, the formula is presented, along with any follow-up treatments.

The third section of each case is called "Reflections and Clarifications." Here the physicians ask questions that delve into the deeper aspects of the case, and Dr. Yu outlines his reasoning. In the discussion he often provides an anecdote about how he learned this treatment strategy from one of his own teachers, or how his teacher came upon it. Just as often the discussion becomes a lesson about a passage from the *Discussion of Cold Damage, Inner Classic,* or other premodern text, with Dr. Yu passing on the interpretation he has received from Dr. Jiang.

This structure allows the reader to witness the process of transmission of Chinese medicine as it has been practiced for centuries. The tension between a culturally reinforced reverence for the past and the human need to adjust to current clinical realities is felt just below the surface of the case-study discussions. This tension is what has continually pulled Chinese medicine into the present tense and prevented it from becoming a static remnant of history. We witness medical knowledge passing from Dr. Jiang to Dr. Yu and on to the participants in the study group—and then to ourselves, the readers.

In the exchanges between Dr. Yu and his students, all of whom are practicing physicians, we can see the intricacies of the process that has characterized the transmission of Chinese medicine through the ages. The scientific revolution of the last few centuries has presented Chinese medicine with its biggest challenges. Modern medicine, with its emphasis on anatomy, biochemistry and microbiology, presents a world view that in many ways contradicts, or at the very least sheds doubt upon, the basic tenets of Chinese medicine. In this text we can see Dr. Yu and his students grapple with these contradictions and doubts as they participate in the traditional transmission of Chinese medicine.

Dr. Yu reminds us many times throughout the book that the proof of the pudding is in the eating. The process of medical transmission includes examining theories and methods, both ancient and modern, with the sole goal of improving clinical outcomes. We become physicians not to argue theoretical convolutions, he argues, but rather, to relieve suffering. Because Dr. Yu's goal is to emphasize the clinical application of knowledge, this text presents cases that not only deepen our understanding of the medicine we practice, but also impart lessons that are immediately applicable in the clinic. We are able to gain insights into many aspects of our practice, and in most instances these insights are applicable to cases that differ substantially from the ones presented.

Dr. Yu's theoretical discussions are always tempered with an emphasis on clinical reality. For example, in answer to a question regarding the theory in traditional medicine that posits that during the course of an externally-contracted disorder, yin patterns transform into cold and yang patterns transform into heat, he states:

> The tenet that pathogens will transform from yin into cold and from yang into heat has a certain utility to it. Nonetheless, when we are discussing the myriad changes of actual diseases, it is extremely difficult to restrict oneself to a limited framework. We have to make general categorizations, as best we can, while recognizing that these cannot capture every incident.

Few of us in the West have the opportunity to study with a doctor who is part of a living lineage. This book sheds light on that tradition, while also providing valuable clinical information that is applicable to our own practices. Because the translation of this book took several years, we had ample opportunity to try out several of Dr. Yu's clinical approaches and specific formulas on ourselves and our patients. The exceptional efficacy we experienced with these formulas and approaches has reinforced our original enthusiasm about the book and amplified our eagerness to present this information to other Western practitioners.

Dr. Yu Guo-Jun

Dr. Yu was born in Sichuan province in 1946. He attended the Southwestern University of Finance and Economics in Chengdu where he majored in economics. Sent down to the countryside during the Cultural Revolution, Dr. Yu learned Chinese medicine there the traditional way—as an apprentice. Dr. Yu studied the fundamentals of Chinese medicine with the well-known Sichuanese practitioner Dr. Jian Yu-Guang. Dr. Jian was a student of the modern-day master of classic formulas, Jiang Er-Xun, with whom Dr. Yu continued his studies. Despite lacking any institutional training in medicine, Dr. Yu became a practitioner at the Leshan Hospital (where he remains active to this day), and over time, took over the advanced seminars that Dr. Jiang had been teaching. As noted above, these seminars were the genesis of this text.

Translation approach

The first step in each translation project is to consider the original text and to develop an approach that will best bring the author's work into the target language. When the source and target languages differ as much as Chinese and English do, this task is particularly important. Early on it became clear to us that this work would require a unique and accommodating translational approach. There were several reasons that a direct word for word or even sentence for sentence translation would fall short. The first and strongest reason is that we felt it was the only way to preserve the colloquial nature and informal tone of the text. Below we discuss some less obvious factors that led us to flexible translation. These factors reflected our decision to consider the target audience, emphasize readability, and take advantage of the internet age.

1. *Considering the target audience*

The target audience for the original book was Chinese practitioners of Chinese medicine. The knowledge base and cultural perspective of this audience differ in important ways from the translated text's target audience of Western practitioners of Chinese medicine.

For example, there are several instances in the text where Dr. Yu or one of the questioning practitioners mentions a theory or concept that is well-known to the Chinese medicine community in China, but perhaps not as well-known to Western-trained practitioners. In these instances we took the liberty to work a brief explanation of the theory or concept into the text of the question or answer. We of course consulted Dr. Yu about this and he wholeheartedly supported this approach. The translators and Dr. Yu all agreed that this was preferable to a footnote or editor's note, as this technique fits the didactic nature of the text and minimizes any disruption in the flow.

2. *Emphasizing readability*

There are many phrases that sound elegant in Chinese, but when strictly translated, give the English reader pause. Some of this is cultural. For example, references to emperors, jade, white tigers, and pagodas elicit quite different things in the Chinese and Western mind.

For the Chinese they draw up clear images and feelings associated with their cultural past. To Westerners they are very foreign and even exotic.

Literal renderings of some Chinese phrases sound quaint or strange in English, or seem to reinforce cultural stereotypes. Most of the time, the phrases themselves are almost like punctuation to the Chinese reader and are seen as "just the way we say things" or "the way educated people write." But when translated into English in a literal fashion, they often appear awkward and, in some cases, pedantic. The educated Chinese person's use of adages serves as a good example.

A Chinese adage (成語 *chéng yǔ*) is a four or eight character saying that has an historical basis and in many cases is a concise allusion to an entire story or a succinct quotation from a literary classic. Adages are used in the same way an English speaker uses a phrase from one of Aesop's fables or a line from a famous poem. Just as "sour grapes" can be used to express the meaning of pretending that one doesn't want something, when in reality that thing is unobtainable to them, and "The best laid plans o' Mice an' Men" can bring to mind thoughts of life's painful ironies, so too can a Chinese adage concisely imply a complex situation or concept.

The difference between Chinese and English in this regard is that Chinese has thousands of these adages and they are the focus of a significant amount of class time in school. It is not uncommon for an educated person to pepper his or her writing with them, even stringing several, one after another, in a four-word cadence that adds emphasis to the point being made.

It takes considerable effort to render consecutive adages into comprehensible English. Even if the effort is somewhat successful at representing the writer's meaning, it can make for stilted English full of mixed metaphors. While we took this as a challenge in some instances, in most cases of multiple contiguous adages in the text, we read the sentence, extracted the meaning, and re-wrote the sentence to make what we hope is smooth English that carries as much of the meaning and tone of the original as possible.

The goal of the translation approach we have utilized here is to place the reader into the room with Dr. Yu and his students. We hope that in this way, author, translator, and reader become linked together in the process of lineage transmission.

3. *Take advantage of the internet age*

In the past, it was rare that the translator of a Chinese medicine text was able to communicate easily with the author of the text. Often the author was no longer alive, or there was great physical distance between the author and the translator. Certainly, translators used traditional mail to pose questions to the author, but correspondence was usually confined to general questions and those that did not require multiple clarifications. With the advent of instant communication through the internet, a translator can now ask for clarification from the author and receive an instantaneous response. The types of questions we had the opportunity to ask of Dr. Yu ranged from queries about suspected typographical errors to issues related to translation or theoretical concepts. Internet communication was immensely helpful in reducing potential errors.

This communication, along with the several visits we made to Leshan (and Dr. Yu's visit to the United States), resulted in many differences between our translation and the original Chinese text. We discussed this with Dr. Yu and he confirmed that we should in no way be confined to the Chinese text. Thus, through our frequent communication, the English version of the text became an updated version of the Chinese one. The original Chinese text was published in 2006. Dr. Yu has undergone over ten years of additional experience since that time and he encouraged us to incorporate what he learned in the meantime into the English version. This meant that we have omitted some things that are in the Chinese text because Dr. Yu instructed us that he no longer used those methods or formulas, and that we have replaced them with his present thinking. Further, several times in the process of explaining a point to us, Dr. Yu mentioned something that, although not in the Chinese text, we felt would add a lot to the book, so we chose to include it. In addition, there were occasions when, as practitioners, we had questions about the material. When Dr. Yu answered our questions we felt that we should share that information with readers, so we included many of these questions and Dr. Yu's answers in the book. For example, in the chapter on the treatment of herpes zoster in the Chinese version, there is no mention of the treatment of post-herpetic nerve pain. We inquired about this, and Dr. Yu then shared with us what he usually did to treat this condition. We entered this question as a practitioner question in the discussion section of the case, and then detailed Dr. Yu's response.

We hope that it is clear that the choices we made in translation and editorial methods were designed to enhance the reader's experience and to bring the Chinese text smoothly into English.

For the translation of technical terms we have, by and large, taken a much more structured approach and followed the glossary of Eastland Press which is available at the 'Resources' tab of the Eastland Press website. Where the text required us to translate a character or phrase that was not in the glossary, or for which the glossary did not have a translation that fit the circumstance, we consulted other glossaries, most notably *A Practical Dictionary of Chinese Medicine* (2nd ed.) by Nigel Wiseman and Feng Ye, or determined our own renderings.

Lastly, for us, the most rewarding aspect of translating this book was the opportunity to work with Dr. Yu. It is hard to describe the enchantment of spending time with a person who is steeped in the culture and history of Chinese medicine and is completely open to sharing his knowledge and experience, someone who treats everyone he meets with care and respect. Dr. Yu's deep regard for the process of transmission of Chinese medicine and culture is evident in everything he does. He clearly delights in the mysteries of the medicine he practices and the world in which he lives. This delight has infected us and we hope it shines through our efforts in this book.

About the title of this book

The Chinese title is:

中醫   師承   實錄

Chinese Medicine   Received from Teacher   Clinical Record

This title has sophistication and clear meaning in Chinese that is extremely difficult to render into English. We decided to use the Chinese title as the English subtitle:

Transmitting a Medical Lineage through Case Records and Discussions

We chose the main title, *A Walk Along the River,* to convey what could not be expressed in the literal translation: the idea that this book is in essence a brief, edifying stroll along the banks of a living Chinese medicine current.

This title seemed particularly apropos to us since a visit with Dr. Yu inevitably includes a walk with him along the picturesque river that cuts through his home town of Leshan. It is a well-known location as, towering over the river on the opposite shore, is the largest statue of Buddha in China.

■ ACKNOWLEDGEMENTS

Andrew Ellis I was surprised when Dan Bensky of Eastland Press agreed to this project, as we had worked together on two previous endeavors. Obviously, he thought that publishing this book would be worth putting up with me for one more effort. For that I am very grateful. My back and forth with Dan during the editing process was great fun and a truly enriching experience. I want to thank Craig Mitchell and Michael FitzGerald for their hard work and for providing enthusiasm and scholarship during the several years it took to complete this project. If they had not signed up for this work you would not be holding this book in your hands. John O'Connor, as always, was a joy to work with; thanks John.

When I discovered this book and brought it to Dan for consideration, I had no idea that it would lead me to develop a close relationship with a gentleman of such high character as Dr. Yu. In the Chinese medicine field it is rare indeed to find a person so willing to share his thoughts and experiences. Furthermore, Dr. Yu took all of us into his life like we were long-lost kin. This truly was a blessing.

Craig Mitchell I would like to thank Andy Ellis for many years of guidance and friendship. You always seem to find the best books! I would like to thank Dan Bensky for his wise counsel and supportive engagement. Your mentoring and friendship have enabled me to succeed. To Michael FitzGerald, well done and on to the next project. To Marguerite, your love and support make all things possible.

Michael FitzGerald I would like to thank Dan and John at Eastland Press for their support of this project, and receptiveness to some of my ideas. Also Andy Ellis, who I have known since the beginning of my journey in Chinese medicine. I am grateful for your support and value your insights and the many discussions we have had over the years about Chinese medicine, both mundane and profound. Craig, it's been great working with you on this project and I hope we have more opportunities to do so in the future. And finally, I would like to thank my wife, whose support I depend on in so many ways.

Preface

Clinical Reasoning in Chinese Medicine[1]

Using Ephedra, Asarum, and Aconite Accessory Root Decoction *(má huáng xì xīn fù zǐ tāng)* to demonstrate approaches to applying classical formulas

Ephedra, Asarum, and Aconite Accessory Root Decoction *(má huáng xì xīn fù zǐ tāng)*, from the *Discussion of Cold Damage (Shāng hán lùn)*, is an effective formula for the treatment of combined *tài yáng* and *shào yīn* disease. Line 301 of that text states: "At the onset of a *shào yīn* disease, if unexpectedly there is feverishness and a sinking pulse, Ephedra, Asarum, and Aconite Accessory Root Decoction *(má huáng xì xīn fù zǐ tāng)* governs." The late 17th-century text *Versified Prescriptions (Tāng tóu gē jué)* notes: "Ephedra, Asarum, and Aconite Accessory Root Decoction *(má huáng xì xīn fù zǐ tāng)* excels at discharging exterior conditions and warming the channels. If one fails to treat exterior and interior simultaneously, one cannot address fever in *shào yīn* disease."

The fundamental pathodynamic of combined *tài yáng* and *shào yīn* disease is an externally-contracted cold pathogen attacking a patient who concurrently suffers from yang deficiency of both the Heart and Kidneys. Ephedrae Herba *(má huáng)* discharges exterior conditions and disperses cold. Aconiti Radix lateralis praeparata *(zhì fù zǐ)* warms the Kidneys and strengthens the Heart. Asari Radix et Rhizoma *(xì xīn)* tracks down and digs out, while warming and dispersing, cold pathogens that have entered deeply into the *shào yīn*.

....

1. *Translators' note:* In this preface, Dr. Yu prepares the reader for what is to come by introducing one of the main concepts he learned from his predecessors: that the efficacy of a formula is related to the underlying pattern for which it is prescribed, and that successful treatment requires accurately targeting the pathodynamic. When the pathodynamic that a formula addresses is properly understood, the practitioner can flexibly use the formula to treat many different, ostensibly unrelated, disorders.

Although the formula contains only three herbs, its elegant construction makes it highly effective. The many opportunities to use this formula in the clinic extend far beyond those few presented in the source text. The formula can be applied to a wide range of conditions in all branches of medicine including pediatrics, gynecology, internal medicine, external medicine and specialties such as eye, ear, nose, and throat.

I have seen two main problems with the application of this formula. First, many physicians are afraid to use it simply because of the harsh nature of the three herbs in the formula. Second, some physicians see a case in which the formula seems appropriate yet insist on adding so many additional substances that it becomes unrecognizable. Is it any wonder that the formula's efficacy is reduced or nonexistent?

These physicians then, instead of considering the error in their own thinking, complain that classical formulas are difficult to use. I say that a carpenter who wants to do good work must first sharpen his tools. In that spirit, I would like to offer a few cases and some discussion of several ways of thinking about the clinical application of this formula in the hopes of sparking further dialogue about its use.

1. *Formula-Pattern Correspondence*

A distinguishing feature of the works of Zhang Zhong-Jing is formula-pattern correspondence, which is also referred to as formula-based pattern identification. The supposition of formula-pattern correspondence is that upon observing specific characteristic symptoms that match those described in the source text, one can directly use the corresponding formula without the limitations and restrictions of modern pattern identification and treatment determination. This method is a way to replicate the clinical experience of Zhang Zhong-Jing and to take a shortcut to effective treatment. The following is an example of this approach.

In March of 1992, I treated a 62-year-old man who, for the previous three days, had felt generalized chills that were most severe on his back. The chills were accompanied by fatigue and a desire to sleep. Falling asleep, however, was difficult. The patient was thin, had an ashen complexion, and a long history of smoking, as well as emphysema. Three years prior, following an X-ray that showed an area of shadow in his lungs, there was concern about a tumor. However, following treatment with antibiotics, the abnormality on the X-ray disappeared. Since that time, three or four times each year he had episodes during which he felt chilled and desired sleep. The symptoms were severe enough that they entailed a hospital stay for two weeks to a month each time. In the hospital he received blood transfusions and intravenous fluids, including treatments with antibiotics, vitamins, and inosine. After such treatment he would gradually recover and be able to leave the hospital. His Western diagnosis was emphysema and severe common cold.

When the current episode began the patient reflected with trepidation upon the thought of the swelling, distention, and discomfort that resulted from having an intravenous line placed in the back of his hand. He decided to treat his illness using Chinese herbs, stipulating that if this was unsuccessful, he would to return to the hospital.

Intake Examination

His temperature was 36.8C (98.2F). He was listless, fatigued, and desired sleep. His appetite was adequate, his tongue was pale with a thin, white coating, and his pulse was sunken and fine.

Line 281 in the *Discussion of Cold Damage (Shāng hán lùn)*, a synopsis of the key characteristics of *shào yīn* disorders, states that *"Shào yīn disease consists of a pulse that is faint and fine with a desire to just sleep."* From the time this patient's illness began, he experienced generalized chills, fatigue, desire to sleep, and his pulse was fine and sunken. This presentation clearly belongs to a pattern of a cold pathogen directly striking the *shào yīn,* and the signs and symptoms correspond to those described in the synopsis.

I had not previously been involved in his care at the hospital, so I was in no way restricted by previous ideas about his presentation or treatment. I decided to follow formula-pattern correspondence. I prescribed Ephedra, Asarum, and Aconite Accessory Root Decoction *(má huáng xì xīn fù zǐ tāng)* to warm the channels and to release the pathogen from the exterior.

Because of his age, infirmity, and the fact that he had been sick for three days, I was concerned about copious sweating damaging the normal qi. Thus, I decided to use prepared Ephedrae Herba *(zhì má huáng)* to gently release the pathogen from the exterior and to add Glycyrrhizae Radix praeparata *(zhì gān cǎo)* in order to support the normal qi.

    prepared Ephedrae Herba *(zhì má huáng)* 10g
    Aconiti Radix lateralis praeparata *(zhì fù zǐ)*
       [precook for 30 minutes] 15g
    Asari Radix et Rhizoma *(xì xīn)*.. 6g
    Glycyrrhizae Radix praeparata *(zhì gān cǎo)* 6g

After one packet, although the patient did not sweat, the chills, fatigue, and desire to sleep all gradually abated. His spirit improved significantly as well. Upon follow-up one year later, the patient reported that the illness had not recurred.

2. *Determining the Method by Observing the Disease Dynamic*

Chapter 74 of *Basic Questions (Sù wèn)* notes: "Carefully monitor the disease dynamics and in each case manage what [signs and symptoms] are associated with it. When [signs and symptoms] are present, investigate them. When [signs and symptoms] are absent, investigate them."

In order to "carefully monitor the disease dynamic" one must first accurately determine what it is. The physician must use all available tools to carefully gather information from the patient using a holistic perspective and considering the results of the four examinations. All of this information must be analyzed to determine the disease dynamic, so that one can then choose an effective formula.

The disease dynamic associated with Ephedra, Asarum, and Aconite Accessory Root Decoction *(má huáng xì xīn fù zǐ tāng)* is Heart and Kidney yang deficiency with a simultaneous externally-contracted cold pathogen. This analysis relates to cases in which there is an externally-contracted illness. In the absence of an externally-contracted illness, the disease dynamic for this formula is yang deficiency and cold congealing internally.

If a physician does a careful investigation of the case, arriving at such a diagnosis is not particularly difficult. In cases in which the patient is not present and the information is received in writing, making the determination is more difficult.

For example, in September 1993, following the publication of an article that I wrote about the treatment of severe calf pain, I received a letter from a Dr. Fan, who is a physician in Jiangsu province. The physician's wife had experienced many years of pain in her right knee, resulting from an injury to the knee more than ten years before. The Western diagnosis was damage to the collateral ligaments of the right knee with evidence of mild bone hyperplasia in the proximal tip of the tibia.

The patient had considered surgery for her knee but in discussions with the surgeon it was determined that because of her age (44), the odds were not good for an optimal surgical outcome. Thus, she decided to try to control her pain through the use of Chinese medicine.

I read the letter many times but still my mind was blank and I had no idea where to begin. Several formulas came to mind but none of them seemed quite right. Nevertheless, I felt compelled to prescribe something and so I turned to a formula that I have frequently used for painful obstruction patterns, Cinnamon Twig, Peony, and Anemarrhena Decoction *(guì zhī sháo yào zhī mǔ tāng)*. I also mentioned to Dr. Fan that, because the information I had was incomplete, there was no way to be entirely clear about the disease dynamic, and therefore, by extension, it was difficult to feel confident about the diagnosis. I hoped that he would be able to continue to gather more information about the patient and her progress.

On October 13th, I received a letter from Dr. Fan informing me that the patient had taken six packets of the formula to no effect. The patient's lower legs were sore and heavy. Her knees were swollen and distended and were particularly painful upon palpation. There was evidence of mild atrophy in the flesh of the right knee. For the previous two days, she had engaged in outside work and had noticed that afterward, walking was difficult. Her complexion lacked luster and her tongue was pale-red with a white coating primarily at the root of the tongue. Her pulse was soggy and lax. The painful areas improved with heat and worsened with cold.

I surmised that the disease dynamic was one of yang deficiency with congealing cold. I decided to prescribe a modified Ephedra, Asarum, and Aconite Accessory Root Decoction *(má huáng xì xīn fù zǐ tāng)* in a large dose.

Ephedrae Herba *(má huáng)*.. 30g
Asari Radix et Rhizoma *(xì xīn)*.. 20g
Aconiti Radix lateralis praeparata *(zhì fù zǐ)*
    [precooked for one hour].. 50g
Rehmanniae Radix praeparata *(shú dì huáng)* 60g

On December 30th, I received another letter from Dr. Fan. He wrote, "The formula that you sent for my wife worked very well! After six packets, the pain in her right knee had disappeared completely and her knee seems like new. Even after intense physical exertion, she experiences no discomfort!" He went on to say, "After having seen several cases, it appears that Ephedra, Asarum, and Aconite Accessory Root Decoction *(má huáng xì xīn fù zǐ tāng)* has exceptional efficacy for lumbar and leg pain." In fact, what Dr. Fan refers to as "exceptional efficacy" is actually just more evidence of how important it is to understand the disease dynamic prior to selecting the formula. A doctor selecting a formula without having a deep understanding of the disease dynamic is akin to a blind person attempting to navigate an unknown path.

3. *Using the Patient's Constitution in Pattern Differentiation*

A person's constitution comprises congenital and post-natal aspects. Also, from a five-phase perspective, each person has strong and weak natural endowments. The *Inner Classic* records that people can be categorized according to the six channels, and also on the basis of the five phases. All of these categorizations can help us understand a person's psychology, physiology, and pathology. These ideas can also assist us in determining the correct course of treatment.

In the *Discussion of Cold Damage (Shāng hán lùn)*, the references to "drinkers," "patients with painful dribbling urination," and "patients with spontaneous external bleeding" should also be considered to be within this category of assessment. Over the generations, many physicians have emphasized the consideration of constitution in pattern differentiation. Zhang Xi-Chun is an example of a modern physician who emphasized the use of patient constitution in the process of pattern differentiation and who wrote about this process with some particularity. Moreover, his work stands up to analysis and testing in the clinic.

In his *Essays on Medicine Esteeming the Chinese and Respecting the Western (Yī xúe zhōng zhōng cān xī lù)* from the early 20th century, Dr. Zhang wrote that:

> When considering patients with an external contraction, we must consider the differences in inherited nature. When two patients contract a seasonal illness, maybe even at the same time or in the same place, they will still manifest differences in the extent to which the disease is tending toward cool or hot. When a patient has accumulated heat or cold within the body, an externally-contracted disease contacting the body will exacerbate that heat or cold respectively.

Patients for whom Ephedra, Asarum, and Aconite Accessory Root Decoction *(má huáng xì xīn fù zǐ tāng)* is appropriate have a constitutional tendency toward yang deficiency. Whenever I treat patients for externally-contracted wind-cold, I keep in mind the concept of a constitutional tendency toward yang deficiency as a possibility. This habit has increased the times that I have effectively utilized Ephedra, Asarum, and Aconite Accessory Root Decoction *(má huáng xì xīn fù zǐ tāng)*.

In the winter of 1991, I treated a 47-year-old man with a month-long recurrent common cold. He had tried formulas such as Ginseng Powder to Overcome Pathogenic Influences *(rén shēn bài dú sǎn)*, Minor Bupleurum Decoction *(xiǎo chái hú tāng)*, Cinnamon Twig Decoction *(guì zhī tāng)*, and Jade Windscreen Powder *(yù píng fēng sǎn)*, all without effect.

INTAKE EXAMINATION

His sleep and food intake were normal. He was able to work. In the afternoon and the evening, however, the middle of his back became cold. He avoided exposing his head and face to wind and had clear nasal discharge. His tongue was pale-red with a thin, white coating.

His pulse was slightly weak. Given that there were no obvious signs of yang deficiency, I did not understand why the formulas mentioned above had been ineffective.

Upon careful questioning, I discovered that not only did he have a persistent backache, but that also he feared exposing his abdomen to cold and that he was averse to eating cold food, even in the summer months. Without a doubt, these symptoms are associated with yang deficiency. I gave him Ephedra, Asarum, and Aconite Accessory Root Decoction *(má huáng xì xīn fù zǐ tāng)*.

> Ephedrae Herba *(má huáng)*... 15g
> Asari Radix et Rhizoma *(xì xīn)*...................................... 15g
> Aconiti Radix lateralis praeparata *(zhì fù zǐ)*
> [precook for 30 minutes[2]].. 30g

After just one packet, all his symptoms resolved.

Thinking back about my time studying in Chengdu thirty years ago, I recall a Professor Liu who was quite good at medicine. Nonetheless, he suffered from persistent insomnia, and although he had tried many formulas, the results were mediocre. Needless to say, he suffered greatly.

We had heard about an older physician in the city who was quite famous. This doctor had been seeing patients for years, and no matter the patient's complaint, no matter the age or the gender, the initial formula always seemed to be Ephedra, Asarum, and Aconite Accessory Root Decoction *(má huáng xì xīn fù zǐ tāng)*. His shop was busy as a market and his clinic was constantly full of patients, often more than a hundred at a time. He was known as the "Fire God Buddha" around town. Professor Liu decided to give him a try. Upon entering the office, the doctor asked to see his tongue. Immediately after observing it, he prescribed Ephedra, Asarum, and Aconite Accessory Root Decoction *(má huáng xì xīn fù zǐ tāng)*. Professor Liu was originally quite angry, but upon further reflection he decided to put it to the test for a packet or two. Surprisingly, that night, after just one packet, he slept soundly.

Because I too was so surprised by this event, I went out and spoke with some of the doctor's other patients. It seemed that although there were some cases in which he was unsuccessful, his efficacy rate was quite high. It turned out that the secret to his success lay in his examination of the tongue. As long as there were no clear signs of heat on the tongue, he would always use Ephedra, Asarum, and Aconite Accessory Root Decoction *(má huáng xì xīn fù zǐ tāng)*. This strategy reminds me of the Ming-dynasty physician Zhang Jie-Bin. As long as there were no obvious signs of heat, he would always use warm, tonifying formulas.

I have related the story of this physician not because I think much of a method that ignores the results of the four examinations and is obviously over-simplified and formulaic, but because it illustrates that the range of applications for Ephedra, Asarum, and Aconite Accessory Root Decoction *(má huáng xì xīn fù zǐ tāng)* is quite large and that there are many opportunities to use it. If one pays careful attention to these methods of clinical analysis, the results will be excellent.

....

2. *Translators' note:* At present, Dr. Yu recommends that this dosage of Aconiti Radix lateralis praeparata *(zhì fù zǐ)* should be precooked for 60 minutes.

INTERNAL MEDICINE

CHAPTER 1

Lung System Disorders

1.1 Colds

A two-month-long cold

Exclusive teachings from a modern master of classical formulas

現代經方大師傳授獨家心法

■ CASE HISTORY

Patient: *39-year-old woman*

Two months prior to coming to the clinic, the patient, after having been exposed to cold temperatures, began having chills and fever. She took medication (first Western drugs and then Chinese herbs) but did not improve. Due to the fact that the external cold pathogen had not resolved, heat gradually began to increase in her interior and her fever rose to 39.2°C (102.6°F). She then went to the hospital where she was given an intravenous drip as well as an oral administration of acetaminophen. She eventually broke a sweat and her fever abated. Shortly afterwards, however, her fever returned and she continued in this state for another seven days.

The patient was then diagnosed by a doctor of Chinese medicine as having a wind-heat common cold and was given three doses of a modified Honeysuckle and Forsythia Powder *(yín qiáo sǎn)*. After taking the formula her temperature dropped to 37.5°C (99.5°F) but she began to sweat profusely, became fatigued, was short of breath, and had loose stools.

The patient sought out a second opinion from another Chinese medicine doctor and was diagnosed as having a qi deficiency common cold. She was given a modification of

Tonify the Middle to Augment the Qi Decoction *(bǔ zhōng yì qì tāng)*, which she said was not markedly effective. As a result, the patient was unwilling to take any more Chinese medicine and simply continued with an intravenous drip coupled with vitamins, inosine, and protein powder. Her temperature fluctuated between 37.3°C and 37.8°C (99.1°F–100°F) for the next two months.

INTAKE EXAMINATION
DATE: August 27, 2002

The patient had a low fever (37.2°C–98.96°F), pale complexion, generalized soreness and weakness, shortness of breath, fatigue, and a slight aversion to wind and cold. She also reported that she was feverish at night, had night sweats, wasn't eating as much as she normally did, had a faint bitter taste in her mouth, and that her bowel movements were somewhat loose. Her tongue was slightly pale, and the coating was thin, white, and greasy. Her pulse was floating and weak, beating five beats per breath.

DIFFERENTIATION OF PATTERNS AND DISCUSSION OF TREATMENT

DR. YU   This patient, whose low fever persisted for two months, can be diagnosed as having a deficiency-type patient's common cold. Such cases involve a deficiency of normal qi, a lingering pathogen, and an inhibited pivot. Treatment centers on a modification of Bupleurum and Cinnamon Twig Decoction *(chái hú guì zhī tāng)*. This assessment is based on the experience of my teacher, Jiang Er-Xun, a modern expert on classical formulas. Forty years ago, when the first graduate students from the Chengdu University of TCM came to our hospital as interns, Dr. Jiang, without the slightest hesitation, passed on to them this jewel of his experience.

PHYSICIAN A   How do we determine if a person is a deficiency-type patient?

DR. YU   A deficiency-type patient is someone whose qi, blood, yin or yang is noticeably deficient. This is the type of person referred to in the *Discussion of Cold Damage (Shāng hán lùn)* when it warns against promoting sweating in those who frequently perspire, have repeated nosebleeds, or who have lost a great deal of blood. It is not difficult to identify patients with such deficiency if a thorough examination employing the four diagnostic methods (observation, inquiry, listening, and palpation) is performed. This is true regardless of whether the deficiency is related to a person's innate constitution or results from long-term illness.

PHYSICIAN B   In reference to the above categories mentioned in the *Discussion of Cold Damage (Shāng hán lùn)*—those who frequently perspire, have repeated nosebleeds, or suffer from blood loss—it seems to me that, practically speaking, those examples refer to unique cases. Furthermore, in this patient's case it is not difficult to identify her deficiency, given that she had a low fever for two months, she took both Western and Chinese medicine without noted improvement, and had a number of signs that indicated she was weak. However, in cases when a patient is in the beginning stages of the common cold, or in any ordinary patient with the common cold, how do we determine whether the individual is or is not a deficiency-type patient?

DR. YU The answer is that you need experience. What kind of experience? First, Chinese medicine etiology can be summed up in the following two tenets:

1. The cause of an illness can be known by how it manifests.

2. Determine the cause of an illness by examining the patterns.

The first principle simply means that the nature and pathway of a contracted pathogen can be deduced from how the illness manifests, develops, and changes. The second principle refers to the search for the cause of an illness and determination of the pattern type through the analysis and organization of information gathered from the four diagnostic methods.

Taking these unique investigative methods of Chinese medicine's approach to etiology and adapting them to Chinese medicine's study of the physical constitution, I coined the following tenets:

1. A person's constitution can be known by how an illness manifests.

2. Determine a person's constitution by examining the patterns.

By developing the ability to understand and differentiate body types, one will gain insight into what is called deficiency. Of course, mastering this kind of thinking takes years of focused clinical observation, noting similarities and differences between patients. One must constantly reflect on the clues gathered and learn to give credence to one's insights. Such abilities certainly don't develop overnight.

TREATMENT AND OUTCOME

The patient was diagnosed with a pattern of deficiency-type patient's common cold, with deficiency of normal qi, a lingering pathogen, and an inhibited pivot. She was given a modification of the formula drawn from the *Discussion of Cold Damage* (*Shāng hán lùn*), Bupleurum and Cinnamon Twig Decoction (*chái hú guì zhī tāng*):

Bupleuri Radix *(chái hú)*	15g
Scutellariae Radix *(huáng qín)*	10g
standard Pinelliae Rhizoma praeparatum *(fǎ bàn xià)*	12g
Cinnamomi Ramulus *(guì zhī)*	15g
Paeoniae Radix alba *(bái sháo)*	15g
Glycyrrhizae Radix *(gān cǎo)*	5g
Zingiberis Rhizoma recens *(shēng jiāng)*	10g
Jujubae Fructus *(dà zǎo)*	10g
Poria *(fú líng)*	20g
Agrimoniae Herba *(xiān hè cǎo)*	50g
Puerariae Radix *(gé gēn)*	30g

After three doses the patient felt much better, was no longer sensitive to wind and cold, and her nighttime feverishness and night sweats had greatly diminished. Her temperature was 36.9°C (98.4°F).

The formula was then changed to Six-Gentlemen Decoction (*liù jūn zǐ tāng*) with Jade Windscreen Powder (*yù píng fēng sǎn*) plus Mori Folium (*sāng yè*) and Agrimoniae Herba (*xiān hè cǎo*), after which the patient fully recovered. She was then given pills of Tonify the Middle to Augment the Qi Decoction *(bǔ zhōng yì qì tāng)* to take for one month to further strengthen her constitution.

Disease	Primary Symptoms	Pattern Differentiation	Treatment Method	Formula
Deficiency-type patient's common cold	Low fever, slight chills, generalized soreness and weakness	Deficient normal qi with a lingering pathogen, and an inhibited pivot dynamic	Resolve the pivot dynamic, support the normal qi and expel the pathogen	Bupleurum and Cinnamon Twig Decoction *(chái hú guì zhī tāng)*

REFLECTIONS AND CLARIFICATIONS

PHYSICIAN A   We students have noticed that the formulas you most frequently use for deficiency-type patients who have a common cold are Ephedra, Asarum, and Aconite Accessory Root Decoction *(má huáng xì xīn fù zǐ tāng)*, Minor Bupleurum Decoction *(xiǎo chái hú tāng)*, and Bupleurum and Cinnamon Twig Decoction *(chái hú guì zhī tāng)*. Since you have already written on the use of Ephedra, Asarum, and Aconite Accessory Root Decoction *(má huáng xì xīn fù zǐ tāng)*, could you please give us a clear overview of your experience using Minor Bupleurum Decoction *(xiǎo chái hú tāng)* and Bupleurum and Cinnamon Twig Decoction *(chái hú guì zhī tāng)*?

DR. YU   Some time ago there was a group of students with a solid grasp of the fundamentals of Chinese medicine who were studying with Dr. Jiang. Often they would candidly ask challenging questions of him. For example, on one occasion a student asked:

> When formula books discuss the treatment of common colds in deficiency-type patients, they center on the patient's deficiency of qi, blood, yin or yang, and suggest treatment that adds substances that boost the qi, nourish the blood, enrich the yin, or assist the yang to commonly used formulas for resolving the exterior. However, you use one formula, Minor Bupleurum Decoction *(xiǎo chái hú tāng)*, to treat all deficiency-type patients suffering from the common cold. What is the reasoning behind this approach?

Dr. Jiang answered:

> The causes and pathodynamics of *shào yáng* disease parallel those found in a deficiency-type patient with a common cold. This is explained by Zhang Zhong-Jing in his discussion of the *shào yáng* pattern in line 97 of the *Discussion of Cold Damage (Shāng hán lùn)*, "If the blood is weak, the qi expended, and the pores and interstices open, pathogenic qi can enter and contend with the normal qi."
>
> In these circumstances inducing sweating is contraindicated, so Minor Bupleurum Decoction *(xiǎo chái hú tāng)* can take care of all such cases. Minor Bupleurum Decoction *(xiǎo chái hú tāng)* contains Ginseng Radix *(rén shēn)* or Codonopsis Radix *(dǎng shēn)*, Glycyrrhizae Radix *(gān cǎo)*, and Jujubae Fructus *(dà zǎo)*. These herbs boost the middle burner Spleen-earth and generate qi and blood. This is the basis for overcoming pathogens. When combined with Bupleuri Radix *(chái hú)*, Scutellariae Radix *(huáng qín)*, standard Pinelliae Rhizoma praeparatum *(fǎ bàn xià)*, and Zingiberis Rhizoma recens *(shēng jiāng)*, these herbs can expel the pathogen from the pivot of *shào yáng* to the exterior

via the qi of the *tài yáng*. This is a subtle and masterly way to simultaneously support the normal qi and expel the pathogen.

In this exchange between Dr. Jiang and his pupil, the student's question was well thought out and cut to the heart of the matter. Dr. Jiang's response was authoritative, citing the *Discussion of Cold Damage (Shāng hán lùn)* to make his point. Chinese medicine contains various schools of thought and there are always differences of opinion about theoretical approaches. That is why Chinese medicine's viability as a treatment modality is dependent on its ability to get results. Consequently, clinical efficacy is the sole standard for evaluating its theories.

PHYSICIAN A   Minor Bupleurum Decoction *(xiǎo chái hú tāng)* is the primary formula for treating *shào yáng* disease and Dr. Jiang said that Minor Bupleurum Decoction *(xiǎo chái hú tāng)* can treat all cases of deficient people with a common cold. Can we then turn that around and say that all deficient people with the common cold have *shào yáng* disease?

DR. YU   Once, one of Dr. Jiang's students posed a similar question: "In most cases, symptoms associated with the early stages of a common cold could be classified as *tài yáng* disease. Why is it that the common cold in a deficiency-type patient is classified as *shào yáng* disease?"

Dr. Jiang responded by saying:

> The protective qi and exterior of a deficiency-type patient are not secure. Consequently, external pathogens can invade and directly enter the interstices and pores. The interstices and pores are within the scope of *shào yáng*. Consequently, even though there are signs of a *tài yáng* exterior pattern, such a pattern is merely the branch of the illness. Even though there may not be signs of a genuine *shào yáng* pattern or of an altered pattern, invariably the interstices and pores are empty and open so there is a struggle between the pathogenic qi and the normal qi. Hence, we can utilize the functions of Minor Bupleurum Decoction *(xiǎo chái hú tāng)* to eliminate the pathogen from the pivot of *shào yáng* out to the qi of *tài yáng*, and consequently, the *tài yáng* branch signs can be eliminated. It is important to remember that Minor Bupleurum Decoction *(xiǎo chái hú tāng)* first appears in the *Discussion of Cold Damage (Shāng hán lùn)* in the chapter on *tài yáng* disease. It can be used to treat the patterns of all channel diseases and isn't just a formula for treating *shào yáng* disease.

PHYSICIAN A   In stating this you are saying that for Dr. Jiang to prescribe Minor Bupleurum Decoction *(xiǎo chái hú tāng)* for deficient people with a common cold, the patient need not have the symptoms that are characteristic of a *shào yáng* pattern such as alternating fever and chills, fullness and discomfort in the chest and lateral costal areas, sullenness and lack of appetite, irritability, and vomiting. It is also not what Zhang Zhong-Jing was referring to at line 101 of the *Discussion of Cold Damage (Shāng hán lùn)*: "[W]hen there is a Bupleurum presentation, if just one sign is present, then that is it; it is not necessary that all be present." Instead, it seems that Dr. Jiang's prescription of Minor Bupleurum Decoction *(xiǎo chái hú tāng)* is based on the etiology and pathodynamic of a common cold in someone who is deficient. This is indeed a unique approach.

How about Bupleurum and Cinnamon Twig Decoction *(chái hú guì zhī tāng)*? Line 146 of the *Discussion of Cold Damage (Shāng hán lùn)* says: "Cold damage for six or seven days with feverishness, slight chills, annoyingly painful joints of the limbs, mild vomiting, and knots of the supports below the heart [mean] that the external pattern has not yet gone: Bupleurum and Cinnamon Twig Decoction *(chái hú guì zhī tāng)* governs it." This passage describes a situation where the pathogen has already entered the *shào yáng* but the external pattern of *tài yáng* has not been resolved. It would seem that if Minor Bupleurum Decoction *(xiǎo chái hú tāng)* can universally treat the common cold in deficient people, then Bupleurum and Cinnamon Twig Decoction *(chái hú guì zhī tāng)*, which is a modification of Minor Bupleurum Decoction *(xiǎo chái hú tāng)*, would be even better suited for treating the same situation. Is this so?

DR. YU   Absolutely! When I treat a deficiency-type patient who has a cold I prefer to use Bupleurum and Cinnamon Twig Decoction *(chái hú guì zhī tāng)*, which is a combination of Minor Bupleurum Decoction *(xiǎo chái hú tāng)* and Cinnamon Twig Decoction *(guì zhī tāng)*. We have already discussed the functions of Minor Bupleurum Decoction *(xiǎo chái hú tāng)*. As for Cinnamon Twig Decoction *(guì zhī tāng)*, the 17th-century author Xu Bin has written, "For external patterns, it resolves the muscle layer and harmonizes the nutritive and protective qi, and for internal patterns, it transforms qi and regulates yin and yang." Thus, it can be seen that Bupleurum and Cinnamon Twig Decoction *(chái hú guì zhī tāng)* is better suited for addressing the etiology and pathology of the common cold in deficient people than either of its component formulas independently.

When I first began using Bupleurum and Cinnamon Twig Decoction *(chái hú guì zhī tāng)* I was concerned that the tonifying quality of the Ginseng Radix *(rén shēn)* or Codonopsis Radix *(dǎng shēn)* in the formula would be obstructive, so I followed the example of the famous Sichuanese physician Pu Fu-Zhou and replaced Codonopsis Radix *(dǎng shēn)* with Adenophorae Radix *(nán shā shēn)* herb grown in Zitong county, my home county, which is called "puffy root" (泡参 *pào shēn*) in Sichuan. This herb, which is also known as Adenophorae Radix *(nán shā shēn* 南沙参) when dried, is light, having holes in it, and doesn't prevent pathogens from being eliminated. However, it does not tonify as strongly as Codonopsis Radix *(dǎng shēn)*. Later, I replaced Adenophorae Radix *(nán shā shēn)* with Agrimoniae Herba *(xiān hè cǎo)*, using about 30-50 grams, and got excellent results. Another name for Agrimoniae Herba *(xiān hè cǎo)* is 脱力草 *tuō lì cǎo*, literally "exhaustion herb." There is a folk custom of stewing it with pork to treat those who are emaciated and weak due to consumptive damage. The well-known contemporary doctor Gan Zu-Wang has said that Agrimoniae Herba *(xiān hè cǎo)* is the "steroid" of Chinese herbal medicine. Unlike Codonopsis Radix *(dǎng shēn)*, Astragali Radix *(huáng qí)* or similar substances, Agrimoniae Herba *(xiān hè cǎo)* supports the normal qi without causing the retention of pathogens. It also lacks any of the side effects associated with steroids.

It is worth mentioning here that there is an eminent doctor from my hometown of Leshan in Sichuan, Chen Si-Yi, who invariably uses a modification of Bupleurum and Cinnamon Twig Decoction *(chái hú guì zhī tāng)* to treat all manner of postpartum illnesses including the common cold, aversion to food, and scant breast milk. His results using this method are consistently good. This is evidence that women who have just given birth fall into the category of deficient people.

PHYSICIAN C   Looking through your case studies where you have used Minor Bupleurum Decoction *(xiǎo chái hú tāng)* or Bupleurum and Cinnamon Twig Decoction *(chái hú guì zhī tāng)* for the treatment of the common cold in those with deficiency, I found that the quantity of Bupleuri Radix *(chái hú)* that you used was from 12 to 24 grams. However, the herb textbooks clearly state that between three and 10 grams is the proper dosage for Bupleuri Radix *(chái hú)*. The textbooks also say that it ascends and discharges and thus this herb is contraindicated in patterns of damage to the true yin or hyperactivity of Liver yang. What is the correct way to reconcile this? Also, the nature of standard Pinelliae Rhizoma praeparatum *(fǎ bàn xià)* is warm and drying and Scutellariae Radix *(huáng qín)* is bitter and cold. Are these herbs appropriate for those who are deficient?

DR. YU   Good question! Indeed, the herb books say that Bupleuri Radix *(chái hú)* is dispersing, raises yang, and has the drawback of plundering yin. Also, standard Pinelliae Rhizoma praeparatum *(fǎ bàn xià)* is said to have a drying quality, and Scutellariae Radix *(huáng qín)* is bitter and cold. It is no wonder that people have concerns about using these three herbs to treat the common cold in those who are deficient.

Dr. Jiang believed that the effects of a compound formula are not simply the sum of the effects of the individual herbs in the formula. Furthermore, the *Divine Husbandman's Classic of the Materia Medica (Shén Nóng běn cǎo jīng)* states that Bupleuri Radix *(chái hú)* governs "cold and hot pathogenic qi," but says nothing about it being dispersing, raising the yang, or plundering the yin. As for standard Pinelliae Rhizoma praeparatum *(fǎ bàn xià)* and Scutellariae Radix *(huáng qín)*, their severe natures appear only when they are used alone. Remember that the *Divine Husbandman's Classic of the Materia Medica (Shén Nóng běn cǎo jīng)* says that Ginseng Radix *(rén shēn)* is slightly cold, so that in Minor Bupleurum Decoction *(xiǎo chái hú tāng)*, the combination of these herbs with the slightly cold nature of Ginseng Radix *(rén shēn)* and the sweet, moderating nature of Glycyrrhizae Radix *(gān cǎo)* and Jujubae Fructus *(dà zǎo)* obviates the harshness of their dry, bitter, and cold properties. Zhang Zhong-Jing used Minor Bupleurum Decoction *(xiǎo chái hú tāng)* to treat *shào yáng* disease where sweating, vomiting, and purgative treatments were contraindicated; in no way does the formula damage yin and consume qi. It is safe to use Minor Bupleurum Decoction *(xiǎo chái hú tāng)* for deficient people who have a common cold.

Examining the *Discussion of Cold Damage (Shāng hán lùn)*, we see that the dosage for Bupleuri Radix *(chái hú)* in Minor Bupleurum Decoction *(xiǎo chái hú tāng)* is half a *jin*, while in Bupleurum and Cinnamon Twig Decoction *(chái hú guì zhī tāng)*, four *liang* are used. Converting these numbers into modern dosages, one half a *jin* equals 24 grams, and four *liang* equals 12 grams. I usually use anywhere from 12 to 24 grams, which is in complete accordance with the standards set out in the *Discussion of Cold Damage (Shāng hán lùn)*. Also, 30 to 60 grams of Bupleuri Radix *(chái hú)* can be used for patients who are not deficient and have a cold or flu together with a very high fever.

Looking further into the functions of Bupleuri Radix *(chái hú)* we find that the *Divine Husbandman's Classic of the Materia Medica (Shén Nóng běn cǎo jīng)* says that it "governs knotted qi in the heart, abdomen, intestines, and stomach; accumulations of food and drink, [treats] hot and cold pathogenic qi; and pushes [out] the old to make way for the new." A thorough reading of the *Divine Husbandman's Classic of the Materia Medica (Shén Nóng běn cǎo jīng)* will reveal that there are 365 different medicinal substances recorded within its pages, but there are only two herbs with the explicit function of "pushing [out] the old to make way for the new": Rhei Radix et Rhizoma *(dà huáng)* and Bupleuri Radix *(chái hú)*. Rhei Radix et Rhizoma *(dà huáng)* is bitter, cold, and has a very potent and harsh nature. Its ability to push out the old to make way for the new exists because of its functions of clearing heat, expelling stasis, and flushing and draining downward. Bupleuri Radix *(chái hú)*, on the other hand, is bitter and balanced and has a mild quality. Its capacity to push out the old and make way for the new is the result of its ability to open and facilitate the qi dynamic and expel pathogens outward. If people took a serious look at Bupleuri Radix's *(chái hú)* ability to push out the old and make way for the new when researching and using Minor Bupleurum Decoction *(xiǎo chái hú tāng)* and its related formulas, the clinical scope of these formulas would be greatly expanded.

1.2 Cough

A three-month-long cough

An outstanding formula for coughs

出類拔萃的止咳專方

■ CASE HISTORY

Patient: *26-year-old woman*

Three months prior to coming to the clinic the patient had been caught in a downpour and came down with a cold. She developed a stuffy, runny nose, chills, generalized aches and pains, and a cough with copious phlegm. She took two doses of Schizonepeta and Saposhnikovia Powder to Overcome Pathogenic Influences *(jīng fáng bài dú sǎn)* combined with Apricot Kernel and Perilla Leaf Powder *(xìng sū sǎn)*. This alleviated all of her symptoms except for the cough. Because she was hoping to get faster results she stopped taking the herbal medicine and began taking Western medication. She took biomedical antivirals and antibiotics for three days but her condition did not improve. She continued these medications with the addition of an intravenous drip for one more week. This also yielded little improvement.

Because her condition had not improved, the patient decided to try Chinese medicine again. She visited a succession of doctors, four in all, and took a total of more than 20 packets of Chinese herbs. Most of the formulas she took consisted of herbs that stop cough and transform phlegm, along with patent medicines that stop cough and expel phlegm such as Snake Bile and Fritillariae Liquid *(shé dǎn chuān beì ye)*, Cough Extract *(ké sou jīng)*, and fresh Bambusae Succus *(zhú lì)*. These treatments did not alleviate her cough.

INTAKE EXAMINATION
DATE: October 13, 1992

The patient reported a tickle in her throat and frequent bouts of coughing (particularly in the morning and evening) that produced a scant amount of phlegm which was difficult to expectorate. The patient also described a mild feeling of tightness in her chest that occurred when she breathed and an occasional hacking cough. Her tongue was verging on pale with a white coating that was slightly thick in the center of the root. Her pulse was fine and carried a quality of slipperiness. A blood test and a chest x-ray did not reveal any abnormalities.

DIFFERENTIATION OF PATTERNS AND DISCUSSION OF TREATMENT

DR. YU   Although cough is one of the most common symptoms of Lung disorders, it can sometimes be difficult to treat. There is a folk saying, "Famous physicians don't treat cough or wheezing." The implication is that famous physicians fear being unable to successfully treat these problems and that such failure would harm their reputations. Though this saying may be an exaggeration, it is nevertheless born from the experience of generations of doctors. Furthermore, because many people consider a cough to be a rather minor health problem, they feel that if a doctor is unable to cure a cough, he or she may be unable to treat more serious illness. I too have had difficulties treating cough and wheezing, so what I present here is learned through the fire of trial and error. Even now, when treating cough, I am reluctant to promise flawless results.

PHYSICIAN A   I agree with you that if treatment fails and the patient's cough lingers on it can be difficult to know how to resolve the situation. In a case such as this one, where the patient had taken Western pharmaceuticals and her cough continued for three months, it would be easy to misdiagnose her case as a pattern of deficiency or a complex of deficiency and excess.

DR. YU   In this case, the patient initially had a pattern of wind-cold with cough. After taking Schizonepeta and Saposhnikovia Powder to Overcome Pathogenic Influences *(jīng fáng bài dú sǎn)* with Apricot Kernel and Perilla Leaf Powder *(xìng sū sǎn)* the patient's general symptoms of common cold markedly improved, but her cough did not.

　　The patient's condition may have improved if, at this point in the treatment, warm, acrid, dispersing herbs had been removed and replaced with herbs to disseminate Lung qi, disperse wind, and promote downward flow of Lung qi, assisted with agents that transform phlegm and stop coughs. Instead, because the patient was anxious to resolve her cough, she began taking Western pharmaceuticals, including expectorants and antibiotics. After those medications failed to improve her situation she went back to Chinese medicine, which included herbs to stop coughs and transform phlegm. Those herbs, however, failed to disseminate Lung qi, disperse wind, and promote the downward flow of qi. Such a treatment cannot drive out pathogens; this allowed the wind pathogen to remain intertwined with the Lung.

　　Let us review the patient's signs and symptoms: cough due to a ticklish sensation in the throat, a sensation of constricted breathing, hacking cough, scant phlegm that is difficult to expectorate, a white tongue coating, and a fine pulse that carries a quality of slipperiness. Together these signs indicate that a wind pathogen is lingering in the Lung and inhibiting the natural dissemination and downward movement of Lung qi. When treating such patients it is wise to heed the ancient precepts: "There is not a 'stopping' [method] for coughs" and "Without [treating to] stop a cough, the cough can stop on its own." The method of disseminating and promoting the downward movement of Lung qi together with dispersing wind is suitable for both chronic and acute coughs. Slavishly adhering to the idea that chronic coughs are usually due to deficiency or internal damage will lead to misdiagnosis and improper treatment.

Even though the patient had a cough for three months she still had a pattern of wind fettering the Lung along with signs that the Lung qi was unable to disseminate and descend.

TREATMENT AND OUTCOME

Treatment involved the use of a modified Inula Powder (jīn fèi cǎo sǎn) which disperses wind-cold and disseminates, clarifies, and promotes the downward flow of Lung qi.

The patient was prescribed two packets of the following formula:

Inulae Flos (xuán fù huā) [separately wrapped] 10g
Paeoniae Radix alba (bái sháo).. 12g
Glycyrrhizae Radix (gān cǎo)... 5g
Schizonepetae Herba (jīng jiè).. 15g
Perillae Folium (zǐ sū yè)... 10g
Peucedani Radix (qián hú) 10g
standard Pinelliae Rhizoma praeparatum (fǎ bàn xià) 10g
Armeniacae Semen (xìng rén) 10g
Sinapis Semen (bái jiè zǐ) 10g
Platycodi Radix (jié gěng) 10g

SECOND VISIT: The ticklish sensation in the patient's throat resolved, her coughing decreased significantly, and expectoration of phlegm had become much easier.

The patient was given three packets of the above formula combined with Stop Coughing Powder (zhǐ sòu sǎn):

Inulae Flos (xuán fù huā) [separately wrapped] 10g
Paeoniae Radix alba (bái sháo).. 10g
Glycyrrhizae Radix (gān cǎo)... 5g
Schizonepetae Herba (jīng jiè).. 10g
Platycodi Radix (jié gěng) 10g
prepared Asteris Radix (zhì zǐ wǎn) 15g
prepared Stemonae Radix (zhì bǎi bù)... 10g
Peucedani Radix (qián hú) 10g
Armeniacae Semen (xìng rén) 10g
Agrimoniae Herba (xiān hè cǎo)[1]... 30g

THIRD VISIT: The patient no longer coughed during the day, but still would occasionally cough at night.

1. For the reason this herb is used, see p. 8

The patient's formula was replaced with a folk formula called Eleven Herbs to Arrest Cough (*zhǐ ké shí yī wèi*) to address her night time cough.

Eleven Herbs to Arrest Cough (*zhǐ ké shí yī wèi*) consists of a decoction of 6g each of the following herbs (the decocted liquid is divided into three doses):

Angelicae sinensis Radix *(dāng guī)*
Chuanxiong Rhizoma *(chuān xiōng)*
standard Pinelliae Rhizoma praeparatum *(fǎ bàn xià)*
Poria *(fú líng)*
Citri reticulatae Pericarpium *(chén pí)*
Glycyrrhizae Radix *(gān cǎo)*
Mori Cortex *(sāng bái pí)*
Citri reticulatae viride Pericarpium *(qīng pí)*
Armeniacae Semen *(xìng rén)*
Schisandrae Fructus *(wǔ wèi zǐ)*
Fritillariae cirrhosae Bulbus *(chuān bèi mǔ)*
　　[grind into fine powder and take with strained decoction] ... 2g per dose

The patient was given two packets of this formula but her cough resolved before she finished the entire prescription.

Disease	Primary Symptoms	Pattern Diagnosis	Treatment Method	Formula
Cough	Cough due to tickle in the throat, scant phlegm that is difficult to expectorate	Wind-cold fettering the Lung, loss of dissemination and descending movement of Lung qi	Disperse wind-cold, disseminate and promote downward movement of Lung qi	Inula Powder (*jīn fèi cǎo sǎn*)

REFLECTIONS AND CLARIFICATIONS

PHYSICIAN A　As I recall, in the standard internal medicine textbooks for universities of traditional Chinese medicine, the formulas recommended for treatment of wind-cold cough vary from one edition to the next. In the second edition, Inula Powder (*jīn fèi cǎo sǎn*) is recommended. However, in the fifth edition, Apricot Kernel and Perilla Leaf Powder (*xìng sū sǎn*), Three-Unbinding Decoction (*sān ǎo tāng*), Stop Coughing Powder (*zhǐ sòu sǎn*), and other formulas are listed as options. This multitude of choices leaves students confused. Would you explain your reasons for using Inula Powder (*jīn fèi cǎo sǎn*)?

DR. YU　There are many formulas that can be employed for any given treatment method. Such a situation can be very confusing for those just beginning to practice and many students will wonder which formula is truly effective. Although it is said that "all roads lead to Rome," surely not all roads are equally direct.

　　My experience confirms that all of the formulas you mention, if properly modified, can treat wind-cold cough. However, there are differences among these formulas, and in my opinion, Inula Powder (*jīn fèi cǎo sǎn*) is the most effective.

PHYSICIAN B　Why is that?

DR. YU Inula Powder *(jīn fèi cǎo sǎn)* is able to disperse wind and scatter cold, and also diffuse and promote the downward flow of Lung qi, as do the other formulas. The key difference lies in three herbs: Inulae Herba *(jīn fèi cǎo)* (nowadays, Inulae Flos [*xuán fù huā*] is more commonly used), Paeoniae Radix alba *(bái sháo)*, and Glycyrrhizae Radix *(gān cǎo)*.

Most ancient and modern documents only mention that Inulae Flos *(xuán fù huā)* has the ability to eliminate phlegm and promote downward flow of Lung qi. This limited understanding may be in part due to a well-known saying: "All flowers rise, Inulae Flos *(xuán fù huā)* alone flows downward." It is certainly true that the ability of Inulae Flos *(xuán fù huā)* to promote the downward flow of Lung and Stomach qi, and to eliminate phlegm and thin-mucus, is quite remarkable. In fact, patients frequently feel a clear sensation that the stagnant qi in their chest and diaphragm is descending after taking the herb.

It shouldn't be forgotten, however, that Inulae Flos *(xuán fù huā)* has other functions as well. It is acrid, and the acrid flavor imparts a dispersing quality and a horizontal movement. Also, this gives the herb the ability to diffuse and disperse Lung qi all the way out to the skin and body hair. It both promotes the downward flow and diffuses Lung qi. Consequently, Inulae Flos *(xuán fù huā)* is able to restore the proper functioning of the Lung. Inulae Flos *(xuán fù huā)* is also said to have a salty flavor, allowing it to enter the Kidneys and promote that organ's function of grasping the qi. Further, it moves the qi downward and returns it to the root (Kidneys). This downward movement of qi stimulates any phlegm, oral-mucus, or thin-mucus in the Stomach to continuously move downward and be eliminated through the turbid pathways[2] so that they don't ascend and attack the Lung. Therefore, the Lung can recover its natural functional state of being clear and empty.

We can see that Inulae Flos *(xuán fù huā)* enables the Lung, Stomach, and Kidneys to keep fluids from bogging down in the body by forming a waterway that promotes the free flow through the three burners.

Paeoniae Radix alba *(bái sháo)* paired with Glycyrrhizae Radix *(gān cǎo)* comprises Peony and Licorice Decoction *(sháo yào gān cǎo tāng)*. Together, sour and sweet transform the yin, and thus the two herbs enrich the Lung's yang fluids and soothe and moderate the Lung qi. Modern pharmacological research has shown that this formula is able to relax spams in the smooth muscle of the bronchioles. Although the dosage of the other herbs in this formula can be changed or even eliminated, Inulae Flos *(xuán fù huā)*, Paeoniae Radix alba *(bái sháo)*, and Glycyrrhizae Radix *(gān cǎo)* are key herbs and thus should not be deleted when the formula is modified.

PHYSICIAN C How was it that you came to realize the profound importance of these three herbs?

DR. YU This was something passed on to me by my teacher, Jiang Er-Xun. When Dr. Jiang was young he was rather weak and often suffered from cough. Each time he successfully treated his cough by using Stop Coughing Powder *(zhǐ sòu sǎn)*, Apricot Kernel and

---

2. *Translators' note:* Turbid pathways (濁道 *zhuó dào*) is a term denoting the pathways by which the dregs of metabolism are led out of the body through urination or defecation.

Perilla Leaf Powder *(xìng sū sǎn)*, and Six-Serenity Decoction *(liù ān jiān)*. One time, however, nothing he tried brought any relief. He had an incessant cough brought on by a constant tickle in his throat. This went on for more than ten days before he discovered a passage in the early 19th-century work *Collection of Medical Writings Following on the Work of Others (Yī xué cóng zhòng lù)*, written by Chen Xiu-Yuan. It read, "In mild cases use Six-Serenity Decoction *(liù ān jiān)*, in severe cases use Inula Powder *(jīn fèi cǎo sǎn)*." Dr. Jiang decided to try the formula and after only one packet both the tickle in his throat and his cough stopped. He was amazed by this so he used the formula with his patients and also got good results. Dr. Jiang used Inula Powder *(jīn fèi cǎo sǎn)* for decades to treat coughs. He preferred to use modifications of this formula regardless of whether the nature of the cough was chronic or acute, external or internal, hot or cold, deficient or excessive. There are many examples of patients cured after a few packets of this formula despite having had coughs of two or three months' duration and extensive treatment with Chinese and Western medicines. I have had patients who passed around copies of the formula to their friends and family who, in turn, also got excellent results with it.

PHYSICIAN D The functions of Inula Powder *(jīn fèi cǎo sǎn)* include dispersing wind-cold and disseminating and clarifying the Lung qi. My understanding is that 'dispersing wind-cold' is a slightly weaker version of 'releasing the exterior' and that both involve inducing sweating. Would not the combination of Inulae Flos *(xuán fù huā)*, Schizonepetae Herba *(jīng jiè)*, and Perillae Folium *(zǐ sū yè)* lead to at least a mild sweat? Is this still appropriate when there are no longer any signs of an exterior condition? Does this make this formula inappropriate for weak patients?

DR. YU This formula does not cause sweating and is very safe in relatively delicate patients. I have used it for quite young children with coughs, often in those as young as a couple of months, and have even used it in infants only a couple of weeks old who otherwise would have been given antibiotics. While this formula may be able to release a very mild exterior condition, its function is really more one of properly disseminating and dispersing the Lung qi and it does not address the systemic signs and symptoms of an exterior condition.

PHYSICIAN E Historically, there are two versions of Inula Powder *(jīn fèi cǎo sǎn)*. One is recorded in the *Book to Safeguard Life Arranged According to Pattern (Léi zhèng huó rén shū)* where the ingredients are:

Inulae Herba *(jīn fèi cǎo)*
Peucedani Radix *(qián hú)*
Schizonepetae Herba *(jīng jiè)*
Asari Radix et Rhizoma *(xì xīn)*
Poria *(fú líng)*
Zingiberis Rhizoma recens *(shēng jiāng)*
Jujubae Fructus *(dà zǎo)*
Glycyrrhizae Radix *(gān cǎo)*

The other is recorded in *Formulary of the Pharmacy Service for Benefiting the People in the Taiping Era (Tàipíng huì mín hé jì jú fāng)* where it consists of the same herbs minus

Poria *(fú líng)* and Asari Radix et Rhizoma *(xì xīn),* and with the addition of Ephedrae Herba *(má huáng)* and Paeoniae Radix alba *(bái sháo).* Also, there is an Inulae Flos Decoction *(xuán fù huā tāng),* recorded in the *Discussion of Illnesses, Patterns and Formulas Related to the Unification of the Three Etiologies (Sān yīn jí yī bìng zhèng fāng lùn),* which is based on the Inula Powder *(jīn fèi cǎo sǎn)* formula from the *Formulary of the Taiping Era* and adds Armeniacae Semen *(xìng rén),* Poria *(fú líng),* and Schisandrae Fructus *(wǔ wèi zǐ).* Which of these formulas does Dr. Jiang use?

DR. YU   Dr. Jiang doesn't strictly adhere to just one of these formulas, but instead makes a formula based on all three. Depending on the pattern involved, he may combine it with Six-Serenity Decoction *(liù ān jiān),* which is Two-Aged [Herb] Decoction *(èr chén tāng)* plus Armeniacae Semen *(xìng rén),* Sinapis Semen *(bái jiè zǐ),* and Platycodon Decoction *(jié gěng tāng).*

   Dr. Jiang has used this formula for decades and has developed a very effective set of modifications based on a patient's patterns. Some of the modifications include formulas within formulas. As is said, a scholar's knowledge grows with time, and Dr. Jiang has greatly expanded the range of this formula. Examples:

- If the patient presents with alternating chills and fever, add Bupleuri Radix *(chái hú)* and Scutellariae Radix *(huáng qín),* as in Minor Bupleurum Decoction *(xiǎo chái hú tāng).*

- For high fever with wheezing, add Ephedrae Herba *(má huáng)* and Gypsum fibrosum *(shí gāo),* as in Ephedra, Apricot Kernel, Gypsum, and Licorice Decoction *(má xìng shí gān tāng).*

- In cases of feverishness with sore throat, add Lonicerae Flos *(jīn yín huā),* Forsythiae Fructus *(lián qiáo),* and Belamcandae Rhizoma *(shè gān),* in the mode of a modification of Honeysuckle and Forsythia Powder *(yín qiáo sǎn).*

- When the patient has copious amounts of sticky phlegm, add Fritillariae thunbergii Bulbus *(zhè bèi mǔ)* and Trichosanthis Semen *(guā lóu rén),* as in Fritillaria and Trichosanthes Fruit Powder *(bèi mǔ guā lóu sǎn).*

- For patients with asthma with a gurgling sound in the throat, add Perillae Fructus *(zǐ sū zǐ)* and Lepidii/ Descurainiae Semen *(tíng lì zǐ),* as in Descurainia and Jujube Decoction to Drain the Lung *(tíng lì dà zǎo xiè fèi tāng).*

- For patients with feverishness, chills, and spontaneous sweating, add Cinnamomi Ramulus *(guì zhī)* and ginger Magnoliae officinalis Cortex *(jiāng hòu pò),* as in Cinnamon Twig plus Magnoliae Decoction *(guì zhī jiā hòu pò tāng).*

- In cases of chronic incessant cough, add Asteris Radix *(zǐ wǎn),* Stemonae Radix *(bǎi bù),* and Eriobotryae Folium *(pí pá yè),* as in Stop Coughing Powder *(zhǐ sòu sǎn).*

- For those with a deficient constitution who frequently catch cold, add Astragali Radix *(huáng qí),* Atractylodis macrocephalae Rhizoma *(bái zhú),* and Saposhnikoviae Radix *(fáng fēng),* as in Jade Windscreen Powder *(yù píng fēng sǎn).*

- When the patient has signs of Spleen deficiency and a poor appetite, or loose stools, add Codonopsis Radix (*dǎng shēn*) and Atractylodis macrocephalae Rhizoma (*bái zhú*), as in Six-Gentlemen Decoction (*liù jūn zǐ tāng*).

- For thin, watery phlegm and oral mucus, dizziness, and epigastric focal distention, add Cinnamomi Ramulus (*guì zhī*) and Atractylodis macrocephalae Rhizoma (*bái zhú*), as in Poria, Cinnamon Twig, Atractylodes, and Licorice Decoction (*líng guì zhú gān tāng*).

__PHYSICIAN A__   It seems that Inula Powder (*jīn fèi cǎo sǎn*) can be modified in numerous ways to make it useful for treating conditions that are externally contracted or internally generated, cold or hot, excessive or deficient. This adaptability makes it difficult for the novice practitioner to get a handle on how to use the formula. Can you give us some simple principles to help us understand how to best make use of this formula?

__DR. YU__   Actually, Dr. Jiang's modifications of this formula aren't limited to what I just listed. Some of his modifications address cases where the patients have been given an improper treatment or received a misdiagnosis, while others are primarily orientated to addressing the patient's constitution. All of Dr. Jiang's modifications come from his clinical experience and the results can be duplicated over and over again in the clinic.

Creating some simple principles to explain this formula would, in my opinion, be like cutting feet to fit the shoes. If forced to simplify things in this way I would say that, at the very least, a practitioner should have a firm grasp on how to treat wind-cold coughs. Most coughs are due to external factors, and of those factors, wind-cold is the most common. When treating coughs due to wind-cold, it is important to select the proper formulas and herbs that can disperse and scatter wind-cold, as well as disseminate and promote the downward flow of Lung qi. In most cases, if this can be accomplished, the effects will be quick. So one may wonder, "If one is able to master the treatment of wind-cold cough, does this make the need for so many modifications of Inula Powder (*jīn fèi cǎo sǎn*) unnecessary?" Unfortunately, the answer is no.

Dr. Jiang once wrote that many doctors, as soon as they see a patient with feverishness (or a high temperature), make a diagnosis of wind-heat or phlegm-heat and begin using Mulberry Leaf and Chrysanthemum Drink (*sāng jú yǐn*) or Honeysuckle and Forsythia Powder (*yín qiáo sǎn*) type formulas and herbs to clear heat and transform phlegm, or even administer antibiotics. In other cases, patients come in with a tickle in the throat, or scant phlegm that is difficult to expectorate, and the doctors immediately declare a diagnosis of wind-dryness or damaged yin and prescribe formulas to moisten dryness or nourish yin. In yet other situations, patients with chronic, incessant coughs are diagnosed with deficiency cough and each patient gets his or her fill of tonifying formulas. The result of such misdiagnosis is that the doctor fails to treat the patient's cough properly with herbs that disperse and scatter wind, and disseminate and promote the downward flow of Lung qi. Hence, the patient's cough drags on without resolving and, in the worst case, develops into what is called a consumptive cough. Zhang Jing-Yue stressed the role of mistreatment by physicians in the development of consumptive disorders. He mockingly noted, "It is commonly said that when colds are not cured they turn into consumption. By what means could a cold [by itself] turn into consumption?"

__PHYSICIAN B__   Roughly what percentage of externally-contracted coughs can be treated using modifications of Inula Powder *(jīn fèi cǎo sǎn)*?

DR. YU   More than 80%.

PHYSICIAN B   And what formula do you use when it is not effective?

DR. YU   In my experience, there are three situations where Inula Powder *(jīn fèi cǎo sǎn)* doesn't produce the desired results. One situation is due to the very bitter and astringent taste of Inulae Flos *(xuán fù huā)*. Some people find it unpleasant to drink and it may lead to vomiting. Consequently these patients are unable to finish the medication. Another situation is that after symptoms have resolved, some patients have a recurrence of coughing, although their symptoms are less severe. The last is because there are always some patients who have what I call the tail end of a cough, as in the case mentioned here, where they will have an intermittent cough.

There is a saying that goes, "A sweet melon has a bitter stem; nothing is perfect." The same holds true for Chinese medicine: are there any herbs or formulas in the world that are perfect? The way I handle these situation is as follows:

- For those who feel nauseous from the formula, I tell them to take the decoction in small amounts over a longer period of time. If they still cannot tolerate the formula, I use Six-Serenity Decoction *(liù ān jiān)* along with a formula created by the 17th-century physician Chen Shi-Duo called Soothe the Lung Decoction *(shū fèi tāng)*:

Cinnamomi Ramulus *(guì zhī)*	10g
Perillae Folium *(zǐ sū yè)*	10g
Platycodi Radix *(jié gěng)*	6g
Glycyrrhizae Radix *(gān cǎo)*	4g
Poria *(fú líng)*	15g
Trichosanthis Radix *(tiān huā fěn)*	15g

- For those who once again develop a cough after having been cured, I prescribe Bupleurum and Cinnamon Twig Decoction *(chái hú guì zhī tāng)* plus prepared Asteris Radix *(zhì zǐ wǎn)*, Cicadae Periostracum *(chán tuì)*, and Oroxyli Semen *(mù hú dié)*.

- For patients with an intermittent cough, I have them continue their treatment using Eleven Herbs to Arrest Cough *(zhǐ ké shí yī wèi)* (see patient's third visit in this case study for a listing of the formula). This formula is a folk remedy that is used to treat cough due to tuberculosis. Twenty years ago I happened to treat a patient with a cough. Once the externally-contracted symptoms had resolved, the patient's cough had diminished but still remained for another ten days or so without resolving. After one dose of this formula the patient's cough ceased. After I began to gain more experience, I started using the formula as a 'finishing' formula. There is nothing special about the herbs in this formula, but when combined, their effects are quite extraordinary. It is difficult to explain how it is that they are so effective.

Something I must mention is that in a very small number of people, even though treatment with modified Inula Powder *(jīn fèi cǎo sǎn)* does alleviate their cough, the follow up with Eleven Herbs to Arrest Cough *(zhǐ ké shí yī wèi)* fails to eliminate the remaining symptoms. Instead, they gradually develop a dry cough, without phlegm, which is worse at night and present a tongue with no coating. In such cases I use a formula that I composed called Stubborn Cough Decoction *(wán ké tāng)*, which contains the following herbs:

Scrophulariae Radix *(xuán shēn)*... 15g
Ophiopogonis Radix *(mài mén dōng)* 15g
Schisandrae Fructus *(wǔ wèi zǐ)* 6g
Glycyrrhizae Radix *(gān cǎo)*... 6g
Platycodi Radix *(jié gěng)* 10g
Agrimoniae Herba *(xiān hè cǎo)*.. 30g
prepared Asteris Radix *(zǐ wǎn)* 30g
Persicae Semen *(táo rén)*... 10g
Carthami Flos *(hóng huā)* 6g
Phragmitis Rhizoma *(lú gēn)* 30g
Untreated Ostreae Concha *(mǔ lì)* 30g

If this merely reduces the cough without completely resolving it, alternating Stubborn Cough Decoction *(wán ké tāng)* with Clear Dryness and Rescue the Lung Decoction *(qīng zào jiù fèi tāng)* should achieve the desired result.

1.2.1 Cough

Hacking cough with a tickle in the throat

Insights from a founder of modern TCM *laryngology*

現代中醫喉科奠基人的創見

■ CASE HISTORY

Patient: *35-year-old woman*

The patient long suffered from chronic throat inflammation for which she had been treated at length without results. Her symptoms included a chronically dry, irritated throat and a slight cough. Two months prior to coming to our clinic she developed a severe cough as a result of a common cold, and was admitted to the hospital for seven days. During that stay she was concurrently given Western pharmaceuticals and Chinese medicinal substances with the result that all of her symptoms fundamentally resolved, except the cough, which showed no improvement.

After leaving the hospital the patient continued to take Chinese medicine. Initially, she took many doses of Inula Powder *(jīn fèi cǎo sǎn)*, but this only aggravated her cough. Following this, she took various formulas including Stop Coughing Powder *(zhǐ sòu sǎn)*,

Clear Dryness and Rescue the Lung Decoction *(qīng zào jiù fèi tāng)*, and Glehnia and Ophiopogonis Decoction *(shā shēn mài mén dōng tāng)*. She took more than ten packets of herbs in all, and, although it seemed at times she experienced some relief, in the end her symptoms did not improve.

INTAKE EXAMINATION
DATE: November 23, 1991

The patient reported a recurring tickle in her throat and complained that the area was dry and irritated. The tickle in her throat would provoke a fit of hacking cough that would go on for an extended period, and the more she coughed, the worse the cough became. She would cough to the point that she would gasp for breath, her face would turn red, and her eyes would well with tears. The patient's phlegm was globular, scant, and extremely difficult to expectorate. Her cough was worse during the day and she seldom coughed at night. However, when she woke in the morning, serious bouts of relentless coughing would begin anew. The patient had an acceptable appetite and her tongue was somewhat pale and lacked moisture. Her pulse had no abnormal characteristics.

DIFFERENTIATION OF PATTERNS AND DISCUSSION OF TREATMENT

DR. YU   A pioneer in modern TCM laryngology with 60 years' experience, Gan Zu-Wang, refers to this type of hacking cough with a tickle in the throat as a 'laryngeal cough.' As the name suggests, the origin and primary disease locale is in the throat and not the Lung. The primary symptoms of laryngeal cough are dry throat and a tickle in the throat that brings on fits of coughing and choking. These symptoms are very distinct from coughs that originate in the Lung or are due to pathology in other organs.

Coughing is a self-protective reaction. It is the body's way of temporarily re-opening the airways by expelling foreign materials or disease by-products. Consequently, coughing generally brings a temporary feeling of relief and comfort to the patient. However, this is not the case with laryngeal cough: the more the patient coughs, the more discomfort he or she feels. This is because repeated coughing of this type leaves the throat drier and more irritated. This makes it more likely for the tickling sensation to develop and provoke another episode of coughing. In this way, a vicious cycle develops.

When I first began treating patients with this type of cough, my thinking was to treat the Lung with formulas such as Stop Coughing Powder *(zhǐ sòu sǎn)*, Clear Dryness and Rescue the Lung Decoction *(qīng zào jiù fèi tāng)*, and Glehnia and Ophiopogonis Decoction *(shā shēn mài mén dōng tāng)*, but this approach yielded poor results. Sometimes I would change formulas seven or eight times and the patient would seem to improve and then not. I'd have exhausted my repertoire and the patients would be left unsatisfied and complaining.

Gan Zu-Wang has written, "If this illness is regarded in the same way as the average cough there will be decided dissatisfaction with the results of treatment. This is because the treatment is directed at the unoffending Lung and not at the location of the pathology: the throat." His words struck me deeply, because I thought these were the words of a man with vast experience and not to be taken lightly.

TREATMENT AND OUTCOME

This led me to consider that perhaps this was a case of laryngeal cough due to wind-dryness damaging the fluids, which deprived the throat of moisture and nourishment. Although the patient had been suffering for two months, and although she didn't have a floating pulse, I thought that because the treatment methods used until now did not yield results, she probably still harbored a superficial pathogen. The proper treatment method would be to dispel wind and moisten dryness, so I prescribed three packets of an augmented version of the formula Six-Ingredient Laryngology Decoction *(hóu kē liù wèi tāng)*:

Schizonepetae Herba *(jīng jiè)* 6g
Saposhnikoviae Radix *(fáng fēng)* 6g
Platycodi Radix *(jié gěng)* 6g
Glycyrrhizae Radix *(gān cǎo)* 6g
Menthae haplocalycis *Folium (bò hé yè)* 6g
Bombyx batryticatus *(bái jiāng cán)* 6g

To this I added the following substances:

Calvatia candida *(bái mǎ bó)* 6g
Belamcandae Rhizoma *(shè gān)* 6g
Cicadae Periostracum *(chán tuì)* 6g
Oroxyli Semen *(mù hú dié)* 15g
Pyri Exocarpium *(lí pí)* [peel of the fresh fruit] 50g

METHOD OF DECOCTION AND ADMINISTRATION: Soak the herbs for one hour in cold water then boil (slow boil) for ten minutes. Remove the liquid and set aside. Add water to the dregs and cook again for ten minutes. Mix the liquid from the two decoctions together. Roughly one liter of liquid should be obtained in total. Drink as tea frequently throughout the day.

SECOND VISIT: The patient's hacking cough and tickling sensation in the throat had improved slightly and the phlegm was easier to expectorate than it had been. Her throat was dry, although her mouth was not, and she said that the frequent drinking of the decoction would only temporarily moisten her throat, which would soon become dry and irritated again. I decided to combine the previous formula with Nourish the Yin and Clear the Lung Decoction *(yǎng yīn qīng fèi tāng)* in hopes of expelling wind, moistening dryness, nourishing yin and engendering fluids.

Schizonepetae Herba *(jīng jiè)* 6g
Platycodi Radix *(jié gěng)* 6g
Glycyrrhizae Radix *(gān cǎo)* 6g
Bombyx batryticatus *(bái jiāng cán)* 6g
Cicadae Periostracum *(chán tuì)* 6g
Moutan Cortex *(mǔ dān pí)* 6g
powdered Fritillariae cirrhosae Bulbus *(chuān bèi mǔ)*
 [3g taken each time with the strained decoction] 6g
Rehmanniae Radix *(shēng dì huáng)* 15g
Ophiopogonis Radix *(mài mén dōng)* 15g
Asparagi Radix *(tiān mén dōng)* 15g
Oroxyli Semen *(mù hú dié)* 15g
Paeoniae Radix alba *(bái sháo)* 15g

dried persimmons *(shì bǐng)* 30g

Pyri Exocarpium *(lí pí)* [peel of the fresh fruit] 50g

The patient said that after taking three packets of this formula, the dryness and tickle in her throat as well as her hacking cough had markedly decreased, and after ten packets, her symptoms had essentially resolved. All that remained was a brief bout of coughing each morning along with the expectoration of a small quantity of sticky phlegm. I changed her formula to a combination of Six-Ingredient Laryngology Decoction *(hóu kē liù wèi tāng)* and Ginseng, Poria, and White Atractylodes Powder *(shēn líng bái zhú sǎn)* to address the remaining symptoms:

Adenophorae Radix *(nán shā shēn)* 10g

Atractylodis macrocephalae Rhizoma *(bái zhú)* 10g

Poria *(fú líng)* 15g

Glycyrrhizae Radix *(gān cǎo)* 6g

Dioscoreae Rhizoma *(shān yào)* 15g

Lablab Semen album *(bái biǎn dòu)* 15g

Platycodi Radix *(jié gěng)* 6g

Puerariae Radix *(gé gēn)* 15g

Agrimoniae Herba *(xiān hè cǎo)* 30g

Condition	Primary Symptoms	Pattern Differentiation	Treatment Method	Formula
Laryngeal cough	Itchy throat, hacking cough, scant phlegm that is difficult to expectorate	Wind-dryness damaging the fluids with a loss of moisture in the throat	Expel wind and moisten dryness	Six-Ingredient Laryngology Decoction *(hóu kē liù wèi tāng)*

REFLECTIONS AND CLARIFICATIONS

DR. YU   In Chapter 23 of the *Basic Questions (Sù wèn)* it states, "As for diseases of the qi of the five [yin organs] … that of the Lung is cough." In order to simplify diagnosis, later generations of physicians divided the causes of cough into two general categories, external contraction and internal damage. Cough due to external contraction means exogenous pathogens have attacked the Lung and the primary treatment principle is to clarify and lead the Lung qi downward. Cough due to internal damage is the result of imbalances in the internal organs, which in turn affect the Lung. The primary treatment principle in such cases is to regulate internal organ function while simultaneously clarifying and leading the Lung qi downward.

This case of laryngeal hacking cough manifested as a pattern of wind-dryness damaging the fluids. Consequently, it is easy to understand why the patient's condition worsened after a few doses of Inula Powder *(jīn fèi cǎo sǎn)*, which leans toward being warm and drying. However, what may not be so easy to comprehend is why, after more than ten doses of formulas such as Stop Coughing Powder *(zhǐ sòu sǎn)*, Clear Dryness and Rescue the Lung Decoction *(qīng zào jiù fèi tāng)*, and Glehnia and Ophiopogonis Decoction *(shā shēn mài mén dōng tāng)*, the patient's condition showed no distinct signs of improvement.

Stop Coughing Powder *(zhǐ sòu sǎn)* is a formula that is warming, moistening, and balanced. It is neither markedly hot nor cold. It disperses wind and dispels phlegm, disseminates Lung qi, and relieves cough. Based on my observations it is effective for both acute and chronic coughs. Clear Dryness and Rescue the Lung Decoction *(qīng zào jiù fèi tāng)* disseminates Lung qi, directs counterflow Lung qi downward, clears dryness, and moistens the Lung. Glehnia and Ophiopogonis Decoction *(shā shēn mài mén dōng tāng)* is sweet and cold. It engenders fluids and clears and nourishes the Lung and Stomach. Although close to correct, none of these formulas is completely suited to treating wind-dryness damaging the fluids. This patient's throat tickle and hacking cough are characteristic of a laryngeal cough, and the location of this type of cough is in the throat and not in the Lung.

PHYSICIAN B   I haven't seen the term 'laryngeal cough' used in any Chinese medicine textbooks. I'm wondering in what book it can be located.

DR. YU   According to Dr. Gan's research, it seems that this term has yet to be found in any ancient text. However, Dr. Gan feels that symptoms described in Chapter 16 (Cough) of the Yuan-dynasty text *Essential Teachings of [Zhu] Dan Xi (Zhū Dān-Xī xīn fǎ)* are very similar to those of this condition. There it states: "Dry cough is difficult to treat. This is part of a pattern of fire-constraint, within which is phlegm-constraint, a pathogen at its center."

The symptoms of dry cough described in the Ming-dynasty book *Comprehensive Outline of Medicine* (Yī xué gāng mù) and *Introduction to Medicine* (Yī xué rù mén), as well as what is described as 'constraint cough' in *Supplemented Collections on Patterns and Treatments* (Zhèng zhì huì bǔ), are all very similar to the symptoms of laryngeal cough. In recent years there has been the occasional report of this type of pattern. In all that I have read, Dr. Gan was the first person whom I recall using the term laryngeal cough. He has written about how he differentiates and treats this condition in *Modern TCM Internal Medicine (Xiàn dài zhōng yī nèi kē xué).*

PHYSICIAN B   In Chinese medicine the throat belongs to the Lung system, so by treating the Lung we can treat the throat. So how can you say that you are "treating the unoffending Lung and not the location of pathology, the throat"?

DR. YU   The phrase "the throat belongs to the Lung system" is not completely accurate. The pharynx is in charge of earth qi and belongs to the Spleen and Stomach. The larynx is in charge of heavenly qi and belongs to the Lung. Speaking in terms of the whole body, by treating the Lung we can indirectly treat the larynx. However, in such cases it is only appropriate to use medicinal substances that discharge and disseminate and not those that direct the Lung qi downward.

Most coughs result from the Lung's inability to disseminate qi and direct it downward. In cases where the Lung qi counterflows upward, treatment should be directed at both dissemination of Lung qi and directing of the Lung qi downward with formulas such as Inula Powder *(jīn fèi cǎo sǎn)*, Apricot Kernel and Perilla Leaf Powder *(xìng sū sǎn)*, and Stop Coughing Powder *(zhǐ sòu sǎn)*. The herbs in these formulas that move Lung qi downward, transform phlegm, and relieve cough such as Inulae Flos *(xuán fù huā)*, Pinelliae Rhizoma preparatum *(zhì bàn xià)*, Armeniacae Semen *(xìng rén)*, Asteris Radix *(zǐ wǎn)*, Stemonae Radix *(bǎi bù)*, and Farfarae Flos *(kuǎn dōng huā)* are inappropriate for treating laryngeal cough. They are inappropriate because the primary pathodynamic of laryngeal cough is wind-dryness damaging the fluids, which causes the throat to lose moisture and nourishment. In this condition, the pathodynamic of Lung qi failing to descend doesn't exist. This is precisely what Dr. Gan has said:

> The primary symptom in all chronic cases of inflammation of the throat is throat dryness. Such dryness is due to yin fluids not nourishing the pharynx and yang fluids not moistening the larynx. There are two distinct causes for this dryness. The first is that lack of moisture leads to pathogenic dryness, which engenders wind, which in turn engenders itching (tickle). It is the tickling sensation that begets this disorder. A second pathway by which parched fluids precipitate itching [is related to the quote from the *Inner Classic,* which says:] "All pain, sores, and itching belong to Heart fire." A lack of moisture leads to pathogenic dryness, pathogenic dryness in turn gives rise to fire, and fire prompts itching. These are the dynamics by which chronic inflammation of the throat leads to laryngeal cough.

Thus we can see that although laryngeal cough has a connection to the Lung, it differs from the common cough in both the location of its pathology and the pathodynamic through which it manifests. Why, then, would we use the same type of treatment for these two disorders?

This makes me think about how people who haven't studied Chinese medicine, and in some cases even those who have, frequently complain that Chinese medicine's etiology and pathology is abstract, vague, or imprecise. Actually, if one takes the time to diligently go through and organize the information, one discovers that much of the content of Chinese medicine can be expressed concretely, clearly, and precisely.

PHYSICIAN C   What would you consider to be the standard formula for treating laryngeal cough?

DR. YU   I would suggest Nourish the Yin and Clear the Lung Decoction *(yǎng yīn qīng fèi tāng)*. This formula was recorded in the 18th-century laryngology text *Jade Key to the Throat* (*Zhòng lóu yù yào*) and was originally used to treat diphtheria disorder owing to yin deficiency. The formula has an excellent ability to nourish and engender fluids, and its scope of treatment can be expanded to include laryngeal cough. Nourish the Yin and Clear the Lung Decoction *(yǎng yīn qīng fèi tāng)* is composed of Increase the Fluids Decoction *(zēng yè tāng)*—containing Rehmanniae Radix *(shēng dì huáng)*, Ophiopogonis Radix *(mài mén dōng)*, and Scrophulariae Radix *(xuán shēn)*—which moistens the Lung and enriches the Kidneys, thus promoting the mutual generation of metal and water and ensuring that the source of the spring is not exhausted. The formula also contains Peony and Licorice Decoction *(sháo yào gān cǎo tāng)*, composed of Paeoniae Radix alba *(bái sháo)* and Glycyrrhizae Radix *(gān cǎo)*. This formula not only enriches the Spleen yin so that the Spleen qi can distribute essence upward to the Lung to moisten the throat, it also relaxes tension, relieves spasms, and alleviates hacking cough. Furthermore, Nourish the Yin and Clear the Lung Decoction *(yǎng yīn qīng fèi tāng)* includes Moutan Cortex *(mǔ dān pí)* to cool the nutritive aspect,

Fritillariae Bulbus *(bèi mǔ)* to transform phlegm, and Menthae haplocalycis Herba *(bò hé)* to disperse knots.

Someone had previously brought up the fact that Clear Dryness and Rescue the Lung Decoction *(qīng zào jiù fèi tāng)* and Glehnia and Ophiopogonis Decoction *(shā shēn mài mén dōng tāng)* are also formulas that nourish yin and engender fluids and thus should be effective in treating the same condition. My experience has shown that unless properly modified, these formulas aren't very effective for treating laryngeal cough, and certainly not as effective as Nourish the Yin and Clear the Lung Decoction *(yǎng yīn qīng fèi tāng)*. It is important to mention that the tickle in the throat and hacking cough associated with this condition is often induced or aggravated by an external contraction. Even though the illness may have persisted for a long time, it often coexists with a superficial pathogen. Consequently, treatment often combines Nourish the Yin and Clear the Lung Decoction *(yǎng yīn qīng fèi tāng)* with a modification of Six-Ingredient Laryngology Decoction *(hóu kē liù wèi tāng)*. Alternatively, a modification of Six-Ingredient Laryngology Decoction *(hóu kē liù wèi tāng)* can be used alone as the vanguard attack, and once the superficial pathogen has been eliminated, Nourish the Yin and Clear the Lung Decoction *(yǎng yīn qīng fèi tāng)* can be used to complete the treatment in a moderate and measured manner.

PHYSICIAN A   Six-Ingredient Laryngology Decoction *(hóu kē liù wèi tāng)* is a formula used to treat wind-cold painful obstruction of the throat. I find it both surprising and difficult to understand how you have effectively used this formula for a pattern of wind-dryness causing damage to the fluids and lack of moisture in the throat.

DR. YU   To use Six-Ingredient Laryngology Decoction *(hóu kē liù wèi tāng)* for a case of painful obstruction of the throat that is truly due to wind-cold, it would be necessary to add acrid and warm medicinal substances to disperse the cold and unbind the painful obstruction. This formula was recorded in the *Arcane Knowledge of Laryngology (Hóu kē mì zhǐ)* and can be modified to treat both red and white (hot and cold) throat disorders in their initial stages. Let's take a closer look at the formula:

> **Schizonepetae Herba** *(jīng jiè)*:
> - acrid and slightly warm; expels wind and resolves the exterior
>
> **Saposhnikoviae Radix** *(fáng fēng)*:
> - acrid, sweet, and slightly warm; dispels wind and resolves spasms
>
> **Platycodi Radix** *(jié gěng)*:
> - bitter and neutral; eliminates phlegm and promotes free flow through the throat
>
> **Glycyrrhizae Radix** *(gān cǎo)*:
> - sweet and neutral; clears fire and resolves toxicity
>
> **Bombyx Batryticatus** *(bái jiāng cán)*:
> - salty, acrid, and neutral; eliminates wind and disperses knots
>
> **Menthae Haplocalycis Herba** *(bò hé)*:
> - acrid and cool; dredges wind and disperses heat and knots

As a whole, the formula has a balanced nature, being neither too hot nor too cold. It disperses wind, dispels phlegm, dissipates knots, and promotes free flow through the throat. Consequently, it can be adapted to treat patterns of wind-cold, wind-heat, and wind-dryness. In cases of wind-cold, add Perillae Folium *(zǐ sū yè)* and Asari Radix et

Rhizoma *(xì xīn)*. For wind-heat, combine with Forsythia and Mentha Decoction *(qiáo hé tāng)*, and for wind-dryness, combine with Nourish the Yin and Clear the Lung Decoction *(yǎng yīn qīng fèi tāng)*.

It is interesting to note that a few years ago a newly-developed formula for treating chronic throat inflammation was widely reported. It was said to be very effective, and many journals wrote articles about it. Looking closely at the formula I was astonished to discover that this "new" formula was in fact Six-Ingredient Laryngology Decoction *(hóu kē liù wèi tāng)*.

CHAPTER 2

Heart System Disorders

2.1 Palpitations

Palpitations for eight years

Thoroughly understanding "evil intentions abide in solitary places"[1]

洞悉 "獨處藏奸"

■ CASE HISTORY

Patient: *40-year-old woman*

Chief complaint: *Palpitations for eight years*

The patient said that for the past eight years she often experienced palpitations accompanied by a feeling of uneasiness, dull pain and stifling sensation in the anterior of the chest, and shortness of breath. These symptoms were exacerbated during the winter and spring as well as during rainy or overcast weather. Whenever the patient felt emotional distress or if she caught cold or was extremely fatigued, she would begin experiencing premature beats and tachycardia (her heart rate sometimes reached 150-180 beats/minute). She frequently had sensations of premature beats just as she was about to enter sleep at night or take an afternoon nap. An electrocardiogram revealed no organic pathology in the patient's heart and she was given a diagnosis of premature atrial contractions and paroxysmal tachycardia.

For an extended period of time the patient was taking such medicines as estazolam,

1. *Translator's note*: "Evil intentions abide in solitary places" is a well-known saying coined by the famous Ming-dynasty physician, Zhang Jing-Yue. It describes the phenomenon of a single symptom revealing the true nature of a disorder.

propranolol, gamma-oryzanol, vitamins, and Compounded Salvia tablets (複方丹參片 *Fù fāng dān shēn piàn*).[2] She had also taken some other patent medicines such as Calm the Spirit and Focus the Resolve Pill *(ān shén dìng zhì wán)*, Restore the Spleen Pill *(guī pí wán)*, Emperor of Heaven's Special Pill to Tonify the Heart *(tiān wáng bǔ xīn dān)*, and Restore the Pulse Pill *(fù mài tāng)*. None of these proved to be particularly effective.

Also of note is that the patient, after the birth of her first child, had three successive abortions. She had also had a history of pyelonephritis and chronic enteritis from which she had gradually recovered.

Intake Examination
DATE: December 25, 1987

The patient was thin and emaciated. Her face looked haggard with dark circles under her eyes and dusky coloring on her cheeks. She complained of lower abdominal menstrual pain and said her menstrual blood was dark and contained clots. Her tongue was red with stasis spots on the sides and tip. The sublingual veins were dark-purple. The tongue coating was yellow and faintly greasy. Her pulse was fine, and on occasion, rapid and irregular.

Differentiation of Patterns and Discussion of Treatment

DR. YU   Palpitations are a common symptom of cardiac disease and can be seen in patterns of both deficiency and excess. Deficient patterns include Heart qi deficiency, Heart yin deficiency, dual deficiency of Heart and Spleen, Kidney yin deficiency, and Kidney yang deficiency. Excess patterns include phlegm (and thin-mucus) and blood stasis.

Palpitations that are part of a pure deficiency or a pure excess pattern are relatively easy to treat. However, most cases seen in the clinic are chronic ones, where the patient presents with a primary pattern of deficiency with some aspects of excess, or a primary pattern of excess with some aspects of deficiency. Naturally, such cases are much more troublesome.

In this case, the patient's deficiency signs were relatively prominent. She had experienced palpitations for eight years. Prior to that she had undergone three abortions, and also had a history of pyelonephritis and enteritis. Her constitution had gradually weakened and this eventually affected her Heart. The patient had previously taken herbal medicines that function to sedate the Heart and calm the spirit and tonify and nourish the Heart and Spleen, as well as formulas that enrich the Heart yin and warmly unblock Heart yang. The results, however, were disappointing. From this we can conclude that the patient's condition was not a simple pattern of deficiency but one of deficiency that includes excess.

PHYSICIAN A   Observing the dark coloring on the patient's cheeks and the suborbital region and the patient's lower abdominal pain, clotted menstrual blood, the stasis spots on her tongue and darkish purple coloring of her sublingual veins, it is obvious the pattern include blood stasis. Nevertheless, you also considered the possibility of phlegm involvement. I'm not clear how you discerned phlegm as a possible pathogen?

....

2. This consists of Salviae miltiorrhizae Radix *(dān shēn)*, Notoginseng Radix *(sān qī)*, and Borneolum *(bīng piàn)*.

DR. YU The patient's overall presentation doesn't suggest that there are any signs of phlegm. However, she had one particularly distinctive symptom: each time she began to fall asleep she was awakened by a sensation of premature beats. This unique symptom is indicative of phlegm and thin-mucus pooling below the Heart. How is this so? The process of falling asleep requires the Heart and Kidneys to interact. Heart yang moves downward to intermingle with the Kidneys and Kidney yin moves upward to intermingle with the Heart in a process known as 'mutual relief of water and fire'. When phlegm and thin-mucus gather in the epigastrium, however, the pathway by which Heart yang descends to interact with the Kidneys becomes obstructed. As a result, Heart yang is hindered in its downward movement and becomes constrained and knotted. It sinks inward, transforming into fire and heat. Fire and heat disturb the Heart-spirit and give rise to insomnia. This is the explanation of the patient's insomnia and pre-slumber experience of premature beats.

Phlegm, thin-mucus, and blood stasis are always intermingled as causes of disease. They are difficult to separate from one another and difficult to resolve. Many notable physicians, both ancient and modern, have highlighted the interrelationship of phlegm and stasis. This is a reminder that when treating palpitations, physicians must not only recognize the importance of blood stasis but also keep in mind the significance of phlegm. Even when there may not be any obvious signs of phlegm, it is advisable to ascertain whether or not any hidden phlegm exists. This means that in these cases, substances that transform phlegm, eliminate (blood) stasis, and unblock the collaterals should be included in formulas that tonify the qi, blood, yin and yang of the Heart. If we consider, then, that this patient's pattern is one of Heart yin depletion and insufficient Heart yang with obstruction of the Heart collaterals by phlegm and stasis, the best course of treatment would be to nourish yin, warm and unblock Heart yang, transform phlegm, eliminate stasis, and unblock the collaterals.

TREATMENT AND OUTCOME

The patient was given six packets of a formula based on modifying a combination of the following three formulas: Generate the Pulse Powder *(shēng mài sǎn)*, Cinnamon Twig and Licorice Decoction *(guì zhī gān cǎo tāng)*, and Warm Gallbladder Decoction *(wēn dǎn tāng)*.

Codonopsis Radix *(dǎng shēn)*	15g
Ophiopogonis Radix *(mài mén dōng)*	20g
Schisandrae Fructus *(wǔ wèi zǐ)*	6g
Cinnamomi Ramulus *(guì zhī)*	15g
Glycyrrhizae Radix preparata *(zhì gān cǎo)*	6g
standard Pinelliae Rhizoma praeparatum *(fǎ bàn xià)*	10g
Poria *(fú líng)*	15g
Citri reticulatae Pericarpium *(chén pí)*	10g
Aurantii Fructus immaturus *(zhǐ shí)*	10g
Bambusae Caulis in taeniam *(zhú rú)*	10g
Sophorae flavescentis Radix *(kǔ shēn)*	10g
Nardostachyos Radix seu Rhizoma *(gān sōng)*	6g
Trogopterori Faeces *(wǔ líng zhī)* [wrapped]	15g

SECOND VISIT: The patient felt that her Heart calmed a bit but that the rest of her symptoms were unchanged. Her pulse was still occasionally rapid and irregular.

Citri reticulatae Pericarpium *(chén pí)* and Bambusae Caulis in taeniam *(zhú rú)* were removed from the previous formula and 20g of Taxilli Herba *(sāng jì shēng)*, 6g of Asari Radix et Rhizoma *(xì xīn)*, and 6g of ground Notoginseng Radix *(sān qī)* (divided into two 3g portions and mixed into the hot decoction) were added, while the amount of Sophorae flavescentis Radix *(kŭ shēn)* was increased to 20g and Nardostachyos Radix seu Rhizoma *(gān sōng)* increased to 12g. Again, six packets were prescribed.

THIRD VISIT: The patient's menses came while she was taking the formula. She reported that her lower abdominal pain and menstrual clotting had both diminished and that she had a notable decrease in palpitations. Her tongue was pink, the stasis spots on the tip and sides of her tongue were less dark, and the color of her sublingual veins had almost returned to normal. Her pulse was fine and no longer rapid and irregular.

Thirty grams of Astragali Radix (huáng qí), 10g of Acori tatarinowii Rhizoma *(shí chāng pŭ)*, and 6g of Polygalae Radix *(yuăn zhì)* were added to the previous formula. A total of six packets were prescribed to be combined, roasted over a low flame until crisp, ground into a fine powder, mixed with refined honey, and made into pills weighing 10g each. The patient was told to take one pill three times a day for 40 days.

FOLLOW-UP REPORT: A year later the patient returned to the hospital (for treatment of unrelated health issues) and said that after finishing the pills her condition had further improved. She then had another two batches of pills made and finished those. In the many months since she was last at the hospital she had no need for Western medicines, and although she did still have occasional premature beats, tachycardia, and brief episodes of palpitations, a slight rest was all she needed to feel better. She also mentioned that her sleep and appetite were good and we could see that her complexion had noticeably improved.

Chief Complaint	Primary Symptoms	Differential Diagnosis	Treatment Method	Formula
Palpitations	Dull pain and stifling sensation in the chest, sensation of premature beats prior to falling asleep	Damaged Heart yin, insufficient Heart yang, phlegm and stasis obstructing the Heart collaterals	Enrich Heart yin, warm and unblock Heart yang, transform phlegm, eliminate stasis, and unblock the collaterals	Generate the Pulse Powder *(shēng mài săn)*, Cinnamon Twig and Licorice Decoction *(guì zhī gān căo tāng)*, and Warm Gallbladder Decoction *(wēn dăn tāng)*

REFLECTIONS AND CLARIFICATIONS

DR. YU   Treatment of palpitations and panicky throbbing with tonification is perfunctory and does not constitute real treatment. When the well-known and eccentric Qing-dynasty physician Chen Shi-Duo treated these disorders, not only did he not rely on tonification of the Heart but instead nourished the Lung, enriched the Kidneys, or fortified the Gallbladder. He did not forget to include agents to transform phlegm, such as Fritillariae Bulbus *(bèi mŭ)*, Bambusae Succus *(zhú lì)*, Sinapis Semen *(bái jiè zĭ)*, Bambusae Caulis in taeniam *(zhú rú)*, or Polygalae Radix *(yuăn zhì)*.

In the case we are discussing, the patient was initially given Generate the Pulse Powder *(shēng mài sǎn)* with Cinnamon Twig and Licorice Decoction *(guì zhī gān cǎo tāng)* to tonify the qi and blood of the Heart, as well as Warm Gallbladder Decoction *(wēn dǎn tāng)* to transform phlegm and pacify the Heart. Trogopterori Faeces *(wǔ líng zhī)* was added to expel stasis and unblock the channels, while Sophorae flavescentis Radix *(kǔ shēn)* was included to improve the Heart's rate and rhythm. Nardostachyos Radix seu Rhizoma *(gān sōng)* was added to awaken the Spleen and enliven the Stomach as well as to counteract the bitter taste and cold nature of Sophorae flavescentis Radix *(kǔ shēn)* and prevent it from damaging the Spleen and Stomach.

PHYSICIAN A Sophorae flavescentis Radix *(kǔ shēn)* is an herb that clears heat and dries dampness, expels wind, kills parasites, and promotes urination. Nevertheless you have used it here to improve the Heart's rate and rhythm. What is this usage based on?

DR. YU Modern research has shown that Sophorae flavescentis Radix *(kǔ shēn)* has the ability to reduce the strength of myocardial contractions, slow down the heartbeat, delay atrial conduction, and decrease sympathetic tone. These qualities make Sophorae flavescentis Radix *(kǔ shēn)* an effective herb for arrhythmia with tachycardia, premature beats, and/or atrial fibrillation/flutter.

Although the ancients could not have known of these properties in such detail, they were not completely ignorant of this herb's effects on the Heart. For example, the *Divine Husbandman's Classic of the Materia Medica (Shén Nóng běn cǎo jīng)* says that Sophorae flavescentis Radix *(kǔ shēn)* "governs qi knotting in the Heart and abdomen." Later, when herb theory established the practice of assigning channels of entry to herbs, Sophorae flavescentis Radix *(kǔ shēn)* was said to enter the channels of the Heart, Liver, Stomach, Large Intestine, and Bladder. The fact that the Heart is at the top of the list is significant. The *Record of One Hundred Herbs from the Classic of Materia Medica (Běn cǎo jīng bǎi zhǒng lù)* says that Sophorae flavescentis Radix *(kǔ shēn)* "specifically treats fire in the Heart channel." In the 3rd-century *Emergency Formulas to Keep up One's Sleeve (Zhǒu hòu bèi jí fāng)* it is written that "3 *liǎng* of Sophorae flavescentis Radix *(kǔ shēn),* 1.5 *shēng* of vinegar, cooked down to 8 *gě* and taken in two doses" treats "Heart pain due to strike [of] noxious [qi]."

After the patient's second visit, we added Taxilli Herba *(sāng jì shēng)*. Traditionally, Taxilli Herba *(sāng jì shēng)* is used only to expel wind-dampness, tonify the Liver and Kidneys, strengthen the tendons and bones, and calm the fetus. However, research has shown that Taxilli Herba *(sāng jì shēng)* is similar in its effects to the calcium channel blocker verapamil and can be specifically effective in treating premature atrial contractions, premature ventricular contractions, and paroxysmal atrial fibrillation/flutter.

The use of Sophorae flavescentis Radix *(kǔ shēn)* and Taxilli Herba *(sāng jì shēng)* in the treatment of this patient's premature atrial contraction and paroxysmal tachycardia is an example of a treatment based on the differentiation of the disease, as opposed to a treatment based on the differentiation of patterns. Experience has shown that when treating arrhythmia, one should differentiate both disease and pattern with emphasis given to differentiation of disease.

PHYSICIAN B Are you referring to diseases as designated by Western medicine or those designated by Chinese medicine?

DR. YU   In this instance I am referring to diseases as designated by Western medicine. In Western medicine, arrhythmia is considered to be either functional or organic. Functional arrhythmia is usually attributable to a dysfunction of the autonomic nervous system, whereas organic arrhythmia is a complication of cardiac disease. Functional arrhythmia is relatively easy to treat while arrhythmia due to organic changes in the heart is considerably more difficult.

Using only the traditional diagnostic methods of Chinese medicine (observation, inquiry, listening, smelling, and palpation) it is impossible to determine with any certainty whether a patient's arrhythmia is functional or organic. To make such a diagnosis it is necessary to perform an electrocardiogram, or, in certain circumstances, an echocardiogram.

PHYSICIAN B   Dr. Yu, I understand the reason you emphasize the necessity of disease differentiation when treating arrhythmia. The importance of a clear understanding of the patient's condition and of having an unambiguous diagnosis cannot be overstated. Such conditions make for a comprehensive treatment strategy and a more accurate prognosis. Nevertheless, it seems to me that you are emphasizing disease differentiation to the extreme, while downplaying the importance of pattern differentiation.

DR. YU   You are absolutely correct! When diagnosing a patient, disease differentiation should come first. It is important to make optimum use of the various diagnostic tools of modern medicine. Nevertheless, we can increase our efficacy by combining the information we gather from disease differentiation and pattern differentiation. In addition, we should integrate macroscopic and microscopic pattern differentiation and combine specific formulas and specific medicinal substances together in a pattern-differentiation based treatment.

In cases where recent laboratory exams aren't available and the patient's palpitations are not part of a long-term illness, but instead are abrupt in nature or occur only periodically, treatment based solely on pattern differentiation or formula-pattern correspondence is acceptable.

Treatment of palpitations based solely on pattern differentiation is exemplified in the following case treated by my teacher, Jiang Er-Xun. Years ago when Dr. Jiang was working among the minority peoples of China, he had a patient from the Yizu tribe, a 28-year-old woman. The woman had severe, intermittent palpitations that were accompanied by uncontrollable shaking. At one point she was bedridden for over a month while undergoing treatment at her local hospital.

One night she had an attack of palpitations so severe that her family literally cried out for someone to help their daughter. Dr. Jiang travelled to see her and when he arrived he saw the young woman curled up on a mattress covered in thick bedding. She was shivering so severely that the bed she lay on shook back and forth. Despite this shivering, she said she didn't feel chilled. Dr. Jiang recalled a passage from the *Discussion of Cold Damage* (*Shāng hán lùn*) in its analysis of True Warrior Decoction (*zhēn wǔ tāng*) that listed symptoms similar to what this patient was experiencing: "palpitations below the Heart, dizziness, generalized twitching, and quivering as if about to fall." He added Fossilia Ossis Mastodi *(lóng gǔ)* and Ostreae Concha *(mǔ lì)* to True Warrior Decoction *(zhēn wǔ tāng)*. That night, after two packets of this formula, the patient's shaking gradually subsided. She took the formula for a few more days to secure the efficacy of the treatment and her symptoms did not return.

PHYSICIAN A   You have said in the past that in addition to the formula you used in this case, there are formulas from Zhang Xi-Chun that you often use for palpitations.

DR. YU   Zhang Xi-Chun has two well-known formulas for treating Heart diseases. One is Stabilize the Heart Decoction *(dìng xīn tāng)*, which treats Heart deficiency with extreme palpitations. The other is Quiet the Ethereal Soul Decoction *(ān hún tāng)*, which treats fright palpitations and insomnia due to the Heart suffering from deficiency impairment of qi and blood along with phlegm and thin-mucus below the Heart. Both of these formulas are quite effective.

Stabilize the Heart Decoction *(dìng xīn tāng)*

Longan Arillus *(lóng yǎn ròu)*	30g
Ziziphi spinosae Semen *(suān zǎo rén)* [dry-fried]	15g
Corni Fructus *(shān zhū yú)*	15g
Platycladi Semen *(bǎi zǐ rén)* [dry-fried]	12g
untreated Fossilia Ossis Mastodi *(lóng gǔ)* [powdered]	12g
untreated Ostreae Concha *(mǔ lì)* [powdered]	12g
Olibanum *(rǔ xiāng)*	3g
Myrrha *(mò yào)*	3g

Stabilize the Heart Decoction *(dìng xīn tāng)* contains Longan Arillus *(lóng yǎn ròu)* to tonify Heart blood, and Ziziphi spinosae Semen *(suān zǎo rén)* and Platycladi Semen *(bǎi zǐ rén)* to tonify Heart qi. Also included is Fossilia Ossis Mastodi *(lóng gǔ)*, which enters the Liver, to calm the ethereal soul, and Ostreae Concha *(mǔ lì)*, which enters the Lung, to stabilize the corporeal soul. Other herbs include Corni Fructus *(shān zhū yú)* to restrain and inhibit dissipation of Heart qi, as well as a small amount of Olibanum *(rǔ xiāng)* and Myrrha *(mò yào)* to harmonize by improving the flow of qi and blood. Over the years I have learned that when a patient has signs of heat, the addition of Sophorae flavescentis Radix *(kǔ shēn)* and Taxilli Herba *(sāng jì shēng)* is particularly effective.

Quiet the Ethereal Soul Decoction *(ān hún tāng)*

Longan Arillus *(lóng yǎn ròu)*	18g
Ziziphi spinosae Semen *(suān zǎo rén)* [dry-fried]	12g
untreated Fossilia Ossis Mastodi *(lóng gǔ)* [powdered]	15g
untreated Ostreae Concha *(mǔ lì)* [powdered]	15g
clear Pinelliae Rhizoma praeparatum *(qīng bàn xià)*	9g
Poria *(fú líng)*	3g
Haematitum *(dài zhě shí)* [ground with a pestle]	12g

Quiet the Ethereal Soul Decoction *(ān hún tāng)* also employs Longan Arillus *(lóng yǎn ròu)* to tonify Heart blood and Ziziphi spinosae Semen *(suān zǎo rén)* to tonify Heart qi. Like Stabilize the Heart Decoction *(dìng xīn tāng)*, it too includes Ostreae Concha *(mǔ lì)* to stabilize the corporeal soul and Fossilia Ossis Mastodi *(lóng gǔ)* to calm the ethereal soul. In addition to this underlying focus on tonification and calming, the formula also includes clear Pinelliae Rhizoma praeparatum *(qīng bàn xià)* and Poria *(fú líng)* to diminish phlegm and thin-mucus, and Haematitum *(dài zhě shí)* to guide Heart yang downward into the yin, thus encouraging the onset of sleep.

You may ask why this formula contains herbs to diminish phlegm and thin-mucus. Zhang Xi-Chun explained:

> Medical books say that when phlegm and thin-mucus have pooled and stagnated below the Heart, the person will often have fright palpitations and be unable to sleep. The Heart [belongs to] fire, while phlegm and thin-mucus [belong to] water. Fire fears water and water torments fire, thus [the patient experiences] fright palpitations leading to insomnia. Phlegm and thin-mucus pooling and stagnating below the Heart is mostly due to excessive thinking. Invariably, it is this excessive thinking that also damages the Heart's qi and blood.

This is Dr. Zhang's explanation of why it is necessary, in cases such as this, to add medicinal substances that eliminate phlegm while also tonifying the qi, blood, yin or yang of the Heart.

PHYSICIAN B   In recent years I have read numerous reports about the efficacy of Prepared Licorice Decoction *(zhì gān cǎo tāng)* for the treatment of arrhythmia, but when I have given it to my patients the results have been unremarkable. Why is this?

DR. YU   The *Discussion of Cold Damage (Shāng hán lùn)* states, "For cold damage with a halting or faltering irregular pulse and Heart-disturbing palpitations, Prepared Licorice Decoction *(zhì gān cǎo tāng)* governs it." This formula is a good choice for cases where the cause of the disorder is dual deficiency of Heart yin and yang.

In addition to properly recognizing patterns, there are two key aspects to using this formula effectively. The first is using the original herb dosages of the formula. The second includes both the method of decocting the herbs as well as the method for taking the decoction.

According to the research of Ke Xue-Fan and others, during the time of Zhang Zhong-Jing's life in the Eastern Han dynasty, one *jin* equaled 250 grams, one *liang* equaled 15.65 grams, and one *sheng* equaled 200 milliliters. Based on various pieces of evidence, they believe that the measurements used in Zhang Zhong-Jing's formulas are also based on these numbers. If this is true, then the amount of herbs used in Prepared Licorice Decoction *(zhì gān cǎo tāng)* is far greater than that commonly used today. For example, the amount of Rehmanniae Radix *(shēng dì huáng)* is listed at one *jin* (250g), while Glycyrrhizae Radix preparata *(zhì gān cǎo)* is listed at four *liang* (62.5g).

The commentary following the formula provides clear instructions for preparation: "For the above nine ingredients, use seven *sheng* of clear wine and eight *sheng* of water. First, boil the eight ingredients [excluding Asini Corii Colla *(ē jiāo)*] to get three *sheng* and remove the dregs. Add Asini Corii Colla *(ē jiāo)* and warm until it is completely dissolved. Take one *sheng* warm, three times a day." I have treated several cases of premature beats with Prepared Licorice Decoction *(zhì gān cǎo tāng)* by strictly adhering to these guidelines and the results were quite good. Caution should be taken, however, in patients with Spleen and Stomach weakness because such large dosages may cause distention, stagnation, or diarrhea.

2.2 **Insomnia**

Insomnia for four years

How to approach a tangle of pathodynamics

病機混雜如何深究

■ CASE HISTORY

Patient: *46-year-old man*

The patient's problems began four years earlier when, due to personal problems, he gradually developed insomnia after becoming discouraged and depressed. In this four-year period the patient frequently took various Chinese patent medicines such as Restore the Spleen Decoction *(guī pí tāng)*, Pill for Nourishing Blood and Calming the Spirit *(yǎng xuè ān shén wǎn)*, Cinnabar Pill to Calm the Spirit *(zhū shā ān shén wán)*, and Arborvitae Seed Pill to Nourish the Heart *(bǎi zǐ yǎng xīn wán)*. In addition, before sleep the patient took diazepam (Valium).

Six months prior to coming into the clinic, the patient's insomnia began to worsen. As a result he increased his dosage of diazepam to 5mg, and although this allowed him to get three to four hours of light sleep per night, his sleep was impaired and full of dreams. He also became apprehensive and easily frightened. Because he chronically suffered from gastritis and cholecystitis, the patient took various herbal patent medications designed to treat these problems. Although these treatments seemed to help temporarily, in truth they were of questionable efficacy and this further increased the patient's distress.

INTAKE EXAMINATION
DATE: October 18, 1996

The patient's face was emaciated and his complexion slightly dusky. He reported having a stifling and full sensation in his epigastric area, but no pain. He also said that he frequently belched, his mouth was bitter and dry, and his stools were dry. His tongue was red with a thick, pasty, yellow coating. His pulse was wiry and sunken.

Differentiation of Patterns and Discussion of Treatment

TREATMENT AND RESULTS

PHYSICIAN A   The many pathodynamics that can lead to insomnia make diagnosis complicated. Modern Chinese medicine textbooks list the possible causative patterns as dual deficiency of Heart and Spleen, failure of interaction between the Heart and Kidneys, Liver yang harassment, Heart deficiency with Gallbladder timidity, and disharmony of Stomach qi. These pathodynamics touch on almost all of the organs.

When a patient comes to be treated for insomnia and only one pathodynamic is involved, treatment is fairly straightforward. However, when two or more pathodynamics are involved, treatment becomes complicated and confusing. Unfortunately, it seems that such cases are the norm.

DR. YU Due to the inherent complexity of many insomnia cases, it is imperative to be very thorough in differentiating all the pathodynamics involved. In addition, there are two aspects of treatment that are important to discuss. One is the importance of avoiding the indiscriminate use of agents that quiet the spirit and settle the emotions. The other is that, aside from addressing the patient's insomnia, one should make sure to give proper attention to treatment of the patient's other longstanding illnesses and accompanying disorders.

In addition to insomnia, this patient also chronically suffered symptoms of gastritis and cholecystitis including epigastric fullness with a stifling sensation, belching, dry mouth with bitter taste, and reduced food intake. It turns out that the pathodynamics behind these symptoms, Gallbladder heat attacking the Stomach and inability of Stomach qi to properly descend, were also among the main pathodynamics involved in the patient's insomnia. Gallbladder heat attacking the Stomach gave rise to heat which produced phlegm; this then developed into a pattern of phlegm-heat harassing the Heart, which in turn gave rise to insomnia.

Clearly, the initial treatment needed to address the patient's longstanding disorders. If the ongoing disorders were not addressed, how could there be any chance for peaceful sleep? Despite having other symptoms, the patient only sought relief from his inability to have a restful night's sleep. By focusing the initial treatment on resolving the disorder's underlying patterns (Gallbladder heat accosting the Stomach and affecting its ability to harmonize and bring about descent), two goals were scored with one kick.

Initially we aimed to clear Gallbladder heat and harmonize the Stomach. Four packets of a modified combination of Warm Gallbladder Decoction with Coptis *(huáng lián wēn dǎn tāng)*, Minor Decoction [for Pathogens] Stuck in the Chest *(xiǎo xiàn xiōng tāng)*, and Pinellia Decoction to Drain the Epigastrium *(bàn xià xiè xīn tāng)* were prescribed as follows:

standard Pinelliae Rhizoma praeparatum *(fǎ bàn xià)* 15g
Poria *(fú líng)* 30g
Bambusae Caulis in taeniam *(zhú rú)* 20g
dry-fried Aurantii Fructus immaturus *(chǎozhǐ shí)* 15g
Coptidis Rhizoma *(huáng lián)* 5g
Scutellariae Radix *(huáng qín)* 10g
Zingiberis Rhizoma *(gān jiāng)* 5g
Trichosanthis Semen *(guā lóu rén)* 15g
Pseudostellariae Radix *(tài zǐ shēn)* 10g
Taraxaci Herba *(pú gōng yīng)* 30g

The patient continued to take diazepam.

SECOND VISIT: The patient reported that he no longer experienced fullness and a stifling sensation in his epigastrium, and his symptoms of belching, dry and bitter mouth, apprehension, and being easily frightened had diminished. His bowel movements were healthy and his sleep showed some slight signs of improvement. The patient was pleased with his progress and was told to continue with the same formula. He decided to stop taking diazepam, but that night he lay awake the entire night and thus felt he had no choice but to resume taking it. After 12 packets of the formula the patient's appetite had returned and the bitterness in his mouth had ceased. Despite these improvements, he was still unwilling to stop taking diazepam because when he did so it became extremely difficult to fall asleep and he felt irritable and restless.

The patient's tongue was still red, but the yellow coating was now thin and slightly dry. The pulse was wiry, deep, and fine. From the patient's current signs and symptoms it was clear that his symptoms of Gallbladder heat and Stomach qi counterflow had resolved and what remained was underlying Liver qi constraint and blood deficiency.

The patient's formula was changed to one based on Sour Jujube Decoction *(suān zǎo rén tāng)*, a formula designed to nourish blood and soothe constraint.

The patient was given three packets of a modified Sour Jujube Decoction *(suān zǎo rén tāng),* as follows:

Ziziphi spinosae Semen *(suān zǎo rén)* 30g
Poria *(fú líng)* 30g
Anemarrhenae Rhizoma *(zhī mǔ)* 12g
Chuanxiong Rhizoma *(chuān xiōng)* 10g
Glycyrrhizae Radix preparata *(zhì gān cǎo)* 10g
Salviae miltiorrhizae Radix *(dān shēn)* 30g
Lilii Bulbus *(bǎi hé)* 30g

The patient also cut his dosage of diazepam in half.

THIRD VISIT: The patient said he had no significant improvement in his sleep, so we added 40g of standard Pinelliae Rhizoma praeparatum *(fǎ bàn xià)*, 30g of Prunellae Spica *(xià kū cǎo)*, and 50g of Sorghum *(gāo liáng mǐ)* to the previous formula.

RESULTS: After three more packets of herbs, the patient was able to fall asleep more quickly and slept peacefully for four to five hours. He then stopped taking diazepam, and after 15 more packets of herbs was falling asleep easily and sleeping restfully for five to six hours. The formula was then made into honey pills and the patient was told to take it regularly. Six months later an inquiry into the patient's condition revealed that his sleep was normal.

Disease Name	Primary Symptom	Pattern Differentiation	Treatment Method	Formulas
Insomnia	Intractable insomnia	1. Gallbladder heat attacking the Stomach 2. Liver constraint with blood deficiency and disharmony of yin and yang	1. Clear the Gallbladder and harmonize the Stomach. 2. Soothe the Liver and nourish blood, facilitate interaction of yin and yang	Warm Gallbladder Decoction with Coptis *(huáng lián wēn dǎn tāng)*, Sour Jujube Decoction *(suān zǎo rén tāng)*

Differentiation of Patterns and Discussion of Treatment

PHYSICIAN A   I find it very interesting that despite the fact that this patient had an extremely difficult case of insomnia, you were in no hurry to use medicinal substances to quiet the spirit, but instead directed your focus on treating the Gallbladder heat that was attacking his Stomach and the resulting failure of Stomach qi to properly descend. You chose to use a modified combination of Warm Gallbladder Decoction with Coptis *(huáng lián wēn dǎn tāng)* combined with Minor Decoction [for Pathogens] Stuck in the Chest *(xiǎo xiàn xiōng tāng)* and Pinellia Decoction to Drain the Epigastrium *(bàn xià xiè xīn tāng)*. Furthermore, it wasn't until after the patient's chronic conditions had markedly improved and his Liver qi constraint and blood deficiency became apparent that you decided to prescribe modified Sour Jujube Decoction *(suān zǎo rén tāng)* to nourish the Liver, soothe constraint, and quiet the spirit. Of course, this patient had already taken spirit-quieting formulas simultaneously with formulas to treat his Gallbladder and Stomach disorders, and that method had proved ineffective.

DR. YU   Insomnia is difficult to treat and relying solely on herb formulas can make successful treatment challenging. There is an old poem that says, "If you meet the master from Hua Mountain, seek not [from him] an immortality formula; seek a sleep formula." Of the many formulas available, it is very challenging to find the one that brings relief.

This case is one of the more successful cases we have treated in the past few years. In addition to the herbal treatments, each time the patient came to the clinic I provided some psychological counseling that I think was beneficial. There is a maxim in Chapter 29 of the *Divine Pivot (Líng shū)* that advises practitioners to inform patients of what can overcome them and speak to them of what is good for them. This refers to communication between doctor and patient that assists the patient in achieving a better understanding of his condition and helps him to gain confidence in the treatment plan. While it is impractical to reveal all the details of everything that I discussed with the patient, I can say that his return to health was the result of a carefully crafted strategy.

PHYSICIAN B   I have often thought that making generalizations about pathodynamics is artificial. Is there any way you could simplify Chinese medicine theory as it relates to the pathodynamic of insomnia? Please point out for us the key points with an emphasis on practicality.

DR. YU   That's an excellent line of reasoning. In the *Inner Classic (Nèi jīng)*, the fundamental pathodynamic behind insomnia is deemed to be disharmony between the protective and nutritive qi. In order to understand the pathodynamic of insomnia, it is important to first explore the pathway to sleep.

Chapter 18 of the *Divine Pivot (Líng shū)* states:

> The protective qi moves within the yang for twenty-five measures and within the yin for twenty-five measures, separated by night and day. Thus, when the qi reaches the yang one arises, when it reaches the yin there one stops. … In the middle of the night [there is] a great meeting, all the people sleep and this is called joining with yin.

This is to say that during the day the protective qi moves in the yang channels and thus people are awake; during the night protective qi moves in the yin channels and thus people sleep. In the middle of the night, during the *zǐ* time (11 p.m.–1 a.m.), the protective qi and the nutritive qi converge and people enter into sleep.

Thinking back to ancient times, productivity was much lower and the people's needs and desires were fewer than they now are. In those days, people followed the rhythms of nature, rising with the sun to work and resting once the sun went down. Insomnia was uncommon. Essentially, insomnia has no other cause than disharmony between nutritive and protective qi. This is what is referred to in Chapter 71 of the *Divine Pivot (Líng shū)*:

> Now as a reversal qi has lodged in the five bowels and six organs, the protective qi only protects the outside and moves through the yang, but cannot enter the yin. As it moves through the yang, the yang qi becomes overly full, and when the yang qi becomes overly full, the *yáng qiāo* becomes full. As [the yang qi] is unable to enter into yin, the yin is deficient and thus the eyes cannot close.

The Qing-dynasty physician Ye Tian-Shi summarized very well the pathodynamic of all types of insomnia when he stated that "Yang is hyperactive and cannot enter the yin, and yin is deficient and cannot be taken in by the yang." The basis of his statement is the aforementioned passage from the *Divine Pivot*.

So how do we treat insomnia? The same chapter of the *Divine Pivot (Líng shū)* mentions Pinellia Decoction *(bàn xià tāng)*, referred to later as Pinellia and Sorghum Decoction *(bàn xià shú mǐ tāng)*:

> Drink one packet of Pinellia Decoction, yin and yang will then communicate with each other freely and sleep will come immediately. ... The formula should be decocted with water that has flowed for more than a thousand *li*. Take eight *shēng* of this water and stir and raise it several thousands of times and take five *shēng* of [the resultant] clear water. Using reeds as fuel to make a fire, boil the water over a high flame, add one *shēng* of sorghum with five *gě* of Pinelliae Rhizoma *(bàn xià)* and continue to cook until one-and-a-half *shēng* of liquid remains. Remove the dregs and start by drinking one small cup of the decoction. Do this three times in one day, increasing the dosage slightly throughout the day until results are seen. If the illness has come about recently, sleep will come after only one cup; once the patient breaks a slight sweat they will be cured. If the illness is chronic, the patient will be cured after taking three doses.

PHYSICIAN A   Is it still possible to get rapid results when using Pinellia and Sorghum Decoction *(bàn xià shú mǐ tāng)* to treat insomnia?

DR. YU   Because of the unique requirements of utilizing water and heating in preparation of this formula, I have not used it by itself. Worth noting, however, is that Zhang Xi-Chun, a prominent physician of the early 20th century known for his emphasis on practical experience and clinical results, held this formula in high regard. He wrote:

> Formulas from the *Inner Classic (Nèi jīng)* are unusually effective. In Pinellia and Sorghum Decoction *(bàn xià shú mǐ tāng)*,[3] Pinelliae Rhizoma preparatum

3. *Translators' note:* As he explains below, Dr. Yu follows Li Shi-Zhen in taking 秫米 *shú mǐ* to be sorghum. Many others take it to refer to millet, Setariae Fructus *(shú mǐ)*, which is why in Eastland Press' *Chinese Herbal Medicine: Formulas & Strategies,* this formula is referred to as Pinellia and Millet Decoction *(bàn xià shú mǐ tāng)*.

(zhì bàn xià) unblocks yin and yang while *shú mǐ* harmonizes the Spleen and Stomach. The opening of yin and yang and harmonization of Spleen and Stomach allows sleep to ensue. This is why the *Inner Classic (Nèi jīng)* says that "sleep will come after only one cup." Its effects are remarkably rapid. Because the formula is simple and ordinary, later generations seldom used it, to the extent that, indeed, a good formula has fallen into disuse.

Zhang Xi-Chun once used a modification of this formula to treat a person who had been sleeping poorly for four months. Because the patient had a stifling, full sensation in the epigastrium, Dr. Zhang modified the formula by making a decoction with 120g of freshly shredded daikon radish. After cooking the radish down to two cups of liquid, he used that liquid to decoct 12g of Pinelliae Rhizoma preparatum *(qīng bàn xià)*. The patient was able to sleep peacefully after taking the decoction.

When I treat difficult cases of insomnia I always add 30-60g of Pinelliae Rhizoma preparatum *(zhì bàn xià)*, 50-100g of Sorghum *(gāo liáng mǐ)*, and 15-30g of Prunellae Spica *(xià kū cǎo)* to whatever formula I have determined appropriate after pattern differentiation. As can be seen from this case, these herbs can truly increase the efficacy of an insomnia formula.

PHYSICIAN A   I have two questions regarding some points that you just raised. In the *Inner Classic (Nèi jīng)* the pathodynamic of insomnia is said to be disharmony of the protective and nutritive qi. However, the formula recommended, Pinellia and Sorghum Decoction *(bàn xià shú mǐ tāng)*, is not a formula that regulates the protective and nutritive qi but instead promotes interaction between yin and yang. Second, based on the pathodynamic described in the *Inner Classic*, can Cinnamon Twig Decoction *(guì zhī tāng)*, a formula which adjusts and harmonizes the protective and nutritive qi, be used to treat insomnia?

DR. YU   In the late 17th-century text *Discussion and Annotation of the Essentials from the Golden Cabinet (Jīn guì yào lüè lùn zhù)*, Xu Bin states that when applied to "an exterior pattern, Cinnamon Twig Decoction *(guì zhī tāng)* resolves the flesh and harmonizes the protective and nutritive qi, and in cases of an interior pattern, it transforms qi and adjusts yin and yang." If this is true, how could it not be an effective formula for insomnia? It is also true that formulas based on Cinnamon Twig Decoction *(guì zhī tāng)* and the many modifications of the formula can be used to treat insomnia as well.

Nutritive and protective qi are nothing more than blood and qi, and blood and qi are nothing more than yin and yang. Pinellia and Sorghum Decoction *(bàn xià shú mǐ tāng)* connects yin and yang and thus can adjust and harmonize the nutritive and protective qi. The theory behind the formula, the methodology of treatment, the construction of the formula, and the nature of the individual herbs that comprise the formula are all consistent with this idea.

PHYSICIAN A   What is the mechanism by which Pinellia and Sorghum Decoction *(bàn xià shú mǐ tāng)* connects yin and yang?

DR. YU   Pinelliae Rhizoma *(bàn xià)* appears in midsummer, around the time of the summer solstice (in the traditional Chinese lunar calendar, this is the middle of summer).

The arrival of summer solstice marks the beginning of the yin part of the year. This is the time in nature when yin and yang converge. If we assume that we can gain an understanding of the nature of things by looking at how they manifest, we can say that Pinelliae Rhizoma *(bàn xià)* can lead yang into yin and by doing so cause yin and yang to converge.

黍米 *shú mǐ* is another name for sorghum, now known as 高粱米 *gāo liáng mǐ*. The color of *shú mǐ* is red; it nourishes the Heart and leads Heart/fire downward. Its fluid is thick; it nourishes the Kidneys and leads Kidney water upward. What makes it remarkable is that its flavor is sweet and can thus fortify the Spleen, harmonize the Stomach, and transform phlegm and thin-mucus. It opens the middle burner, leaving it unobstructed, and thus makes it easier for Heart fire to connect below with Kidney water and vice versa. When the Heart and Kidneys are in a state of continuous interaction with one another, this resembles the state described by hexagram 63 ䷾ in the *Book of Changes (Yì jīng)*, "Completion" (既濟 *jì jì*), in which the inner trigram is water and the outer fire, and sleep becomes naturally restful.

Regarding Prunellae Spica *(xià kū cǎo)*, the *Comprehensive Outline of Materia Medica (Běn cáo gāng mù)* cites Zhu Dan-Xi's discussion of the herb: "After the summer solstice this herb begins to wither. It is endowed with pure yang qi, but when yin arrives, it begins to wither." This reveals that the nature of Prunellae Spica *(xià kū cǎo)* is one that moves from yang to bring about yin; thus it can facilitate the interaction of yin and yang. When this herb is combined with Pinelliae Rhizoma preparatum *(zhì bàn xià),* the two herbs reinforce one another, thus increasing their ability to promote interaction between yin and yang.

PHYSICIAN B Speaking of the pathodynamics of insomnia, physicians from later eras thoroughly complicated the topic, but they were also basing their ideas on theory from the *Inner Classic (Nèi jīng)*. Would you agree with this assessment, Dr. Yu?

DR. YU Yes I would. There was considerable discussion of the pathodynamic of insomnia by later generations of physicians. These discussions were an extension and development of the theory of the five spirits and their corresponding yin organs.

Chapter 47 of the *Divine Pivot (Líng shū)* states, "The five yin organs store essence, spirit, blood, qi, the ethereal soul, and the corporeal soul." Specifically, "The Heart stores the spirit, the Liver stores the ethereal soul, the Lung stores the corporeal soul, the Spleen stores the intention, and the Kidneys store resolve." These five spirits are part of the higher mental activities of the central nervous system. Since this is the case, a functional imbalance in any of the five yin organs can affect a person's mental activities and lead to problems with sleep.

Some people say that discussing such ideas is a waste of time because there is no scientific evidence to support them and they are based on speculation or imagination. However, modern Western medicine itself acknowledges that it is unclear what part excitatory and inhibitive mechanisms of the central nervous system play in insomnia. Even the mechanisms behind normal sleep are far from clear.

We have discussed the five spirits and the yin organs, but we have yet to talk about the six yang organs. Influenced by the statement in the *Inner Classic (Nèi jīng)*, "The

Gallbladder governs decision making", the Qing-dynasty physician Shen Jin-Ao wrote, "When a person suffers from Heart and Gallbladder timidity, they become easily frightened, have copious confused dreams, deficiency irritability, and insomnia." In reference to the Stomach, the *Inner Classic* says, "Stomach disharmony leads to restless sleep." Meng Qing-Yun, who works on various intersections between Chinese and Western medicines at the China Academy of Chinese Medicine in Beijing, points to researchers from Harvard University who discovered that muramic acid within the macrocells lining the walls of the colon has the ability to facilitate sleep as well as boost the immune system. In other words, low levels of muramic acid in the large intestine increase the incidence of insomnia and weaken the immune system. These are just a few examples of the relationship of the yang organs' involvement in the pathodynamic of insomnia.

Theory, however, is only theory. In recent years the patterns I most commonly see in patients with insomnia include Liver constraint with blood deficiency associated with Sour Jujube Decoction *(suān zǎo rén tāng)*; phlegm-heat disturbing the Heart associated with Warm Gallbladder Decoction with Coptis *(huáng lián wēn dǎn tāng)*; and Heart and Spleen deficiency associated with Restore the Spleen Decoction *(guī pí tāng)*. Less common is the pattern associated with pathogenic heat in the *shào yīn*, as treated by Coptis and Ass-Hide Gelatin Decoction *(huáng lián ē jiāo tāng)*.

In addition to these patterns are two other unique ones that deserve mention. The first is the pattern associated with Calm the Ethereal Soul Decoction *(ān hún tāng)*. This pattern manifests with the patient falling asleep easily, but then waking after being frightened by bad dreams. After waking, falling back to sleep is extremely difficult. Zhang Xi-Chun says this is a pattern of damage to the qi and blood of the Heart, and if the patient wakes with fright and palpitations, this is owing to thin-mucus pooling below the Heart. Decoction to Quiet the Ethereal Soul *(ān hún tāng)* includes 18g of Longan Arillus *(lóng yǎn ròu)* and 12g of Ziziphi spinosae Semen *(suān zǎo rén)* to tonify Heart qi, 15g of both Fossilia Ossis Mastodi *(lóng gǔ)* and Ostreae Concha *(mǔ lì)* to calm both the ethereal and corporeal souls, 9g each of Pinelliae Rhizoma preparatum *(zhì bàn xià)* and Poria *(fú líng)* to transform phlegm and thin-mucus, and 12g of unprepared Haematitum *(shēng dài zhě shí)* to lead the Heart yang downward to be stored within the yin. I have used this formula many times and it is effective. Its efficacy is increased by combining it with Pinellia and Sorghum Decoction *(bàn xià shú mǐ tāng)* and Prunellae Spica *(xià kū cǎo)*.

The other pattern involves children who don't sleep well, toss and turn during the night, prefer to sleep on their stomach, and kick off their blankets. Mostly this is due to food accumulation and stagnation. Treatment should include dispersing food accumulation and guiding out stagnation while also supporting the Spleen's transportive function and harmonizing the Stomach, such as Preserve Harmony Pill *(bǎo hé wán)*. A small amount of Uncariae Ramulus cum Uncis *(gōu téng)* and Cicadae Periostracum *(chán tuì)* can be added to calm the Liver.

In cases where all efforts fail, blood stasis is often the culprit. I use Wang Qing-Ren's Drive out Stasis from the Mansion of Blood Decoction *(xuè fǔ zhú yū tāng)* to invigorate blood and transform stasis. This formula can achieve remarkable and unexpected results. I found it to be useful in several cases in which hope had been lost.

■ Supplement

On the question of toxicity and dosage of Pinelliae Rhizoma *(bàn xià)*

Since the publication of the insomnia case study I have received a steady stream of letters from readers offering comments or asking questions. A number of these readers expressed their concerns regarding the 40g dose of standard Pinelliae Rhizoma praeparatum *(fǎ bàn xià)* given to the patient on his third visit.

One letter, from a Dr. Xia of Jinhua city in Zhejiang, was typical of the many questions that I received:

> Dr. Yu, after reading your case study on the man with insomnia, coincidentally, a man came to me who had a similar condition. This man had suffered from insomnia for the last year and had been treated many times before without results. The patient, a 47-year-old man, also suffered from chronic cholecystitis and chronic gastritis. He had also sought treatment for these two ailments from numerous sources.
>
> The man had taken various patent Chinese medicines. These preparations approached treatment of acute cholecystitis and atrophic gastritis through clearing heat, resolving dampness, tonifying the Spleen, and regulating qi. At the time he came to see me he was taking an extract of Drive out Stasis from the Mansion of Blood Decoction *(xuè fǔ zhú yū tāng)* and 5mg of diazepam, which enabled him to sleep 2-3 hours a night.
>
> Since my patient's condition was so similar to the one in your case study, I decided to take the bold step of prescribing for him the formula you wrote for your patient. After five packets of the formula the patient reported that the results were better than anything he had taken previously. He was very happy and thanked me profusely. I showed him your article. He said he wanted to continue taking herbs, so I gave him seven more packets of the same formula. After finishing the prescription the patient was able to sleep 4-5 hours a night when he didn't take diazepam, and 7-8 hours a night when he took 2.5mg.
>
> At this point the patient asked me if I thought it would be possible for him to sleep normally without taking sedatives. His symptoms of Gallbladder heat attacking the Stomach had already been resolved and he appeared to be exhibiting signs of blood deficiency and qi stagnation. Consequently, I gave him the same formula you gave your patient on his third visit: Sour Jujube Decoction *(suān zǎo rén tāng)* combined with Pinellia and Sorghum Decoction *(bàn xià shú mǐ tāng)*.
>
> I was surprised to learn that the hospital pharmacist refused to dispense the formula; she felt that the dose of standard Pinelliae Rhizoma praeparatum *(fǎ bàn xià)* was too large. She said that she had been a pharmacist for half of her life and had never before seen anyone prescribe 40g of standard Pinelliae Rhizoma praeparatum *(fǎ bàn xià)*. I was very embarrassed. She was a senior pharmacist and was speculating that perhaps the magazine had misprinted the dosage. I am writing to confirm with you the facts of the situation. This will not only help me to address the pharmacist's questions but also to explain to my patient the best path for treatment.

In my response to Dr. Xia the first thing I made clear was that the dose of standard Pinelliae Rhizoma praeparatum *(fǎ bàn xià)* mentioned in the article was not a misprint. More importantly, I felt that I needed to respond to the more pertinent issue: is Pinelliae Rhizoma *(bàn xià)* toxic, and can it be used in large doses?

As most practitioners know, Pinelliae Rhizoma *(bàn xià)* is divided into unprocessed Pinelliae Rhizoma *(shēng bàn xià)* and Pinelliae Rhizoma preparatum *(zhì bàn xià)*. Unprocessed Pinelliae Rhizoma *(shēng bàn xià)* is toxic. When using 40g, one must pay careful attention to pre-cook it for at least an hour in order to destroy its toxic ingredients. Nowadays, however, even 40g of standard Pinelliae Rhizoma praeparatum *(fǎ bàn xià)*, which is well processed, is rejected at the pharmacy. This state of affairs in Chinese medicine has created a confusing atmosphere for beginning practitioners.

There is a historical basis for this experienced pharmacist's position as various materia medica throughout history, including Li Shi-Zhen's *Comprehensive Outline of the Materia Medica (Běn cǎo gāng mù)*, have expressed this view. There is not one source that doesn't obfuscate the issue of the toxicity of Pinelliae Rhizoma *(bàn xià)*. Even the present-day standardized textbooks perpetuate the same problem and record the accepted dose as 5-10g.

A commonly used materia medica textbook has this to say about the toxic properties of Pinelliae Rhizoma *(bàn xià)*:

> The toxic components of Pinelliae Rhizoma *(bàn xià)* have an intensely irritating effect on local tissue. When consumed raw it can cause numbness, swelling and pain of the tongue, throat and oral cavity, as well as drooling, and difficulty opening the mouth. In severe cases it can lead to vomiting and even asphyxiation.

Indeed, unprocessed Pinelliae Rhizoma *(shēng bàn xià)* is extremely toxic and these warnings should be taken seriously.

However, it is important to note that these warnings refer to what could happen when consuming unprocessed Pinelliae Rhizoma *(shēng bàn xià)* directly, that is, without cooking. Those who do consume the raw herb, often do so mistakenly. What about consuming it after it has been cooked? The same textbook goes on to say, "These toxic substances are not easily dissolved in water and can be broken down after extended heating." Thus, after being cooked, unprocessed Pinelliae Rhizoma *(shēng bàn xià)*, or the liquid made from decocting it, ought to be essentially non-toxic. Oddly, however, the conclusion that the textbook comes to is that "unprocessed Pinelliae Rhizoma *(shēng bàn xià)* is toxic and generally is not used internally." Very confusing indeed!

This materia medica textbook goes on to clarify that the toxicity of unprocessed Pinelliae Rhizoma *(shēng bàn xià)* "cannot be broken down with ginger juice alone, but can be eliminated by Alumen *(bái fán)*." It can be seen then that Pinelliae Rhizoma *(bàn xià)*, which has been processed in complete accordance with processing standards, is not toxic.

Given the above information we can draw a few conclusions:

1. Pinelliae Rhizoma preparatum *(zhì bàn xià)* is not toxic. Unprocessed Pinelliae Rhizoma *(shēng bàn xià)* is toxic, but extended cooking can eliminate its toxicity.

2. Properly processed Pinelliae Rhizoma *(zhì bàn xià)* can be used in large doses, and does not need to be pre-decocted. Unprocessed Pinelliae Rhizoma *(shēng bàn xià)* should be pre-decocted for at least a half an hour in order to eliminate its toxicity. If using between 30-60g, it should be pre-decocted for at least an hour.

3. If, when using large doses (30g or more), the practitioner is concerned that the Pinelliae Rhizoma preparatum *(zhì bàn xià)* was possibly not processed in accordance with strict standards and thus may still retain some toxicity, the Pinelliae Rhizoma preparatum *(zhì bàn xià)* should be precooked for 30 minutes as a precautionary measure.

I will end my comments on Dr. Xia's questions here, but I would like to add some thoughts about Pinelliae Rhizoma *(bàn xià)* for fellow travelers on the path of Chinese medicine.

1. The *Discussion of Cold Damage (Shāng hán lùn)* contains a great many formulas that use Pinelliae Rhizoma *(bàn xià)*. In each of them it is clearly noted that Pinelliae Rhizoma *(bàn xià)* should be washed. That is, unprocessed Pinelliae Rhizoma *(shēng bàn xià)* is to be decocted after washing it clean with water. This is completely different from the custom of later generations who used ginger, Zingiberis Rhizoma recens *(shēng jiāng)*, and Alumen *(bái fán)* to make various forms of Pinelliae Rhizoma preparatum *(zhì bàn xià)*.[4]

   The well-known, early 20th-century physician Zhang Xi-Chun often used processed Pinelliae Rhizoma *(zhì bàn xià)*, but loathed using any Pinelliae Rhizoma preparatum *(zhì bàn xià)* that had been processed improperly and contained too much Alumen *(bái fán)*. He explained:

   > [When] overly processed, it has absolutely no acrid flavor and instead tastes like Alumen *(bái fán)*, which causes retching and vomiting. The clear Pinelliae Rhizoma praeparatum *(qīng bàn xià)*, prepared by the pharmacies, also contains Alumen *(bái fán)*, which is acceptable if using it to resolve dampness. However, it is inappropriate if used to arrest retching and vomiting, or if used to treat vomiting of blood, or nosebleeds. When I treat such problems, I need to wash the clear Pinelliae Rhizoma praeparatum *(qīng bàn xià)* many times with mildly warm water before I use it. Such multiple washings diminish the potency of the herb, thus I am forced to increase the dose.

2. There are many opportunities for the use of Pinelliae Rhizoma preparatum *(zhì bàn xià)* and the key to using it effectively is in the amount prescribed. For drying dampness and transforming phlegm, 6-8g is sufficient. If using it to settle counterflow qi and check vomiting, 15-20g is not excessive. To sedate and quiet the spirit, a dose of 30-60g must be used.

3. Untreated Pinelliae Rhizoma *(shēng bàn xià)* is a very powerful herb. When intractable phlegm and chronic blood stasis lead to illness, as in pain related to cancer, processed Pinelliae Rhizoma *(zhì bàn xià)* is not strong enough. In such circumstances it is necessary to use large doses of unprocessed Pinelliae Rhizoma *(shēng bàn xià)*, remembering to pre-decoct it for an extended time in order to eliminate its toxicity.

....

4. *Translators' note:* When harvested, the rhizome of Pinelliae has a thin skin covering, not unlike the outer skin on an onion. The herb should be soaked in water and this skin removed. The slimy, sticky substance just beneath the skin contains a large amount of the irritating component of the herb. This is why Zhang Zhong-Jing stipulated that the herb be washed before decoction. Note that most unprocessed Pinelliae Rhizoma *(shēng bàn xià)* on the market nowadays has had the skin removed and has been washed.

CHAPTER 3

Spleen and Stomach System Disorders

3.1 Epigastric pain

Dull epigastric pain lasting three years

Skill is apparent in the subtleties

細微之處見功夫

■ **CASE HISTORY**

Patient: *42-year-old woman*

For three years prior to her examination the patient experienced dull epigastric pain exacerbated by hunger. The pain was especially severe 3-4 hours after breakfast, and it was relieved by warmth, pressure, and eating. The accompanying symptoms included acid regurgitation, indefinable epigastric discomfort, intestinal rumbling, and black stools.

After an endoscopic examination, she was diagnosed with active peptic ulcer of the duodenal bulb accompanied by duodenitis and chronic superficial gastritis. For more than a year, she tried many medications including cimetidine, hericium mushroom, and furazolidone without any lasting effect.

A doctor of Chinese medicine diagnosed her with deficiency cold in the Spleen and Stomach for which he prescribed Astragalus Decoction to Construct the Middle *(huáng qí jiàn zhōng tāng)* plus Alpiniae officinarum Rhizoma *(gāo liáng jiāng)*, Piperis longi Fructus *(bì bá)*, and Amomi Fructus *(shā rén)* combined with Cuttlefish and Frittelaria Powder *(wū bèi sǎn*).[1] After more than ten packets, the patient's pain, acid regurgitation, indefinable epigastric discomfort, and intestinal rumbling were greatly improved. However, because of side effects such as dry mouth and throat and bleeding gums, she stopped taking the formula and came in for a consultation.

INTAKE EXAMINATION
DATE: August 25, 1994

Her primary presentation was as described above. Although food intake moderated the intensity of the pain temporarily, it also led to epigastric fullness with a stifling sensation. The patient had a lusterless complexion and was fatigued. She slept poorly, had many dreams, experienced black stools and, although her mouth was dry, she had no desire to drink. Her tongue was slightly pale and had a thin, yellow coating that lacked moisture. Her pulse was weak and slightly rapid.

Differentiation of Patterns and Discussion of Treatment

DR. YU   Upon examining this patient and considering the presenting symptoms such as lusterless complexion, fatigue, and sub-par, dream-disturbed sleep, we felt that the pattern differentiation pointed to deficiency of Spleen qi and Heart blood. We could point to the Spleen failing in its transportive function as being responsible for the patient's epigastric fullness and stifling sensation. However, in this instance, because the Spleen and Stomach are interdependent and chronic diseases can enter the collaterals, this situation caused stasis in the Stomach collaterals, which in turn led to a loss of harmonious downward movement in the Stomach and the resulting epigastric fullness and stifling sensation.

PHYSICIAN A   Spleen-Stomach deficiency-cold Stomach and duodenal ulcers are fairly common. In the 1950s, Qin Bo-Wei popularized the treatment of peptic ulcers with yang-warming, qi-augmenting, and center-building Astragalus Decoction to Construct the Middle *(huáng qí jiàn zhōng tāng)*. Since that time, many people in the medical community have respected this methodology and found it effective.

Considering this case of duodenal ulcer accompanied by duodenitis and chronic superficial gastritis in which the symptoms worsen with hunger but improve with heat and pressure, and noticing that these symptoms are greatly alleviated with a modified Astragalus Decoction to Construct the Middle *(huáng qí jiàn zhōng tāng)*, we can conclude that the primary disease dynamic is deficiency cold in the Spleen and Stomach. This finding is not contradicted by the fact that after more than ten bags of the formula some heat symptoms appeared. Yet, upon seeing the patient, you differentiated the pattern as one of Heart and Spleen deficiency and stasis in the Stomach collaterals. What is the logic of that?

DR. YU   The previous physician, upon seeing the primary symptoms (dull epigastric pain that worsened with hunger and improved with warmth and pressure, temporarily so

....

1. *Translators' note:* This is a modern formula comprised of 255g of Sepiae Endoconcha *(hǎi piāo xiāo)* and 45g of Fritillariae thunbergii Bulbus *(zhè bèi mǔ)*. The two are ground together into a powder with 1.5-3g taken 2-3 times a day with warm water on an empty stomach.

after eating), diagnosed the patient with deficiency cold in the Spleen and Stomach, which he treated with Astragalus Decoction to Construct the Middle *(huáng qí jiàn zhōng tāng)*. Of course, this made perfect sense. My assertion that deficiency cold in the Spleen and Stomach may not be the primary disease dynamic, but instead an accompanying dynamic, was the result of considering the efficacy of the formula and the appearance of the side effects.

There are three points to consider when thinking about the side effects of dry mouth and throat and bleeding gums in this case:

1. Spleen-Stomach deficiency cold was not the primary disease dynamic, but was an attendant dynamic.

2. "Overdoing is as bad as not doing enough"— the extended use of acrid, hot herbs created a situation in which, before the cold disorder resolved, a heat disorder arose.

3. In cases of blood in the stool, one should be extremely cautious about the use of warm, dry, blood-stirring herbs such as Cinnamomi Ramulus *(guì zhī)*, Alpiniae officinarum Rhizoma *(gāo liáng jiāng)*, and Piperis longi Fructus *(bì bá)*.

PHYSICIAN B   It seems that you are, on the one hand, agreeing that the diagnosis of Spleen-Stomach deficiency cold made perfect sense, yet on the other hand, suggesting that Spleen-Stomach deficiency cold may not be the primary disease dynamic. Isn't this a contradiction?

DR. YU   It would seem that it is a contradiction; however, in the language of Western medicine, this is known as an 'amended diagnosis.' Furthermore, in clinical practice, this type of situation is a common occurrence. Because of the deep influence of traditional Chinese culture and ways of thinking on Chinese medicine as it developed into the modern era, Chinese medicine is considered a phenomenological medical science. In clinical practice, Chinese medical diagnosis emphasizes phenomena and proceeds according to the tenets of "All internal [phenomena] must take form on the outside" and "Upon seeing the external correspondence, one can know the interior." In this context, "outside" or "external" refers to external manifestations of the disease, whereas "internal" or "interior" refers to the internal nature of the disease.

The nature of the disease and the manifestations are essentially an antithetical pair, and the full revelation of the nature of the disease is actually a process. Remember the words of Karl Marx: "All science would be superfluous if the form of appearance of things directly coincided with their essence." Because practicing physicians will sometimes be unable to quickly determine the nature of a disease, it is difficult to avoid reaching different conclusions at different points in the process.

The notion of this pain being due to blood stasis in the collaterals can be traced back to an idea of the famous 17th-century physician Ye Tian-Shi. He observed that long-standing pain must involve the collaterals. Often, as is the case here, long-standing pain that does not respond to other types of treatment can be considered as stasis affecting the collaterals. Considering that the pattern is one of Heart-Spleen deficiency and stasis in the Stomach collaterals, the treatment should be to strengthen the Spleen, nourish the Heart, unblock the collaterals, and harmonize the Stomach.

Treatment and Outcome

We selected Restore the Spleen Decoction *(guī pí tāng)* to strengthen the Spleen, nourish the Heart, augment the qi, and tonify the blood, and combined it with Salvia Drink *(dān shēn yǐn)* to move the qi, transform stasis, unblock the collaterals, and harmonize the Stomach.

Here is the formula, as modified:

Astragali Radix *(huáng qí)* 30g
Codonopsis Radix *(dǎng shēn)* 15g
Atractylodis macrocephalae Rhizoma *(bái zhú)* 15g
Glycyrrhizae Radix praeparata *(zhì gān cǎo)* 6g
Acori tatarinowii Rhizoma *(shí chāng pǔ)* 6g
processed Polygalae Radix *(zhì yuǎn zhì)* 6g
dry-fried Ziziphi spinosae Semen *(suān zǎo rén)* 12g
Aucklandiae Radix *(mù xiāng)* 15g
Angelicae sinensis Radix *(dāng guī)* 10g
Poria *(fú líng)* 15g
Salviae miltiorrhizae Radix *(dān shēn)* 30g
Notoginseng Radix *(sān qī)* [powder and take with strained decoction] ... 5g

The patient was advised to take three packets, and if there were no side effects, to continue taking more. She was also given a version of Stop Bleeding Powder *(zhǐ xuè sǎn)* made up by our hospital. This is a formula composed of Sepiae Endoconcha *(hǎi piāo xiāo)*, Bletillae Rhizoma *(bái jí)*, and Notoginseng Radix *(sān qī)*.

SECOND VISIT: After taking 12 bags, the patient's dull epigastric pain still appeared occasionally, but her acid regurgitation, indefinable epigastric discomfort, and intestinal rumbling had greatly decreased. The epigastric fullness and stifling sensation had resolved. Her spirit, physical strength, and sleep had all improved. Although her stool was no longer black, laboratory exam still revealed occult blood. The patient's tongue was pale-red with a thin coating and her pulse was moderate and weak.

To the previous formula, we added pills made of four packets of the following:

Lilii Bulbus *(bǎi hé)* 30g
Nelumbinis Semen *(lián zǐ)* 30g
Bletillae Rhizoma *(bái jí)* 30g

Instructions: Roast these herbs until crisp using a low flame then grind them to a fine powder. Mix with refined honey and make into pills, each pill weighing 10g. Take one pill three times per day.

Result: Upon follow-up after eight months, the patient reported that she was unwilling to undergo another endoscopy, but that her epigastric pain along with all the other symptoms

Disease	Primary Symptoms	Pattern Differentiation	Treatment Method	Formulas
Epigastric pain (duodenal ulcer)	Dull epigastric pain, worsens when hungry	Deficiency of Heart and Spleen, stasis in the Stomach collaterals	Strengthen the Spleen, nourish the Heart; unblock the collaterals, harmonize the Stomach	Restore the Spleen Decoction (guī pí tāng) and Salvia Drink (dān shēn yǐn)

had resolved. Furthermore, laboratory tests showed that her stool was negative for blood.

Reflections and Clarifications

PHYSICIAN C   What is the rationale behind your usage of Restore the Spleen Decoction (guī pí tāng) for the majority of cases of deficiency-type epigastric pain resulting from duodenal ulcer?

DR. YU   This usage comes from the experience of my teacher, Jiang Er-Xun. He came to this understanding by reading about the treatments of the mid-Qing physician Chen Xiu-Yuan for 'deficiency pain of the epigastrium.' In *Excellent Usage of Contemporary Formulas (Shí fāng miào yòng)*, Chen wrote that

> Deficiency pain is [the same as] palpitations and pain. The pulse is deficient, fine, and small or short and rough, and there are epigastric palpitations. The pain is relieved with pressure or food intake. The bowels and urination are normal. It is appropriate to use Restore the Spleen Decoction (guī pí tāng) plus one *qián* of Acori tatarinowii Rhizoma (shí chāng pǔ).

Epigastric pain arising from duodenal ulcer is typically dull, long-term, occurs with hunger, is ameliorated by warmth and pressure, and is somewhat relieved by food intake. It undoubtedly belongs to the category of deficiency pain.

Furthermore, a pattern of Spleen and Heart deficiency is indicated by the presence of lingering pain, poor appetite, weakened Spleen transport, difficult transformation of food and fluids, and deficiency of qi and blood. This pattern often presents with a lusterless complexion, palpitations, shortness of breath, insomnia, and poor memory.

Due to the Heart and Spleen insufficiency with deficiency of qi and blood, the locus of the ulceration loses normal warming and nourishment. As it is said, "Without nourishment, there is pain." Therefore, the pain persists for an extended period of time and the lesions are difficult to heal.

One must sever and interrupt this vicious cycle. Dr. Jiang considered Restore the Spleen Decoction (guī pí tāng) as a particularly effective formula to strengthen the Spleen, nourish the Heart, augment and tonify the qi, and thereby interrupt the vicious cycle.

Observation in the clinic has revealed that after a patient has taken several packets—up to about ten—of Restore the Spleen Decoction (guī pí tāng), if their pain has decreased and their appetite has increased, then the palpitations, shortness of breath, insomnia, and forgetfulness will generally also improve greatly. The converse is also true, that is, if the palpitations, insomnia, etc. improve first, the pain will decrease later.

Dr. Jiang pointed out that the efficacy of Restore the Spleen Decoction *(guī pí tāng)* for this type of disease cannot be attributed solely to the fact that it is a sweet, warming formula that tonifies deficiency, because there are many other formulas of this type. He quoted Zhang Jing-Yue: "In patients where qi and blood are deficient and cold and unable to nourish the Heart and Spleen, there are often patterns of pain in the epigastrium and abdomen. This disease is inevitably seen in those who have experienceed long-term overwork, over-thinking, and lack of fulfillment." There is some similarity between this perspective and that of modern medicine with regards to the dynamic that produces ulcers in the digestive system.

Dr. Jiang further stressed that this disease is intimately connected to the seven emotions. When worry and over-thinking injure the Heart and Spleen, the Stomach certainly will also meet with disaster. Taking this further, he concurred with the brilliant teaching of Chen Xiu-Yuan that "the method to restore the Spleen aims at the double yang." ("Double yang" refers to the foot *yáng míng* Stomach.) The hidden meaning of this phrase is that soothing the emotions with Restore the Spleen Decoction *(guī pí tāng)* is the way to restore the highest level of function to the central nervous system.

PHYSICIAN A   Can you explain how to modify and use the formula?

DR. YU   Dr. Jiang emphasized that when modifying ancient formulas, we should not attach too much importance to the specific functions of individual herbs. Generally, we should not build formulas by addressing specific symptoms, but instead should aim at the pathodynamic and make any changes on that basis. We must do our best to consider the entire formula and the way that the individual ingredients work together. At the same time, we should not be too rigid and should realize that some modifications of a base formula can increase its efficacy. For example, taking Restore the Spleen Decoction *(guī pí tāng)* as a base, the following additions can be very useful:

- If the disease is accompanied by Liver constraint, add Bupleuri Radix *(chái hú)* and Paeoniae Radix alba *(bái sháo)*, recalling Rambling Powder *(xiāo yáo sǎn)*.

- If the pain is distinct or accompanied by fullness and a stifling sensation, modify with Salviae miltiorrhizae Radix *(dān shēn)*, as was done in this case, which is reminiscent of Salvia Drink *(dān shēn yǐn)*.

- To address acid regurgitation, add Sepiae Endoconcha *(hǎi piāo xiāo)* and Fritillariae Bulbus *(bèi mǔ)*, as in Cuttlefish and Fritillaria Powder *(wū bèi sǎn)*.

- For blood in the stools, include Sepiae Endoconcha *(hǎi piāo xiāo)*, Bletillae Rhizoma *(bái jí)*, and Notoginseng Radix *(sān qī)*, evoking Stop Bleeding Powder *(zhǐ xuè sǎn)*.

- If there is a lot of blood in the stool, increase Ginseng Radix rubra *(hóng shēn)*.

- For cold, add Zingiberis Rhizoma preparata *(páo jiāng)*, suggestive of Regulate the Middle Pill *(lǐ zhōng wán)*.

- If there is also heat, add Moutan Cortex *(mǔ dān pí)* and Paeoniae Radix alba *(bái sháo)*.

- For dampness, add Pogostemonis/Agastaches Caulis *(huò xiāng gĕng)* and Eupatorii Herba *(pèi lán).*

- For focal distention, pain, and belching, add Inulae Flos *(xuán fù huā)* and Haematitum *(dài zhĕ shí),* evoking thoughts of Inula and Haematite Decoction *(xuán fù dài zhĕ tāng).*

- And if addressing abdominal fullness, include ginger Magnoliae officinalis Cortex *(jiāng hòu pò)* and Pinelliae Rhizoma preparatum *(zhì bàn xià),* as in Magnolia, Fresh Ginger, Pinellia, Licorice, and Ginseng Decoction *(hòu pò shēng jiāng bàn xià gān căo rén shēn tāng).*

PHYSICIAN B   If epigastric deficiency pain is the result of a peptic ulcer, can we still use Restore the Spleen Decoction *(guī pí tāng)?*

DR. YU   The formula can still be used, but you must differentiate the pattern carefully and then flexibly modify the formula. Dr. Jiang held that although stomach and duodenal ulcers belong to the category of peptic ulcers, and the pain characteristics and accompanying symptoms have some similarity, there are also some important differences. Both conditions produce pain that is typically long-term, dull, and improves with pressure. However, stomach-ulcer pain typically occurs 30-60 minutes after meals; thus, it is referred to as 'satiation pain,' which is connected with the pathodynamic of a failure of downward movement of the Stomach qi. In contrast, duodenal ulcer pain typically occurs about three hours after meals; thus, it is referred to as 'hunger pain.' It is rarely coupled with excess.

Furthermore, at the onset of pain the qi knots in the channels; after some time the blood is damaged and enters into the collaterals. As a result, both types of ulcers can cause blood in the stool, evidence that a deficient Spleen is failing to control the blood. However, peptic ulcers tend to produce vomiting of blood because of the previously mentioned connection with a failure of the downward movement of Stomach qi. Vomiting of blood is very rarely encountered in duodenal ulcer cases.

Careful consideration of these similarities and differences can assist us when we think about the usage of Astragalus Decoction to Construct the Middle *(huáng qí jiàn zhōng tāng)* in the treatment of peptic ulcers. Dr. Jiang believed that among the herbs in the formula, Cinnamomi Ramulus *(guì zhī)* is most able to stir the blood and thus, in patients with vomiting of blood or blood in the stool, it should be used cautiously, if at all. When Dr. Jiang treated peptic ulcers that belonged to the category of deficiency cold in the Spleen and Stomach, and bleeding was present, he preferred to use Restore the Spleen Decoction *(guī pí tāng),* adding Zingiberis Rhizoma preparata *(páo jiāng)* which, being blackened, stops bleeding. This combination brings to mind Licorice and Ginger Decoction *(gān căo gān jiāng tāng)* combined with Regulate the Middle Pill *(lĭ zhōng wán).* In cases where there was no bleeding, he used Restore the Spleen Decoction *(guī pí tāng)* with Cinnamomi Ramulus *(guì zhī)* and Paeoniae Radix alba *(bái sháo),* which is reminiscent of Astragalus Decoction to Construct the Middle *(huáng qí jiàn zhōng tāng).*

3.2 Focal distention and fullness

Focal distention, fullness, and dull epigastric pain for six months

Differentiating primary and secondary concerns in order to avoid "errors at the outset"

辨主次避免 "開手便錯"

■ CASE HISTORY

Patient: *55-year-old man*

For six months prior to coming to the clinic the patient had been experiencing focal distention, fullness, and dull epigastric pain. Endoscopy revealed evidence of the following:

- chronic superficial gastritis (affecting the gastric body and antrum)
- bile-reflux gastritis (also known as reactive or chemical gastropathy)
- duodenitis
- distal esophagitis

The patient had been continuously taking both prepared Chinese medicines and Western medicines (metoclopramide, amoxycillin, hericium mushroom, and motilium) for several months. Although these medications had reduced the severity of the symptoms, as soon as the patient stopped taking them, the focal distention and pain returned just as before. However, further endoscopy showed that the inflammatory conditions had in fact decreased; thus, the patient was perplexed.

INTAKE EXAMINATION
DATE: November 5, 1998

The patient's facial complexion was slightly dark and yellowish. His affect was depressed. He reported that he experienced focal distention, fullness, and dull pain in his epigastrium. His accompanying symptoms included poor appetite, belching, an indeterminate gnawing sensation, and acid reflux. The patient's tongue was dark and dull with a thin, yellow, and greasy coating. His pulse was wiry and soggy.

When the patient was queried more specifically about the feeling in his epigastrium, he replied that the predominant symptom was focal distention and fullness; the dull pain was secondary.

Differentiation of Patterns and Discussion of Treatment

DR. YU   Pathological changes in the stomach and duodenum (including inflammatory and ulcerative conditions) are categorized by some contemporary Chinese medicine physicians as belonging wholly to the category of stomach and epigastric pain, but this does not seem congruent with clinical reality. For example, in the present case of focal distention, fullness, and dull pain, the symptom that the patient found least tolerable was not the pain, but the feeling of fullness, oppression, and blockage. This is in accord with the focal distention patterns described in the *Discussion of Cold Damage (Shāng hán lùn)*.

There are those who refer to line 149 of that text, which clearly states that "if it is only fullness and not pain, this constitutes focal distention." This suggests that focal distention patterns should be completely devoid of pain, to the extent that if pain is present, then the pattern cannot be one of focal distention. This bears further consideration.

First, it is my opinion that the phrase "only fullness and not pain" is meant to distinguish focal distention from chest knotting, which is described as "epigastric fullness, hardness, and pain." Second, we need to consider if pain is truly completely absent in focal distention patterns. Consider the lines from the *Discussion of Cold Damage (Shāng hán lùn)* that discuss focal distention. At line 154, the description of the pattern for Rhubarb and Coptis Decoction to Drain the Epigastrium *(dà huáng huáng lián xiè xīn tāng)* is "epigastric focal distention that is soft when pressed," which is to say that it is mushy when pressed and may not be painful. However, at lines 157 and 158 describing the patterns associated with Fresh Ginger Decoction to Drain the Epigastrium *(shēng jiāng xiè xīn tāng)* and Licorice Decoction to Drain the Epigastrium *(gān cǎo xiè xīn tāng)*, the finding is described as "epigastric hard focal distention," which suggests that the area is tense and resistant when pressed, and not necessarily completely painless. Furthermore, we frequently see patients with pathological changes in the stomach and duodenum who manifest with varying degrees of both pain and focal distention.

For physicians to grasp these patterns, they must carefully question the patient in order to clearly distinguish the relative severity of pain in relation to the focal distention. Only in this way can one avoid "making a mistake right at the beginning of the task."

PHYSICIAN A   The view that you have described happens to coincide with that of Western medicine. While in Western medicine, treatment follows the diagnosis of specific diseases, in the treatment of inflammatory and ulcerative conditions of the stomach and duodenum it is necessary to clearly differentiate pain from distention.

Pronounced pain occurs when excessive peristalsis leads to spasms and should be treated with medicines that relieve spasms and pain; pronounced fullness and distention occurs when insufficient peristalsis leads to motility disorders and should be treated with medicines that stimulate the force of peristalsis, such as domperidone. If you are saying that there is similarity between fullness and distention and the specific pattern of focal distention, would it be reasonable to say that Pinellia Decoction to Drain the Epigastrium *(bàn xià xiè xīn tāng)*, which relieves focal distention and eliminates distention, is similar to Western medicines that stimulate peristalsis?

DR. YU   There is a certain logic to what you have said. However, there are two lines from the classics that relate to Pinellia Decoction to Drain the Epigastrium *(bàn xià xiè xīn tāng)*. One, line 149 of the *Discussion of Cold Damage (Shāng hán lùn)*, states:

> When cold-damage exists for five or six days with retching and fever and the presence of all the Minor Bupleurum Decoction *(xiǎo chái hú tāng)* presenta-

tion has been purged with other medicines, if the Minor Bupleurum Decoction *(xiǎo chái hú tāng)* presentation is still present, Minor Bupleurum Decoction *(xiǎo chái hú tāng)* can still be given. ... If the epigastrium is only full and not painful, this constitutes focal distention. It is not right to give them Bupleurum [formulas]; Pinellia Decoction to Drain the Epigastrium *(bàn xià xiè xīn tāng)* is appropriate.

Does it not seem that this line is referring to an inhibition of peristaltic force, leading to insufficient peristalsis?

Conversely, the other line, from Chapter 17 of the *Essentials from the Golden Cabinet (Jīn guì yào lüè)*, which discusses retching, vomiting, and diarrhea, states: "When [there is] retching and intestinal rumbling, and epigastric focal distention, Pinellia Decoction to Drain the Epigastrium *(bàn xià xiè xīn tāng)* governs." So we see that the formula treats focal distention, yet it also treats intestinal rumbling. How can we explain that? Doing so by citing a peristaltic action of the formula is inherently contradictory. However, from the perspective of Chinese medicine, the basic pathodynamic of focal distention involves a heat-cold complex, mixed deficiency and excess, and irregular ascent and descent. Therefore, using Pinellia Decoction to Drain the Epigastrium *(bàn xià xiè xīn tāng)* and its related formulas to disperse focal distention and dispel fullness by regulating heat and cold, deficiency and excess, and ascent and descent is a flawless example of the fundamental relationship between principles, strategies, formulas, and medicinal substances.

PHYSICIAN A   There are five related formulas in the *Discussion of Cold Damage (Shāng hán lùn)*: Rhubarb and Coptis Decoction to Drain the Epigastrium *(dà huáng huáng lián xiè xīn tāng)*, Aconite Accessory Root Decoction to Drain the Epigastrium *(fù zǐ xiè xīn tāng)*, Pinellia Decoction to Drain the Epigastrium *(bàn xià xiè xīn tāng)*, Fresh Ginger Decoction to Drain the Epigastrium *(shēng jiāng xiè xīn tāng)*, and Licorice Decoction to Drain the Epigastrium *(gān cǎo xiè xīn tāng)*. When you say Pinellia Decoction to Drain the Epigastrium *(bàn xià xiè xīn tāng)* and the related formulas, am I correct in assuming you are referring to the latter three?

DR. YU   That is correct. These three formulas are named after the chief ingredient in each formula. In fact, only one ingredient differs among the three formulas. There are seven herbs in common: Pinelliae Rhizoma *(bàn xià)*, Zingiberis Rhizoma *(gān jiāng)*, Scutellariae Radix *(huáng qín)*, Coptidis Rhizoma *(huáng lián)*, Ginseng Radix *(rén shēn)*—which is frequently replaced at present with Codonopsis Radix *(dǎng shēn)* or Pseudostellariae Radix *(tài zǐ shēn)*—Glycyrrhizae Radix *(gān cǎo)*, and Jujubae Fructus *(dà zǎo)*.

In the formula, Pinelliae Rhizoma *(bàn xià)* and Zingiberis Rhizoma *(gān jiāng)* disperse cold with acridity and unblock with warmth. Scutellariae Radix *(huáng qín)* and Coptidis Rhizoma *(huáng lián)* clear heat via their bitter flavor and descending, cold, and draining natures. Ginseng Radix *(rén shēn)*, Glycyrrhizae Radix *(gān cǎo)*, and Jujubae Fructus *(dà zǎo)* tonify Spleen and Stomach qi deficiency with sweetness and warmth. Thus, cold and heat, ascending and descending, and tonifying and draining are used simultaneously in order to disperse focal distention and dispel fullness.

The pattern associated with Pinellia Decoction to Drain the Epigastrium *(bàn xià xiè xīn tāng)* is the result of erroneous purgation of a Minor Bupleurum Decoction *(xiǎo chái hú tāng)* pattern. Because retching is prominent, Pinelliae Rhizoma *(bàn xià)*, which directs counterflow qi downward and relieves retching, is the chief. According to the Qing-dynasty scholar Ke Yun-Bo, Pinellia Decoction to Drain the Epigastrium *(bàn xià xiè xīn tāng)*

> is Minor Bupleurum Decoction *(xiǎo chái hú tāng)* minus Bupleuri Radix *(chái hú)* with the addition of Coptidis Rhizoma *(huáng lián)* and Zingiberis Rhizoma *(gān jiāng)*. … [Further, the dosage of] Pinelliae Rhizoma *(bàn xià)* is doubled and Zingiberis Rhizoma recens *(shēng jiāng)* is removed [thereby] slightly changing the half-exterior treatment [strategy] of Bupleuri Radix *(chái hú)* to emphasize the *shào yáng* half-interior idea.

Fresh Ginger Decoction to Drain the Epigastrium *(shēng jiāng xiè xīn tāng)* is Pinellia Decoction to Drain the Epigastrium *(bàn xià xiè xīn tāng)* with a reduced dose of Zingiberis Rhizoma *(gān jiāng)* and the addition of a large dose of Zingiberis Rhizoma recens *(shēng jiāng)*, which serves as the chief. It treats a pattern in which water-qi in the epigastrium and abdomen is not transformed, or as it is described in the source text at line 157: "disharmony in the Stomach, epigastric focal distention and firmness, dry belching with the stench of [undigested] food, water-qi below the ribs, thunderous rumblings in the abdomen, and diarrhea."

Licorice Decoction to Drain the Epigastrium *(gān cǎo xiè xīn tāng)* is Pinellia Decoction to Drain the Epigastrium *(bàn xià xiè xīn tāng)* with a large dose of Glycyrrhizae Radix *(gān cǎo)*, which serves as the chief. It treats a Spleen-Stomach deficiency pattern with sinking of the clear yang, or as it is described in the source text at line 158: "the person [will experience] diarrhea more than ten times per day with undigested food, thunderous rumblings in the abdomen, epigastric fullness and hard focal distention, dry heaves, irritability in the chest, and inability to repose."

Treatment and Outcome

FIRST VISIT: This patient was diagnosed with a focal distention pattern. We gave a modification of Pinellia Decoction to Drain the Epigastrium *(bàn xià xiè xīn tāng)* in the hopes of using its acrid-opening and bitter-downward directing properties to transform stasis and unblock the collaterals in order to eliminate focal distention and alleviate pain.

Here is the formula:

standard Pinelliae Rhizoma praeparatum *(fǎ bàn xià)* 20g
Zingiberis Rhizoma *(gān jiāng)*... 10g
Scutellariae Radix *(huáng qín)*... 6g
Coptidis Rhizoma *(huáng lián)*... 6g
Pseudostellariae Radix *(tài zǐ shēn)* 15g
Taraxaci Herba *(pú gōng yīng)*... 30g
Salviae miltiorrhizae Radix *(dān shēn)* 30g
Aucklandiae Radix *(mù xiāng)* 10g
Mume Fructus *(wū méi)*... 15g

Instructions: Decoct the herbs three times to obtain about 600ml of liquid. Take 100ml warm before each meal. After taking one packet, if there are no problems, take several more packets.

SECOND VISIT: After taking the herbs, the patient experienced a comfortable feeling in his stomach. After six packets, the focal distention and fullness the patient had felt in his stomach was greatly reduced. The patient's belching, indeterminate gnawing sensation, and acid reflux had also become mild. His food intake was improving. He experienced occasional dull pain.

A local physician changed the patient's formula to Minor Decoction [for Pathogens] Stuck in the Chest (xiǎo xiàn xiōng tāng) with the addition of Aurantii Fructus immaturus (zhǐ shí), Lonicerae Flos (jīn yín huā), Curcumae Radix (yù jīn), Cyperi Rhizoma (xiāng fù), and Dalbergiae odoriferae Lignum (jiàng xiāng). Afterward, the patient's epigastrium again felt uncomfortable and his stools became thin and loose. After continuing to take three packets, his stools were semiliquid and sometimes contained undigested food. The focal distention, fullness, and dull pain in the epigastrium all worsened. He then ceased taking that formula and promptly came to discuss his treatment with me.

The patient's tongue continued to be dull and pale and was covered with a thick, pale yellow, greasy coating. His pulse was wiry and soggy.

This case illustrates the overuse of cold, bitter, and draining herbs, which led to Spleen and Stomach qi deficiency and irregularity of ascent and descent.

We prescribed a modification of Licorice Decoction to Drain the Epigastrium (gān cǎo xiè xīn tāng) in the hopes of harmonizing the Stomach, supporting the Spleen, eliminating focal distention, and stopping diarrhea.

Here is the formula:

Glycyrrhizae Radix preparata (zhì gān cǎo)	12g
Scutellariae Radix (huáng qín)	5g
Coptidis Rhizoma (huáng lián)	3g
standard Pinelliae Rhizoma praeparatum (fǎ bàn xià)	20g
Zingiberis Rhizoma (gān jiāng)	15g
Jujubae Fructus (dà zǎo)	15g
Codonopsis Radix (dǎng shēn)	15g

THIRD VISIT: After four packets of the formula the diarrhea ended and the stool was formed. The focal distention and fullness in the epigastrium had become mild, but he still experienced occasional dull pain. We then switched his formula to a powder form, as follows:

standard Pinelliae Rhizoma praeparatum (fǎ bàn xià)	200g
Zingiberis Rhizoma (gān jiāng)	50g
Coptidis Rhizoma (huáng lián)	50g
Pseudostellariae Radix (tài zǐ shēn)	150g
Taraxaci Herba (pú gōng yīng)	200g
Salviae miltiorrhizae Radix (dān shēn)	300g
Aucklandiae Radix (mù xiāng)	100g
Mume Fructus (wū méi)	150g

Lilii Bulbus *(bǎi hé)*.. 200g

Linderae Radix *(wū yào)*... 100g

Atractylodis macrocephalae Rhizoma *(bái zhú)*......................... 150g

Poria *(fú líng)*.. 150g

Glycyrrhizae Radix preparata *(zhì gān cǎo)*............................. 50g

Citri reticulatae Pericarpium *(chén pí)*................................... 100g

Astragali Radix *(huáng qí)*.. 300g

Puerariae Radix *(gé gēn)*... 200g

Instructions: This group of sixteen herbs, a modified combination of Pinellia Decoction to Drain the Epigastrium *(bàn xià xiè xīn tāng)*, Six-Gentlemen Decoction *(liù jūn zǐ tāng)*, and Lily Bulb and Lindera Decoction *(hé wū tāng)*,[2] were toasted until crisp over a low flame and then ground to a fine powder. The patient mixed the powder with boiled water and took 6g before each meal.

The patient took the formula continuously for more than two months and the dull pain he had felt in his epigastrium gradually diminished and then disappeared. He still experienced occasional focal distention, fullness, and dull pain after emotional upset or intemperate food intake, but the symptoms were mild and easily resolved by taking a few packets of Pinellia Decoction to Drain the Epigastrium *(bàn xià xiè xīn tāng)* combined with Salvia Drink *(dān shēn yǐn)*.

Disease	Main Symptoms	Pattern Identification	Treatment Method	Formula
Focal distention pattern (chronic gastritis)	Fullness and stifling sensation in the epigastrium, blockage, and dull pain	Heat-cold complex, mixture of deficiency and excess, and loss of regulation between ascending and descending functions	Open with acridity and promote downward movement with bitterness, transform stasis and unblock the collaterals	Pinellia Decoction to Drain the Epigastrium *(bàn xià xiè xīn tāng)*

REFLECTIONS AND CLARIFICATIONS

PHYSICIAN A   In this example, Pinellia Decoction to Drain the Epigastrium *(bàn xià xiè xīn tāng)* was originally effective and then the erroneous use of Minor Decoction [for Pathogens] Stuck in the Chest *(xiǎo xiàn xiōng tāng)* led to undigested food in the stool. At the time of the second visit, Licorice Decoction to Drain the Epigastrium *(gān cǎo xiè xīn tāng)* was given, and after four packets, the diarrhea ceased. The ingenuity of the Drain the Epigastrium Decoction *(xiè xīn tāng)* formula is clearly visible. However, I still have two questions about the use of medicinal substances in this case. The first is that in the last formula there is a large dose of Taraxaci Herba *(pú gōng yīng)*. Perhaps this is being used to kill *Helicobacter pylori?* If not, why use a cooling herb in a case of Stomach cold? The second question is about acid reflux. This symptom indicates that the patient had an excess of stomach acid yet you added Mume Fructus *(wū méi)*, which is extremely sour, to the patient's formula. This is hard to understand.

....

2. This is a formula devised by the mid-Qing physician Chen Xiu-Yuan and is made up of Lilii Bulbus *(bǎi hé)* 30g and Linderae Radix *(wū yào)* 9g.

DR. YU   Taraxaci Herba *(pú gōng yīng)* is an edible wild herb, which can be both eaten and used as a medicine. Though sweet and cold, it does not injure the Stomach qi and is especially good for treating Stomach heat. In this case, although the Stomach is cold, the Gallbladder is hot. Taraxaci Herba *(pú gōng yīng)* clears the Gallbladder and harmonizes the Stomach. Further, it enriches the Kidneys, dredges the Liver, and can moderate flaring of Liver fire. Finally, I relied on the sweet, cold, enriching nature of Taraxaci Herba *(pú gōng yīng)* to provide relief from the acrid dryness of standard Pinelliae Rhizoma praeparatum *(fǎ bàn xià)* and Zingiberis Rhizoma recens *(shēng jiāng)*, as well as the bitter dryness of Coptidis Rhizoma *(huáng lián)* and Scutellariae Radix *(huáng qín)*.

As for the rationale of using the very sour Mume Fructus *(wū méi)* in a case with acid reflux, my patients frequently ask this question as well. Although the flavor of Mume Fructus *(wū méi)* is very sour, taking it in a formula is not equivalent to increasing stomach acid. In this pattern, the Spleen is deficient and the Liver fire is exuberant. The extreme sourness of Mume Fructus *(wū méi)* restrains the Liver in order to support the Spleen, because sourness drains the Liver by restraining it. When used in a large dose, within its restraining action, there is also a major unblocking and dredging force, which can disperse focal distention, eliminate fullness, and relieve pain. The clinical effects can be quite outstanding. In the past, my colleagues and I discussed quick, effective treatments utilizing Mume Pill *(wū méi wán)* for intractable periumbilical pain. You may refer to the notes from that meeting *(see pages 70-76)*.

PHYSICIAN B   Dr. Yu, I recall that you have said that the treatment principle of "open with acidity and direct downward with bitterness" that is associated with Pinellia Decoction to Drain the Epigastrium *(bàn xià xiè xīn tāng)* has a specific connotation that is different from the ideas associated with this principle in modern texts. In the *Selected Explanations for the Technical Terms of Chinese Medicine (Zhōng yī míng cí shù yǔ xuǎn zé)*, this principle is explained as follows:

> Use acrid-flavored medicinal substances to open and unblock phlegm-dampness in the chest and diaphragm; use bitter-flavored medicinal substances to treat damp-heat in the chest and diaphragm. Using these two together treats symptoms such as focal distention, stifling sensation, distention, fullness, nausea, and vomiting resulting from phlegm-dampness, and heat obstructing the chest and gastric cavity. Acrid-flavored herbs include ginger Magnoliae officinalis Cortex *(jiāng hòu pò)*, bran-fried Aurantii Fructus *(fū chǎo zhǐ ké)*, Zingiberis Rhizoma recens *(shēng jiāng)*, Pinelliae Rhizoma preparatum *(zhì bàn xià)*, and Citri reticulatae Pericarpium *(chén pí)*. Bitter-flavored herbs include Coptidis Rhizoma *(huáng lián)* and Scutellariae Radix *(huáng qín)*.

What is the basis for this type of explanation?

DR. YU   It is possible that this type of explanation for "open with acridity and direct downward with bitterness" comes from a work of the early Qing-dynasty physician Ye Tian-Shi, entitled *Case Records as a Guide to Clinical Practice (Lín zhèng zhǐ nán yī àn)*. When Ye Tian-Shi treated damp-heat obstructing the middle burner by using Pinellia Decoction to Drain the Epigastrium *(bàn xià xiè xīn tāng)*, he removed Glycyrrhizae

Radix *(gān cǎo)* and Jujubae Fructus *(dà zǎo)*. In some cases, he even removed Ginseng Radix *(rén shēn)*. He added acrid, aromatic, transforming herbs such as Aurantii Fructus immaturus *(zhǐ shí)*, Armeniacae Semen *(xìng rén)*, Citri reticulatae Exocarpium rubrum *(jú hóng)*, and ginger Magnoliae officinalis Cortex *(jiāng hòu pò)*. As far as the efficacy of Dr. Ye's modifications, we cannot verify the outcomes. In any case, I think that for removing those herbs from Pinellia Decoction to Drain the Epigastrium *(bàn xià xiè xīn tāng)* to be effective, the pattern must be one of excess and not of deficiency or even mixed deficiency and excess.

PHYSICIAN B Focal distention can be part of a deficiency pattern?

DR. YU Yes. Focal distention occurring in a patient with a pale tongue, a weak pulse, and a complexion that lacks luster, or focal distention and fullness that is aggravated after taking a formula that opens with acridity and directs downward with bitterness, is assuredly part of a deficiency pattern.

The pathodynamic for deficiency focal distention was described by the Ming-dynasty physician Zhang Jing-Yue as follows: "When a deficient Spleen does not transport, it leads to focal distention that is plugged and cannot be opened up." The treatment should focus primarily on strengthening the transportive function of the middle burner by opening with acridity and directing downward with bitterness. However, regardless of whether the focal distention is completely owing to excess or deficiency, neither pattern is in exact accordance with the true meaning of focal distention. Strictly speaking, focal distention is part of a mixed pattern of deficiency and excess, with more deficiency than excess. This is represented by the Pinellia Decoction to Drain the Epigastrium *(bàn xià xiè xīn tāng)* pattern. Similarly, strictly speaking, opening with acridity and directing downward with bitterness refers to the complete process of supporting normal qi, harmonizing heat and cold, and regulating ascent and descent. From this perspective, if one treats focal distention without supporting the normal qi, it is not opening with acridity and directing downward with bitterness!

PHYSICIAN B Past generations of physicians refer to the fundamental pathodynamic of the Pinellia Decoction to Drain the Epigastrium *(bàn xià xiè xīn tāng)* pattern as a heat-cold complex, a mixture of deficiency and excess, and loss of regulation between ascent and descent. Modern textbooks also use this language. I am simply a clinician and have always felt that this pathodynamic was too abstract, leaving me unable to make heads or tails of it. So my question is whether or not it is possible to take this abstract pathodynamic of heat-cold complex, mixed deficiency and excess and irregular ascent and descent, and make it concrete in terms of the organs?

DR. YU Why not? Given that the six channel patterns are a product of the trinity of organs, channels, and qi transformation, of course we can make it concrete in terms of the organs. In my opinion, heat-cold complex refers to Stomach cold and Gallbladder heat; mixed deficiency and excess refers to Spleen deficiency and Liver exuberance; and loss of regulation between ascent and descent refers to the Spleen's failure to properly bear the clear upward and the Stomach's failure to properly bear the turbid downward.

PHYSICIAN B   Your way of making this concrete is truly something that I have never heard before. Is there some foundation for these ideas?

DR. YU   In the *Discussion of Cold Damage* (*Shāng hán lùn*), focal distention patterns are the result of inappropriate purging, which, of course, damages the Spleen and Stomach. Once the Spleen and Stomach are damaged, ascent and descent lose their mutual regulation and inescapably affect the Liver and Gallbladder.

Why do I say this? The Spleen and Stomach inhabit the middle burner and are the pivot of the ascending and descending functions of the qi dynamic. Only when Spleen qi ascends can it transport and transform the essence of liquids and grains in order to spread it throughout the body. Only when the Stomach qi descends can it receive and decompose liquids and grains and transfer waste outside the body. When you look at it from this perspective, the physiologic phenomenon of Spleen ascent and Stomach descent is not only characteristic of the basic normal function of the Spleen and Stomach, but also of the Liver and Gallbladder. The Qing-dynasty physician Huang Kun-Zai observed that "Liver qi should ascend and Gallbladder fire should descend. Without the upward movement of the Spleen qi, Liver qi does not ascend; without the downward directing of the Stomach qi, Gallbladder fire does not descend."

The cause of focal distention is not limited to inappropriate purging. For many diseases of the digestive system, such as chronic gastritis, duodenitis, bile reflux gastritis, chronic cholecystitis, and chronic pancreatitis, there may a focal distention pattern without a history of inappropriate purging. Many of these patients incur injury to the Spleen and Stomach as a result of emotional problems, overwork, and dietary intemperance.

There is a saying these days, "For major diseases, go to the hospital and for minor ones, go to the herb shop." Upon entering an herb shop one is immediately confronted with a wide variety of medicines for stomach disorders. Without distinguishing between pain and distention, patients purchase medicines. Chinese and Western prepared medicines are dispensed carelessly, thereby harming the Spleen and Stomach. Spleen and Stomach function gradually diminishes and over time develops into a focal distention pattern. The primary pathodynamic here falls within the parameters of Stomach cold and Gallbladder heat; Spleen deficiency and Liver exuberance; and failure of the Spleen to bear the clear upward and failure of the Stomach to bear the turbid downward.

PHYSICIAN C   I noticed that you often change a patient's formula into powder or pill form at the stage of the disorder where one's goal is to consolidate the treatment and prevent recurrence. Why is the change made?

DR. YU   Often, by this time in the treatment the inconvenience and trouble of cooking and drinking decoctions has become quite tedious. A formula in powder or pill form is more suited for long-term treatment and has obvious advantages for the patient's lifestyle. Decoctions are faster-acting and are thus ideally suited for acute or sub-acute situations.

3.3 **Gastric prolapse**

Two cases of chronic gastric prolapse

The side of the "road" is still the road

"路" 的旁邊還是路

■ CASE HISTORY #1

Patient: *36-year-old woman*

The patient had a five-year history of mild gastric prolapse[3] with the angular notch of the lesser curvature of the stomach being 4.5cm below the level of the iliac crest. For a long time, she had taken Tonify the Middle to Augment the Qi Pill *(bŭ zhōng yì qì wán)* along with an empirical herb formula, but this proved ineffective.

INTAKE EXAMINATION

The patient was thin and frail and her complexion had a dark-green and yellowish hue. She belched and experienced abdominal distention with a sense of prolapse, which was worse after meals. Her stools were sometimes dry and sometimes loose. The tip and sides of her tongue were red and the coating was greasy and mixed white and yellow. Her pulse was wiry and weak.

■ CASE HISTORY #2

Patient: *38-year-old woman*

The patient had a seven-year history of mild gastric prolapse. The angular notch of the lesser curvature of the stomach was 4cm below the level of the iliac crest. She had taken Chinese herbs to no effect.

INTAKE EXAMINATION

The patient was thin and frail and her complexion was greenish, yellow, and slightly dusky. She experienced abdominal distention that worsened after meals. She also complained of fullness and a stifling sensation in the chest and lateral costal region, irritability, and irascibility. Her mouth was dry and she was constipated. She had a red tongue with a thin, yellow coating and lacked moisture. Her pulse was wiry, fine, and slightly rapid.

Differentiation of Patterns and Discussion of Treatment

DR. YU   Gastric prolapse is a biomedical disease name. In this disease, when the person

---

3. *Translators' note:* This diagnosis is no longer recognized by mainstream medicine in most Western countries. When it is diagnosed it describes an abnormal elongation of the stomach and not an actual prolapse.

is standing, the angular notch of the lesser curvature of the stomach descends below the iliac crest. It is an organic disease and the moderate and severe presentations are relatively difficult to treat.

By saying difficult to treat, I mean that it is challenging, solely using Chinese herbs, to induce the stomach to return to its normal position. But this is not to say that it is difficult to ameliorate or eliminate the presenting symptoms of this condition.

PHYSICIAN A   At the present time, it seems that there is no disease in Chinese medicine that is generally agreed upon to correspond to gastric prolapse, probably because the symptoms are so varied. The main symptom associated with gastric prolapse is abdominal distention that worsens after meals. This symptom may be accompanied by others such as poor appetite, stomach pain, watery stool or constipation, shortness of breath, and lack of strength. Thus, it is very difficult to find one disease name in Chinese medicine that completely matches this condition.

Investigating the modern medical literature of Chinese medicine, gastric prolapse is placed in the categories of abdominal distention, abdominal pain, or stomach pain, and differentiation and treatment proceeds from there. This categorization is cumbersome. There are many vague discussions of the matter and ultimately it is difficult to know how to approach the subject. Further, there are those who simply draw equivalence between gastric prolapse and downward sinking of the middle burner qi, as described by Li Dong-Yuan, and then propose the use of Tonify the Middle to Augment the Qi Decoction *(bǔ zhōng yì qì tāng).*

DR. YU   In the past when I treated a case of gastric prolapse, I limited myself to considering the Spleen and Stomach. With this artificial limitation in place it was difficult to avoid reaching the limits of what I could do. However, by drawing on the lessons of my predecessors and learning from the skills of contemporary physicians, I was able to think about things from a different perspective.

First, let's consider the primary symptom of gastric prolapse: abdominal distention that worsens after meals. Medical books categorize this as the failure of the Spleen to transport and transform food. Why does the Spleen fail to transport and transform? It is because the Liver is flaring and encroaches on the Spleen. The *Basic Questions (Sù wèn)* states that "Arrival of *jué yīn* qi causes swelling and distention." The main aspect of the contradiction here is the pathological changes of *jué yīn* Liver-wood and not those of the Spleen-Stomach.

Second, let's consider the location of the disease. Is the location of gastric prolapse only the Spleen and Stomach? Gastric prolapse, as defined in Western medicine, is equivalent to 'Stomach descending' and 'Stomach laxity' in Chinese medicine. In the *Divine Pivot (Líng shū)* it states that "in Stomach descending, the lower tube is restricted and inhibited." What exactly is the "lower tube?" Modern anatomical dissection has shown that it is the gastrophrenic ligament and the hepatogastric ligament. Gastric prolapse occurs when these ligaments become slack and then prolapse.[4] The ligaments have insufficient strength to support the stomach in position. Since ligaments belong to sinews in Chinese medicine and the Liver governs the sinews, we should treat the Liver.

....

4. *Translators' note:* As noted above, a frank prolapse of the stomach, where it would be separated from the diaphragm, does not occur and the term "gastric prolapse" in Western medicine refers to an over-elongation of the stomach.

Third, we should consider gastric prolapse from the perspective of body type. This symptom often occurs in patients who are thin and weak with a facial complexion that is greenish and carries a slightly yellow color, all of which imply the wood body type.

If the considerations above are not in error, it can be argued that it would be logical to treat gastric prolapse starting with the Liver, or at least by placing emphasis on the Liver.

PHYSICIAN A The primary location of disease in gastric prolapse is the Spleen and Stomach, yet you place the Liver at the center of the treatment and your treatments are effective. The explanation that you gave above is quite new to me and I do not really know what you mean when you speak about a wood body type.

DR. YU The concept of a wood body type comes from the study of body types in Chinese medicine. In the *Divine Pivot*, five phase theory is applied to constitutional or body type assessment. People are divided into five types (wood, fire, earth, metal, and water) on the basis of skin hue, physical form, physical strength, intellect, and psychology.

The skin hue and physical form of the wood body type is described as follows in Chapter 64 of that book: "Similar to Cang Di [one of the five mythological emperors of antiquity] the person will have a dark-green complexion, a small head, a long face, a straight back, large shoulders, a small body, and good hands and feet." The physical strength, intellect, and psychology are described as follows: "[These people] are talented, they like to work with their minds, they are not physically strong, they frequently worry and they toil over things."

From years of observation I have noticed that patients who have the thin and weak body with a complexion that has a dark green and slightly yellowish hue characteristic of a wood body type have a greater tendency to contract chronic diseases of the Liver, Gallbladder, Spleen, and Stomach. Perhaps in these people, the Liver qi tends to flare, and thus the qi dynamic, qi transformation, and self-regulatory functions easily become erratic.

PHYSICIAN A According to Western medicine, gastric prolapse is also seen more commonly in tall, thin patients who lack strength. This body type seems to fit with the concept of the wood body type of Chinese medicine. Patients with gastric prolapse, in some cases, also have prolapse of the liver or kidneys and Western medicine has no particular treatment. In Chinese medicine, when treating patients with gastric prolapse, aside from giving substances that patients take internally, we can also use acupuncture, dietary therapy, and physical exercises in order to increase the treatment effect. What do you think about that?

DR. YU That's correct!

PHYSICIAN B I have also been pondering your way of approaching and treating patients with gastric prolapse. The primary symptom of gastric prolapse is abdominal distention that worsens after eating. You categorize this as a wood-earth disharmony.

The wood-earth disharmony that you discuss is not simply a disharmony of the Liver and Spleen, but contains a rich and diverse set of ideas.

For example, in the first case, the Liver is flaring and the Spleen is deficient, while the

Gallbladder is hot and the Stomach is cold. In the second case, the yin of the Liver and Spleen is exhausted, the Gallbladder is constrained, and the Stomach is dry. Thus the Liver, Spleen, Gallbladder, and Stomach have all lost their regular functionality. We have to consider the entire situation in order to understand how to regulate their functions.

Furthermore, it is Mume Pill *(wū méi wán)* from the *Discussion of Cold Damage (Shāng hán lùn)* that ultimately fits this treatment methodology. Mume Pill *(wū méi wán)* combines hot and cold, firming and softening, tonifying and draining, and ascending and descending. It drains the *jué yīn*, harmonizes the *shào yáng,* and protects the *yáng míng*. Especially important is the large dosage of Mume Fructus *(wū méi)*, which restrains the Liver in order to drain the Liver (disperse the Liver to tonify; restrain it to drain). Further, combined with Cinnamomi Ramulus *(guì zhī)*, it calms the Liver (in nature, no trees, i.e., wood, grow near cinnamon trees, so it is said that cinnamon withers wood.) Within this combination's sour restraint there is a strong unblocking force. For this reason, when treating abdominal distention caused by wood-earth disharmony, you especially like to use large doses of Mume Fructus *(wū méi)*.

In the second case, aside from the symptoms associated with gastric prolapse, the patient also suffers from a stifling sensation in the chest and lateral costal regions, irritability, bad temper, dry mouth, and constipation. These symptoms indicate wood-earth disharmony from exhaustion of Liver and Spleen yin with Gallbladder constraint and Stomach dryness. Thus, you combined Linking Decoction *(yī guàn jiān)* and Frigid Extremities Powder *(sì nì sǎn)* to nourish the Liver, augment the Spleen, soothe the Gallbladder, and enrich the Stomach.

I think that in the clinic we will certainly encounter other disease patterns and we should learn from the cases presented here in order to flexibly address other presentations.

DR. YU   Absolutely! We must not diminish the importance of pattern differentiation and treatment theory, and we also should not ignore the importance of disease differentiation as we choose medicinal substances.

Treatment and Outcome

CASE #1

We considered this case to be a wood-earth disharmony with a pattern of Liver exuberance, Spleen weakness, Gallbladder heat, and Stomach cold.

We prescribed a modification of Mume Pill *(wū méi wán)*.

Mume Fructus *(wū méi)*	40g
Zanthoxyli Pericarpium *(huā jiāo)*	10g
Aconiti Radix lateralis preparata *(zhì fù zǐ)*	10g
Cinnamomi Ramulus *(guì zhī)*	10g
northern Asari Radix et Rhizoma *(běi xì xīn)*[5]	10g

5. *Translators' note:* This is Asari Radix et Rhizoma *(xì xīn)* from Liaoning province, *Asarum heterotropoides f.* var. mandshuricum (MAXIM.) KITAG. Not only is it considered to be the best quality, it also often contains the lowest concentration of the suspected nephrotoxin, aristolochic acid.

Zingiberis Rhizoma *(gān jiāng)*..30g
dry-fried Aurantii Fructus *(chǎo zhǐ ké)*.....................................30g
Atractylodis Rhizoma *(cāng zhú)*..30g

Instructions: Divide the liquid from the decoction of one packet of herbs into three doses and take one dose before each meal.

The patient was also instructed to lie on her right side for 30 minutes after each meal in order to assist the stomach to assume its normal position.

After six packets, the patient's abdominal distention was greatly reduced. Her tongue appeared more normal and its white-yellow, greasy coating was reduced by more than half. After 18 packets, all symptoms had gradually resolved. Through the use of a barium swallow, it was determined that the patient's stomach had returned to its normal position.

CASE #2

This case is wood-earth disharmony with a pattern of exhausted Liver and Spleen yin, Gallbladder constraint, and Stomach dryness.

We prescribed a modified combination of Linking Decoction *(yī guàn jiān)* and Frigid Extremities Powder *(sì nì sǎn)*.

Glehniae Radix *(bêi shā shēn)* 30g
Ophiopogonis Radix *(mài mén dōng)* 30g
Polygonati Rhizoma *(huáng jīng)* 30g
dry-fried Trichosanthis Semen *(chǎo guā lóu rén)*..........................20g
Rehmanniae Radix *(shēng dì huáng)*..15g
Bupleuri Radix *(chái hú)*..10g
Paeoniae Radix alba *(bái sháo)*..30g
dry-fried Aurantii Fructus *(chǎo zhǐ ké)*.....................................30g
dry-fried Cassiae Semen *(chǎo jué míng zǐ)*.................................30g
wine-prepared Cistanches Herba *(jiǔ cōng róng)*..........................30g
Armeniacae Semen *(xìng rén)* 15g
Astragali Radix *(huáng qí)*...30g
Atractylodis Rhizoma *(cāng zhú)*..30g

The instructions for decoction, dosing, etc. were the same as in the case above.

After six packets, the patient's abdominal distention was greatly reduced and her bowels were moving freely.

After removing dry-fried Cassiae Semen *(chǎo jué míng zǐ)* and Rehmanniae Radix *(shēng dì huáng)*, and adding Hordei Fructus germinatus *(mài yá)* 30g, the formula was given for 12 more packets. All symptoms gradually resolved and a subsequent barium swallow revealed that her stomach had returned to its normal position.

Reflections and Clarifications

DR. YU   In recent years, I have dismissed the idea that one must treat gastric prolapse just from the perspective of pathological changes in the Spleen and Stomach. Instead I have placed more emphasis on the role of the Liver. While I have certainly had some patients who did not do well, I have also successfully treated many patients. I have provided the two cases here for everyone's reference.

PHYSICIAN A   In thinking about the two cases that you provided, I noticed that the first case was considered a *jué yīn* disease and treated with the main formula for *jué yīn* disease, Mume Pill *(wū méi wán),* with the additions of Astragali Radix *(huáng qí),* bran-fried Aurantii Fructus *(fū chǎo zhǐ ké),* and Atractylodis Rhizoma *(cāng zhú).* The second case was considered one of exhaustion of Liver and Spleen yin with Gallbladder constraint and Stomach dryness. It was treated with a combination of Linking Decoction *(yī guàn jiān)* and Frigid Extremities Powder *(sì nì sǎn)* with the same additions. It seems as though the use of these three substances is an example of letting the biomedical disease differentiation guide the choice of medicinal substances.

DR. YU   That is correct. According to modern pharmacologic research, bran-fried Aurantii Fructus *(fū chǎo zhǐ ké)* stimulates the smooth muscle of the stomach and has the function of lifting prolapsing organs. However, a large dose of bran-fried Aurantii Fructus *(fū chǎo zhǐ ké)* can also break up and consume the qi. Thus, using an equal amount of Astragali Radix *(huáng qí),* which lifts and tonifies the source qi, mitigates this potential harm. In cases of Stomach dryness is it wise to use Atractylodis Rhizoma *(cāng zhú)?* Not to mention using a large dose of it! Clinical experience has shown that large doses of Atractylodis Rhizoma *(cāng zhú)* can harmonize the Stomach, direct turbidity downward, improve the Spleen's transportive function, preserve essence, and yet not increase dryness.

PHYSICIAN A   I mentioned earlier that there are some who consider gastric prolapse to be identical to the pattern of middle qi sinking downward, described by Li Dong-Yuan, and then will only use Tonify the Middle to Augment the Qi Decoction *(bǔ zhōng yì qì tāng).* I have tried this myself in several cases and not only was it ineffective, but the abdominal distention actually got worse.

DR. YU   It is true that gastric prolapse and middle qi sinking downward are not equivalent, yet there are patients with gastric prolapse who certainly fit the pattern of a loss of normal ascending and descending functions in the Spleen and Stomach. You can use Tonify the Middle to Augment the Qi Decoction *(bǔ zhōng yì qì tāng)* for these patients, giving them 30-60g of Astragali Radix *(huáng qí)* to tonify the Spleen qi and cause it to ascend. You can also add dry-fried Aurantii Fructus *(chǎo zhǐ ké)* 30g and Atractylodis Rhizoma *(cāng zhú)* 30g in order to harmonize the Stomach and direct the turbid downward. The effect is satisfactory.

PHYSICIAN A   Gastric prolapse indicates that the Stomach qi is excessively descending, so we should use uplifting substances. In your application of Tonify the Middle to Augment the Qi Decoction *(bǔ zhōng yì qì tāng),* you added 30g each of dry-fried Aurantii Fructus *(chǎo zhǐ ké)* and Atractylodis Rhizoma *(cāng zhú)* to harmonize the Stomach and direct turbidity downward. Bran-fried Aurantii Fructus *(fū chǎo zhǐ ké)* strongly opens, breaks and directs qi downward, and has only a very slight lifting action. Including an herb that sinks and directs downward in the treatment of gastric prolapse is difficult to understand.

DR. YU   By stating that gastric prolapse indicates excessive descent of Stomach qi, you have made an equivalence between gastric prolapse and the descent of the Stomach qi. The

Spleen and Stomach inhabit the middle burner and are the pivot of ascent and descent. Because Spleen qi ascends, movement and transformation occurs and fine essence is distributed throughout the body. Because Stomach qi descends, food is received, decomposition occurs, and waste is transferred out of the body.

Thus, the ascending and descending actions of the Spleen and Stomach reflect normal physiological activity. It is incorrect to speak of pathology in terms of excessive ascent of Spleen qi or excessive descent of Stomach qi.

Gastric prolapse does not represent the excessive descent of the Stomach qi; in fact, it is exactly the opposite. When the Stomach is stagnant, the qi dynamic becomes chaotic, and although the Stomach qi should descend, it does not. In other words, in this situation the problem is the inability to maintain the functions of Spleen ascent and Stomach descent. And further, the inability to maintain the normal physiologic state in which when the stomach is full, the intestines are empty, and when the intestines are full, the stomach is empty. Once you have understood this principle, you are more than halfway there!

3.4 **Abdominal distention**

Abdominal distention lasting a year

Mulling over a case in which many formulas were tried unsuccessfully

思之再三 , 連拟數方,皆不如意

■ CASE HISTORY

Patient: *48-year-old woman*

The patient reported frequent periumbilical distention for the previous year. The distention was worse at night and when it was severe she would toss and turn and have difficulty sleeping. Sometimes, although she was extremely tired and felt sleepy, every night around 2-3 a.m. she would feel that the abdominal wall around the umbilicus was distended, extremely tense, and the area would seem inflated. This feeling was unbearable and so she would throw on her clothes and sit up or get up and go for a walk, all the while massaging her own abdomen. After a long time, this would bring some relief and then she could gradually get back to sleep.

She had undergone blood tests, ultrasound, x-rays, and colonoscopy, but no pathology was found. She had tried both Western and Chinese medicines to no avail.

This patient had taken many different prepared medicines, such as Bupleurum Powder to Dredge the Liver (*chái hú shu gān săn*), Three-Substance Decoction with Magnolia Bark (*hòu pò sān wù tāng*), and Magnolia Bark, Fresh Ginger, Pinellia, Licorice, and Ginseng Decoction (*hòu pò shēng jiāng bàn xià gān căo rén shēn tāng),* which dredge the Liver and move and break up qi; Six-Gentlemen Decoction with Aucklandia and Amomum *(xiāng shā liù jun zǐ tāng)* combined with Preserve Harmony Pill *(băo hé wán)*, one to tonify and one to disperse; and Tonify the Middle to Augment the Qi Decoction *(bǔ zhōng yì qì tāng)*, which was used on the basis of the principle of treating blockage by blocking (塞因塞用 *sāi yīn sāi yòng*, i.e., treating stagnation with tonification). She had taken more than forty packets of herbs in total without any effect.

INTAKE EXAMINATION
DATE: October 20, 1992

Her symptoms were as described above. The patient's complexion had a slight green-ish-yellow hue. She complained of bitter taste in the mouth, dry throat, and poor appetite. Her stools were unformed and difficult to pass. She reported that her menstrual cycle was irregular. Her tongue was slightly red with a thin, yellow coating and her pulse was wiry, slightly rapid, and faded away with heavy pressure.

Differentiation of Patterns and Discussion of Treatment

PHYSICIAN B   This patient presented with persistent periumbilical distention that had resisted numerous treatment approaches and continued for more than a year. One must consider that the cause of abdominal distention, especially in those cases where the distention is substantial, must include an element of internal qi stagnation. Thus, moving and breaking up qi should be a primary treatment. The intractable nature of this case is evident from the fact that not only was the application of the principle of dredging the Liver, moving qi, reducing accumulations, and breaking up qi ineffective, but that employment of the opposite principle, tonifying to treat the blockage, was equally ineffective.

DR. YU   Strictly speaking, this type of intractable abdominal distention is referred to by the classical term 'bloating and distention' (膜胀 *chēn zhàng)*. This is a wood-earth disharmony in which there is a complete loss of normal regulation in the relationship between the Liver-Gallbladder and the Spleen-Stomach.

More specifically, first, the distention is focused on the sides of the umbilicus; this clearly relates to the Liver channel. Second, consider that according to the stems and branches, 2-3 a.m. is the time when the Liver channel governs. The patient's abdominal distention is at its worst during the time when the Liver is the most exuberant and takes advantage of and intimidates the Spleen. Third, the patient's complexion was darkish yellow, and she experienced a bitter taste in the mouth and a dry throat. This indicates exuberant counterflow of Liver qi and upward blazing of constrained Gallbladder fire. Fourth, poor appetite and difficult bowel movements with unformed stools indicate that wood is overwhelming earth, leading to deficiency cold.

In summary, the pattern is one of Liver qi exuberance, constrained Gallbladder fire, and Spleen-Stomach deficiency.

Treatment and Outcome

I remembered a case from ten years earlier that was quite similar. So I decided to try Mume Pill *(wū méi wán)* as a decoction. I followed the ratio of the dosage of the ingredients in the original pill version of the formula:

Mume Fructus *(wū méi)*. 40g

northern Asari Radix et Rhizoma *(běi xì xīn)*[6] 9g

Zingiberis Rhizoma *(gān jiāng)*. 15g

Coptidis Rhizoma *(huáng lián)*. 6g

Aconiti Radix lateralis preparata *(zhì fù zǐ)* [pre-cooked]. 9g

Angelicae sinensis Radix *(dāng guī)*. 6g

scorched Phellodendri Cortex *(jiāo huáng bǎi)* 9g

Cinnamomi Ramulus *(guì zhī)*. 9g

Ginseng Radix rubra *(hóng shēn)*. 9g

Zanthoxyli Pericarpium *(huā jiāo)* 6g

Instructions: three packets

Results: That evening the patient took the first dose of the formula. She did not experience the customary increase in severity of distention in the middle of that night. The following morning, she felt that the distention was greatly reduced. After three packets, the symptoms had resolved completely. Four years later, she had experienced no recurrences.

Disease	Main Symptoms	Pattern Identification	Treatment Method	Formula
Bloating and distention	Periumbilical distention, worse at 2-3 a.m. and accompanied by abdominal bloating	Exuberant Liver qi, constrained Gallbladder fire, deficiency of Spleen-Stomach	Restrain the Liver, clear the Gallbladder, harmonize the Spleen-Stomach	Mume Pill *(wū méi wán)*

Reflections and Clarifications

PHYSICIAN B   In this case, you used the original formula for Mume Pill *(wū méi wán)*, observing the original ratios of the ingredients, and after the first dose, there was significant effect. After three packets, the abdominal distention had resolved completely. It is no wonder that Jiang Er-Xun [Dr. Yu's teacher] frequently said that Mume Pill *(wū méi wán)* had unexpected efficacy. Yet since the formula does not contain even one herb that moves the qi or breaks up the qi, how is it that it worked so well?

DR. YU   In my experience, this type of abdominal distention is a mixture of heat and cold, and deficiency and excess. From the perspective of six-channel theory, it touches on *jué yīn*, *shào yáng*, *tài yīn*, and *yáng míng*. From the perspective of organ theory, it involves the Liver, Gallbladder, Spleen, and Stomach. If one does not explore deeply, but instead sees only a broad case of wood-earth disharmony and then employs formulas that simply move and break up the qi, or that tonify and disperse, or treat blockage with blocking, one would miss a deeper understanding of the case. It is just for this reason that it is not at all easy to deploy a formula that matches the presentation of this disorder! Fortunately, the formula Mume Pill *(wū méi wán)* includes a variety of tastes

6. *Translators' note:* This is Asari Radix et Rhizoma *(xì xīn)* from Liaoning province, *Asarum heterotropoides f.* var. mandshuricum (MAXIM.) KITAG. Not only is it considered to be the best quality, it also contains the lowest concentrations of the toxic aristolochic acid.

and thus fits the present pattern well.

The formula contains a high dose of Mume Fructus *(wū méi)*, which is exceptionally sour in flavor and very softening in nature. It enters the Liver channel to restrain and to drain the Liver (disperse the Liver to tonify; restrain it to drain). The formula also contains warm, acrid, firming, and drying herbs: Zanthoxyli Pericarpium *(huā jiāo)*, Asari Radix et Rhizoma *(xì xīn)*, Zingiberis Rhizoma *(gān jiāng)*, Aconiti Radix lateralis preparata *(zhì fù zǐ)*, and Cinnamomi Ramulus *(guì zhī)*, which are combined with the cold, bitter herbs Coptidis Rhizoma *(huáng lián)* and Phellodendri Cortex *(huáng bǎi)*. This combination uses hot and cold, and firming and softening, to drain the *jué yīn* and harmonize the *shào yáng*. In addition, Ginseng Radix *(rén shēn)* and Angelicae sinensis Radix *(dāng guī)*, which are sweet and warm, are employed to warmly tonify the *yáng míng*.

In summary, when you consider Mume Pill *(wū méi wán)* as a whole, it is one of the best formulas for regulating patterns of disharmony between wood and earth. So, in treating this case of recalcitrant abdominal distention, the effects were quite rapid and exceptional.

PHYSICIAN C   It seems that whenever you yourself treat distention patterns related to congestion of the qi dynamic, whether involving the abdomen, lateral costal areas, or even the shoulders and back, if you don't actually use Mume Pill *(wū méi wán)*, you definitely add a large dosage of Mume Fructus *(wū méi)* (30-60g) to whatever formula you choose, and you achieve excellent effects. From a theoretical perspective, it is difficult to understand how restraining and binding medicinal substances treat distention patterns.

DR. YU   In modern times, Mume Fructus *(wū méi)* is clearly placed in the category of herbs that restrain and bind. Its efficacy in restraining the Lung, binding the intestines, generating fluids, and quieting roundworms is noted. What is absent in these descriptions is any mention of this herb's ability to open, unblock, and promote free flow.

Let's consider the traditional literature. In the *Divine Husbandman's Classic of the Materia Medica (Shén Nóng běn cǎo jīng)*, Mume Fructus *(wū méi)* is said to drive qi downward. In *Emergency Formulas to Keep Up One's Sleeve (Zhǒu hòu bèi jí fāng)*, Mume Fructus *(wū méi)* is said to treat and cure distending pain in the Heart, that is, the epigastric region. The *Comprehensive Outline of the Materia Medica (Běn cǎo gāng mù)* records an experiential formula from the Gong family in which Mume Fructus *(wū méi)* is used to treat plum-pit and diaphragm qi. Given these examples of its usage, how can we say that Mume Fructus *(wū méi)* does not unblock and promote free flow in the qi dynamic? Given these classical citations and the clinical efficacy of Mume Fructus *(wū méi)*, how we can we doubt this?

PHYSICIAN B   I noticed that you used an unfamiliar disease name in our earlier discussion. In what text does the term 'bloating and distention' (䐜脹 *chēn zhàng*) first appear?

DR. YU   The term first appears in the *Yellow Emperor's Inner Classic: Basic Questions (Huáng Dì nèi jīng: sù wèn)*. "Arrival of the *jué yīn* qi causes bloating and distention," and "When turbid qi is in the upper body, it produces bloating and distention." In the *Sea of Words (Cí Hǎi)*, a well-respected encyclopedic dictionary, the definition is consistent with this meaning. The character 䐜 *chēn* is defined as "distended, full, and swollen like a drum."

For some people, the statement "When turbid qi is in the upper body it produces bloating and distention" is easy to understand, whereas "arrival of the *jué yīn* qi causing bloating and distention" is more difficult to understand. The best way to make sense of these two phrases is to understand that the first phrase refers to outcome, whereas the second refers to the cause.

Let's consider this in practical terms. *Jué yīn* belongs to the Liver, which is the organ of wind-wood. When *jué yīn* Liver qi is exuberant, it combines with *shào yáng* Gallbladder fire and invades *yáng míng* earth. This invasion causes a deficiency of earth, which then fails to properly manage the ascent of the clear and the descent of the turbid. The rising counterflow of turbid qi causes bloating and distention. This explanation integrates cause and effect as well as the etiology and symptoms.

PHYSICIAN A   Although you have stressed that Mume Pill *(wū méi wán)* is perhaps the best formula for regulating wood-earth disharmony patterns, this notion is completely new to me. It seems that for most physicians, Mume Pill *(wū méi wán)* is considered a specialized formula for the treatment of roundworm inversion. Furthermore, roundworm inversion, as described in Chinese medicine, is very similar to the pattern of biliary tract roundworms, as described in Western medicine. This seems to have greatly limited the clinical application of this classical formula.[7]

DR. YU   More than a few physicians over the centuries have viewed Mume Pill *(wū méi wán)*, just as you said, as a specialized formula for roundworm inversion. They say that the formula contains bitter, sour, and acrid herbs and that "the roundworms are quieted by sourness, moved downward by bitterness, and subdued by acridity." This way of speaking sounds reasonable and almost as if you can see it yourself. The fact of the matter is that it is conjecture and hypothesis.

In the *Discussion of Cold Damage (Shāng hán lùn)*, the Mume Pill *(wū méi wán)* entry ends with the phrase, "Also governs long-term diarrhea." The Qing-dynasty medical scholar Ke Yun-Bo, an expert on this text, wrote that "We can see that the various *jué yīn* symptoms match this formula. Taking '[If] one purges there will be unremitting diarrhea' [from line 326] and 'also governs long-term diarrhea' together, then Mume Pill *(wū méi wán)* is the main formula for the *jué yīn*, not just a formula for roundworm inversion." Ke also noted that

> [Zhang] Zhong-Jing took this formula originally as a method for the various symptoms of *jué yīn* [diseases]. [Wang] Shu-He edited it so that it was placed in the line about roundworms, causing people to forget that it was the main formula for the *jué yīn*. When one looks at how the herbs match the various symptoms, how could one possibly limit it only to [treating] vomiting of roundworms!

....
7. *Translators' note:* In Chinese medicine, the term 蛔厥 *huí jué*, which we translate as 'roundworm inversion,' is a disease name that originated in the *Discussion of Cold Damage (Shāng hán lùn)* as described at line 338, discussed below. In modern Chinese, these same two characters can be used as one name for the biomedical disease 'roundworm infestation,' so there is often confusion between the larger concept expressed in the classical texts and the narrow meaning from Western medicine.

Modern university textbooks on the *Discussion of Cold Damage (Shāng hán lùn)* not only completely adopt this idea, but they go one step further in citing other Qing-dynasty commentaries from the *Golden Mirror of the Medical Tradition (Yī zōng jīn jiàn)* and by Zhang Xu-Gu that emphasize Mume Pill *(wū méi wán)* as the governing formula for the basic pattern of the *jué yīn*. This fits both the spirit of the formula composition and clinical reality.

The formula contains a large dose of Mume Fructus *(wū méi)*, which enriches and drains the Liver. Sour and sweet collectively enrich the yin, whereas sour and bitter employed together drain heat. These actions represent the basic goals of the formula. Acrid and sweet in concert warm yang, whereas the combination of acrid and bitter unblock and direct downward. Thus, the formula is appropriate for *jué yīn* diseases with damage to yin and yang and internal blazing of wood fire (Liver-Gallbladder fire).

PHYSICIAN B   Thinking of Mume Pill *(wū méi wán)* as a specialized formula for roundworm inversion actually goes against Zhang Zhong-Jing's original intention. I seem to remember that Dr. Jiang wrote some articles in the early 1980s pointing out that many later physicians' conceptions of roundworm inversion deviated from Zhang Zhong-Jing's original ideas.

DR. YU   Dr. Jiang advocated taking the original text as the benchmark when approaching the works of Zhang Zhong-Jing . If you carefully examine it word by word and sentence by sentence, its whole truth will come to light.

Let us look at line 338 in the source text:

> When cold damage with a faint pulse and inversion lasts up to seven or eight days with cold skin, and the patient is restless without any periods of ease, this is visceral inversion, not roundworm inversion. In roundworm inversion the patient should vomit up worms. If now the patient is quiet, but then periodically becomes irritable, this is the organs being cold. Roundworms ascend and enter the diaphragm and so there is irritability, but in an instant these symptoms will stop again. After getting food there is vomiting and irritability again. This is because the roundworms smell the food's odor and emerge. Such a patient will frequently and spontaneously vomit roundworms. For roundworm inversion, Mume Pill *(wū méi wán)* governs. It also governs enduring diarrhea.

Successive generations of physicians have explained the pattern of roundworm inversion as presenting with symptoms of vomiting of roundworms and abdominal pain, accompanied by cold extremities. This description has led modern physicians to make a direct correlation to biliary ascariasis.

Dr. Jiang treated many patients with roundworm inversion, and they did not have abdominal pain or vomit roundworms, nor did they have icy cold extremities. In fact, these patients matched quite well the vivid description in the source text of being "quiet, but then periodically becoming irritable … but in an instant these symptoms will stop again."

For example, Dr. Jiang treated an 18-month-old child with recurrent irritability following recovery from measles. The initial diagnosis for the child was residual heat from the measles and herbs were given to nourish yin and to clear the Heart. Not only were these ineffective, but the irritability actually worsened in severity and frequency. Each time the family would eat a meal of noodles, as soon as the child ate, he would become very irritable and restless. He would crawl around everywhere, crying and yelling, until after about a minute, he would settle down.

After witnessing this scene, Dr. Jiang promptly exclaimed, "Is this not roundworm inversion?!" In the description of this pattern, the text describes, "If now the patient is quiet, but then periodically becomes irritable. ... Roundworms ascend and enter the diaphragm and so there is irritability, but in an instant these symptoms will stop again. After food intake there is vomiting and irritability again. This is because the round-worms smell the food's odor and emerge." This description seemed to closely match this child's situation.

Dr. Jiang prescribed Mume Pill *(wū méi wán)*, removing the warm, drying herbs: Cinnamomi Ramulus *(guì zhī)*, Aconiti Radix lateralis preparata *(zhì fù zǐ)*, Zingiberis Rhizoma *(gān jiāng)*, and Asari Radix et Rhizoma *(xì xīn)*. He also added the following anti-parasitic herbs: Toosendan Fructus *(chuān liàn zǐ)*, Arecae Semen *(bīng láng)*, and Carpesi abrotanoidis Fructus *(hè shī)*. The day after taking the first packet, the child's bowel movement was like sludge and it contained countless pinworms, some alive and some dead. Afterward, he was no longer irritable.

In another case, Dr. Jiang treated a five-year-old boy, also with intermittent irritabili-ty and restlessness following measles. When symptomatic, he would actually bite people and would sometimes even bite his own fingers and hands. As a result of biting himself, he had infections on both hands. He was admitted to the hospital and diagnosed with post-measles encephalitis. He was given sedatives for more than ten days without any effect. The irritability and restlessness also followed ingestion of food and would quiet after a short period of time. Dr. Jiang diagnosed him with roundworm inversion and gave him a modification of Mume Pill *(wū méi wán)*. Afterward, he passed many tens of roundworms for a few days and was no longer irritable or restless.

If Dr. Jiang had not been able to so thoroughly remember the source text, or if he had remembered it but in clinic had "presented a decoction of medicine promptly after just facing the patient,"[8] how would he have been able to recognize the true image of roundworm inversion? Dr. Jiang said that every time he pondered the text for the Mume Pill *(wū méi wán)* pattern, his mind would go back to that ancient time. He thought that if Zhang Zhong-Jing had not personally observed this specific pattern in a patient, how could he have described it with such vivid specificity?

Dr. Jiang was also quick to point out that the explanations for roundworm inversion over the centuries have their own logic, as well, and should not be simply dismissed. However, he emphasized that in the source text there is a distinction between visceral inversion, in which "the patient is restless without any periods of ease," and roundworm inversion, in which "the patient is quiet, but then periodically becomes irritable ... but in an instant these symptoms will stop again." The source text mentions irritability and restlessness; there is no mention of pain or cold limbs. If every time we see the character 厥 *jué* (inversion) in the text we assume that it means fainting or collapse, we will be

....

8. *Translators' note:* This quotation is from the preface to the *Discussion of Cold Damage (Shāng hán lùn)* in which Zhang Zhong-Jing admonishes his contemporaries for not taking the time to do their job correctly.

way off. And given the first case above, obviously, not all patients with a diagnosis of roundworm inversion actually have roundworms. If Dr. Jiang had not had all of this direct experience, how could he have made these discoveries?

PHYSICIAN C   In reading your cases from the last twenty years, it appears that in many of them, you did not use the original formula, but made modifications to Mume Pill *(wū méi wán)*. For example, you used Zanthoxylum and Mume Decoction *(jiāo méi tāng)*[9] to treat damage to the Liver yin in children with chronic diarrhea, and Coptis and Mume Decoction *(lián méi tāng)* to treat damage to Kidney yin in children with chronic diarrhea.

Is it the case that in your early years you were strongly influenced by the works of Ye Tian-Shi and Wu Ju-Tong such that you generally followed their convention? Thus, when you used Mume Pill *(wū méi wán)* you did not include Cinnamomi Ramulus *(guì zhī)*, Asari Radix et Rhizoma *(xì xīn)*, or Phellodendri Cortex *(huáng bǎi)*?

DR. YU   That is correct. When Ye Tian-Shi treated malarial or dysenteric disorders due to wood accosting earth, he would always use a modification of Mume Pill *(wū méi wán)*, generally without Cinnamomi Ramulus *(guì zhī)*, Asari Radix et Rhizoma *(xì xīn)*, and Phellodendri Cortex *(huáng bǎi)*. Wu Ju-Tong followed this same line of thought.

In the early years of my practice, I followed this idea blindly. Also, I warily sought proof when searching for theoretical foundations. Since those three herbs did not enter any of the relevant channels—*jué yīn* (Liver), *shào yáng* (Gallbladder), *tài yīn* (Spleen), or *yáng míng* (Stomach)—I thought that there was no benefit to using them.

However, with the passage of time, having deepened my understanding of fundamental theory and revisited these ideas, I would say that it is generally best to use these three herbs, especially Cinnamomi Ramulus *(guì zhī)* and Asari Radix et Rhizoma *(xì xīn)*.

I once treated an elderly woman with a long history of abdominal distention, indefinable epigastric discomfort, and intense heartburn. She had tried many formulas with little success, so I tried Mume Pill *(wū méi wán)*. Because her heat signs were relatively prominent, I removed Cinnamomi Ramulus *(guì zhī)*, Aconiti Radix lateralis preparata *(zhì fù zǐ)*, Zingiberis Rhizoma *(gān jiāng)*, and Asari Radix et Rhizoma *(xì xīn)*. After three packets, there were no noticeable results. At that point, I added the Aconiti Radix lateralis preparata *(zhì fù zǐ)* and Zingiberis Rhizoma *(gān jiāng)* and gave her two more packets. These additions also did not improve things. I then added Cinnamomi Ramulus *(guì zhī)* and Asari Radix et Rhizoma *(xì xīn)* and gave her one packet of the formula in its original form. This one packet produced a clear effect.

Since that time, whenever I use Mume Pill *(wū méi wán)*, regardless of the presence or absence of heat signs, I use the formula in its original form, without modification.

According to the theory of channel entry, neither Cinnamomi Ramulus *(guì zhī)* nor Asari Radix et Rhizoma *(xì xīn)* enters the Liver channel; clinical experience, however,

....

9. *Translators' note:* This formula, listed in the *Systematic Differentiation of Warm Pathogen Diseases,* consists of Coptidis Rhizoma *(huáng lián)* 6g, Scutellariae Radix *(huáng qín)* 6g, Zingiberis Rhizoma *(gān jiāng)* 6g, Paeoniae Radix alba *(bái sháo)* 9g, dry-fried Zanthoxyli Pericarpium *(chǎo huā jiāo)* 9g, Mume Fructus *(wū méi)* 9g, Ginseng Radix *(rén shēn)* 8g, Aurantii Fructus immaturus *(zhǐ shí)* 4.5g, and Pinelliae Rhizoma praeparatum *(zhì bàn xià)* 6g.

would seem to suggest otherwise.

In my hospital, I once treated a woman in her 60s who had chronic adrenal insufficiency. Her state of health was very poor, and to make matters worse, she experienced frequent distention in the lower abdomen. She had taken a variety of herbal formulas including those to eliminate food accumulation and move the qi, dredge the Liver and relieve constraint, and warm the yang and tonify the Kidneys. As none of these had been of any use, she had lost faith that there were treatments that could help her. Her pulse was wiry, fine, and tight. Her tongue was pale purple. I thought that this might be cold stagnation in the Liver channel and so I gave her Tangkuei Decoction for Frigid Extremities plus Evodia and Fresh Ginger *(dāng guī sì nì jiā wú zhu yú shēng jiāng tāng)*. In this formula I used 30g of Cinnamomi Ramulus *(guì zhī)* and 20g of Asari Radix et Rhizoma *(xì xīn)* and had her pre-cook these herbs for 30 minutes. After taking just two packets, her lower abdominal distention had completely resolved. Over the last ten years, any occasional recurrences of this symptom were quickly treated with a packet or two of this same formula.

I think it is clear that Cinnamomi Ramulus *(guì zhī)* and Asari Radix et Rhizoma *(xì xīn)* enter the Liver channel after they are taken by patients, even though, according to channel entry theory, neither does. There is a proverb from the West that says, "Grey, dear friend, is all theory, And green the golden tree of life."[10] In China, we say, "Genuine knowledge comes from practice." There is no more than this, how could it be otherwise?

3.5 Vomiting

Retching and vomiting for two months

Concise and simple formulas address severe illnesses

精方簡藥起大症

■ CASE HISTORY

Patient: *52-year-old woman*

For the past five years the patient has experienced recurrent stomach pain, accompanied by retching and vomiting. She had been hospitalized multiple times. After an endoscopic exam she was diagnosed with chronic superficial gastritis.

Two months ago after getting chilled, her stomach pain worsened and began to radiate to her back. The pain was accompanied by nausea and vomiting. She self-prescribed Patchouli/Agastache Liquid to Rectify the Qi *(huò xiāng zhèng qì shǔi)* and metoclopramide; neither of these medications relieved her symptoms, so she was again admitted to the hospital.

After receiving intravenous fluids, antispasmodics, analgesics, and Chinese herbal med-

10. *Translators' note:* Mephistopheles to his student in Goethe's *Faust,* Lines 2038-9.

icines, the patient's stomach pain gradually resolved and her nausea and vomiting were mitigated. However, she was still afraid to eat since, when she did so, she would vomit repeatedly about 30 minutes later.

She had tried many different formulas, such as Liver-Transforming Decoction (*huà gān jiān*),[11] Minor Pinellia plus Poria Decoction *(xiǎo bàn xià jiā fú líng tāng)*, Six-Gentlemen Decoction with Aucklandia and Amomum *(xiāng shā liù jūn zǐ tāng)*, Warm Gallbladder Decoction *(wēn dǎn tāng)*, and Inula and Haematite Decoction *(xuán fù dài zhě tāng)*. However, after ingesting a small amount of these formulas she would often vomit the decoction back up, so she was fearful of taking any more.

A second endoscopic examination confirmed the presence of superficial gastritis.

INTAKE EXAMINATION
DATE: April 6, 1988

The patient was gaunt, her complexion lacked luster, and her cheeks were sunken. She was fatigued, lacked strength, was short of breath, and her voice was weak. Within 30 minutes of eating, she would vomit up mucus and a small amount of food. She had a dry mouth with a bitter taste and her stool was scant and only passed with difficulty. Her urine was yellow. Her tongue was pale-purple with a coating that was slightly yellow, thin, and greasy. Her pulse was wiry, fine, and slightly rapid.

Differentiation of Patterns and Discussion of Treatment

PHYSICIAN A   In view of the fact that so many different formulas were given to treat this patient's vomiting, it seems as though no one completely got a handle on the pathodynamic, don't you agree?

DR. YU   Perhaps that is true. In general, the pathodynamic of vomiting is not hard to grasp. In fact, we can sum it up in three words: Stomach qi counterflow.

The Stomach governs intake, as well as food decomposition, so its natural direction of movement is downward. In this case, after food intake, but prior to decomposition, the food was regurgitated. Management of normal downward movement of the Stomach qi failed and so qi counterflowed upward.

The main method of treatment is therefore to harmonize the Stomach and to direct counterflow qi downward. Once we determine what is causing the Stomach qi to counterflow, we can decide on the specific treatment strategy. For example, if the cause is cold, we should use a warming strategy; for heat, a clearing strategy; for food accumulation, a dispersing strategy; and for deficiency, a tonifying strategy.

However, in this case of vomiting, the pathodynamic was not so simple. For one thing, the disease course was relatively long. For another, the patient was relatively weak. Finally, this was a complex of heat and cold, as well as deficiency and excess, so none of the many formulas tried were effective.

PHYSICIAN B   So, in this case, what is the pathodynamic?

11. From Zhang Jing-Yue: Citri reticulatae viride Pericarpium *(qīng pí)*, Citri reticulatae Pericarpium *(chén pí)*, Paeoniae Radix *(sháo yào),* each 6g; Moutan Cortex *(mǔ dān pí)*, Gardeniae Fructus *(zhī zǐ)*, Alismatis Rhizoma *(zé xiè)*, each 4.5g, Fritillariae Bulbus *(bèi mǔ)* 6-9g.

DR. YU   Line 359 of the *Discussion of Cold Damage (Shāng hán lùn)* states:

> If the physician again induces vomiting and purges cold damage [in a patient] who originally had cold diarrhea, a cold barricade [will result]. If again they are adversely [treated with] vomiting and purging, they will vomit as soon as any food enters the mouth, Ginger, Scutellaria, Coptis, and Ginseng Decoction *(gān jiāng huáng qín huáng lián rén shēn tāng)* masters it.

I believe that the pathodynamic in this case is cold barricade and heat harassment in addition to wood taking advantage of a defeated earth.

PHYSICIAN B   Can you explain that a bit more concretely?

DR. YU   'Cold barricade' means that when the Stomach qi is deficient and cold, food and drink make a barricade. Even if you force the person to eat, the cold makes it impossible for the Stomach to decompose the food and so it is then ejected. 'Heat harassment' indicates constrained heat in the Gallbladder organ. When the Gallbladder is constrained by heat, not only does it fail to assist the Stomach in the decomposition of food, but it actively harasses the Stomach, causing chaos in the intake and decomposition of food; this leads to vomiting.

If there is long-term vomiting, Stomach function is gradually weakened, leaving it open to invasion by Gallbladder heat. This creates a vicious cycle that is referred to as 'wood taking advantage of defeated earth.'

This case is cold barricade, heat harassment, and earth overwhelmed by wood encroachment, all of which gives rise to difficulty ingesting herbs.

Treatment and Outcome

Ginger, Scutellaria, Coptis, and Ginseng Decoction *(gān jiāng huáng qín huáng lián rén shēn tāng)* plus Zingiberis Rhizomatis Succus *(jiāng zhī)*:

Zingiberis Rhizoma *(gān jiāng)*	3g
Scutellariae Radix *(huáng qín)*	3g
Coptidis Rhizoma *(huáng lián)*	3g
Codonopsis Radix *(dǎng shēn)*	5g

Preparation: Place the herbs in enough cold water to cover them by a centimeter. Soak for 30 minutes and then bring to a boil and simmer for 30 minutes. Remove 200ml of the decoction. Separately, peel and crush 30g of Zingiberis Rhizoma recens *(shēng jiāng)*. Soak it in 30ml of cold water for 30 minutes and then remove the ginger mash from the water and press out the juice.

Administration:

1. Take 50ml of the warm decoction and add to it 5ml of the Zingiberis Rhizomatis Succus *(jiāng zhī)*. Take this dose in small sips, once every two hours.

2. Amomi Fructus rotundus *(bái dòu kòu)* 5g: Prior to taking the decoction, chew two of the fruits and spit out the dregs.

3. Ginseng Radix rubra *(hóng shēn)* 10g: Slice this into thin pieces and hold 2-3 at a time in the mouth until they soften, then chew and swallow.

Results: After one packet, the vomiting ceased. In order to secure the treatment effect the patient was given a second packet.

After that, we switched to a modified Six-Gentlemen Decoction plus Bupleurum and Peony *(chái sháo liù jūn zǐ tāng)* to dredge the Liver, improve the Spleen's transportive function, harmonize the Stomach, and direct counterflow qi downward.

Bupleuri Radix *(chái hú)*	10g
Paeoniae Radix alba *(bái sháo)*	10g
Codonopsis Radix *(dǎng shēn)*	10g
Atractylodis macrocephalae Rhizoma *(bái zhú)*	10g
Poria *(fú líng)*	12g
Glycyrrhizae Radix *(gān cǎo)*	3g
standard Pinelliae Rhizoma praeparatum *(fǎ bàn xià)*	5g
Citri reticulatae Pericarpium *(chén pí)*	5g
Zingiberis Rhizoma *(gān jiāng)*	3g
Zingiberis Rhizoma recens *(shēng jiāng)*	3g
Coptidis Rhizoma *(huáng lián)*	3g

The patient took 26 packets of this formula over the course of one month. She also chewed 3g of Ginseng Radix rubra *(hóng shēn)* slices each day, as described above.

One year later, she had experienced no recurrences of stomach pain or vomiting and her overall health had improved.

PHYSICIAN A   In this case of chronic superficial gastritis, the patient vomited mucus and a small amount of food shortly after eating. Many formulas were tried without success and the patient was quite debilitated. You used a simple formula, Ginger, Scutellaria, Coptis, and Ginseng Decoction *(gān jiāng huáng qín huáng lián rén shēn tāng)* plus Zingiberis Rhizomatis Succus *(jiāng zhī)*, with few ingredients and small dosage, and not only achieved rapid results, but the effect also was maintained a year after the treatment. I hope that I can learn from your experience. You have frequently said that "concise and simple formulas address severe illnesses" and truly seeing something once is better than hearing about it a hundred times.

DR. YU   This formula was selected because of its functionality. Zingiberis Rhizoma *(gān jiāng)* warms the Stomach and dispels cold; Scutellariae Radix *(huáng qín)* and Coptidis Rhizoma *(huáng lián)* disperse heat; and Codonopsis Radix *(dǎng shēn)* (in place of Ginseng Radix *(rén shēn)*) supports the normal qi. This formula was selected to address the pathodynamic; it was not a case of observing vomiting and then selecting a formula that treats that one specific symptom.

Disease	Main Symptoms	Pattern Identification	Treatment Method	Formula
Stubborn retching and vomiting	Vomiting of mucus and food after eating	Deficient and cold Stomach qi, constrained heat in the Gallbladder	Warm the Stomach, clear the Gallbladder	Ginger, Scutellaria, Coptis, and Ginseng Decoction *(gān jiāng huáng qín huáng lián rén shēn tāng)* plus Zingiberis Rhizomatis Succus *(jiāng zhī)*

REFLECTIONS AND CLARIFICATIONS

PHYSICIAN A The analysis of the pathodynamic and the selection of the formula was clearly influenced by line 359, which states that:

> In cold damage originally there was spontaneous cold diarrhea, yet the physician [used] vomiting and precipitation so [there is] cold barricade. [After] further adverse [treatment] [through] vomiting and precipitation, if [there is] immediate vomiting after food enters the mouth, Ginger, Scutellaria, Coptis, and Ginseng Decoction *(gān jiāng huáng qín huáng lián rén shēn tāng)* governs.

However, most textbooks and many experts explain this pathodynamic as upper-body heat and lower-body cold barricading each other. What is the basis for your description of this pattern as Stomach cold and Gallbladder heat?

DR. YU In fact, I have drawn on others' ideas of understanding of this line. Still, my understanding of it is a bit different.

First, using terms like 'a mutual barricade of heat and cold' or 'upper-body heat and lower-body cold barricading each other' to describe the pathodynamic here is needlessly general and vague. This description does not help one to arrive at a true understanding of the pattern.

Second, in the passage above, the patient is described as originally having deficiency-cold diarrhea. Then the physician employed formulas that cause purging and vomiting. Where in the world would we find such a clueless physician? This conflict is why the *Golden Mirror of the Medical Tradition (Yī zōng jīn jiàn)* states that

> The character "下" [*xià,* down] [which is taken to mean diarrhea] should actually be the character "格" [*gé,* barricade], which fits the meaning of the line. Many commentators explain that there is Stomach cold with diarrhea, but this does not fit the line, nor is it compatible with the use of Scutellariae Radix *(huáng qín)* and Coptidis Rhizoma *(huáng lián).*

Third, in classical texts, the character 關 [*guān,* shut] and the character 格 [*gé,* barricade] are opposites. 'Shut' indicates blockage of urinary flow and bowel movements. 'Barricade' indicates refusal of food or immediate vomiting of ingested food. At line 359 "cold barricade" has this meaning; it is not some kind of barricade between heat and cold where each repels the other.

If we reconsider this case, there are clear symptoms of constrained heat in the Gallbladder organ: dry mouth, bitter taste in the mouth, inhibited and scanty bowel movements, yellow urine, a pale-purple tongue body with a thin, slightly yellow, and greasy coating, and a pulse that is wiry, fine, and slightly rapid. It is not my intention to use this case of vomiting as a way of explaining line 359, as the circumstances here are not the same as those in the original text. I am simply offering a discussion of my clinical reasoning to illustrate how one can use an understanding of the underlying pathodynamic to arrive at an effective treatment.

PHYSICIAN B Ginger, Scutellaria, Coptis, and Ginseng Decoction *(gān jiāng huáng qín huáng lián rén shēn tāng)* treats vomiting of food when that vomiting occurs immediately after eating, but in this case, the patient vomited 30 minutes after eating. Why is this formula still suitable?

DR. YU   In my opinion, vomiting within about 30 minutes still fits this pattern. 'Immediate vomiting after food enters the mouth' is actually an opposing symptom in relation to either 'vomiting in the evening of food eaten in the morning' or 'vomiting in the morning of food eaten in the evening.' These latter types of vomiting indicate pure deficiency-cold of the Spleen and Stomach, whereas the former pattern of vomiting immediately after eating is one in which constrained heat is intermingled.

PHYSICIAN C   In using this formula, the dosages were very small, except for a large dose of Zingiberis Rhizoma recens *(shēng jiāng)*. Were you not concerned about the potential of aggravating the heat?

DR. YU   This type of vomiting, in which there is a cold barricade and heat harassment in addition to earth overwhelmed by wood encroachment and difficulty in ingesting the decocted herbs, is a very difficult situation for which to write a formula. If you have the patient sip a small formula in a concentrated decoction, it increases the likelihood that the patient will be able to keep the formula down. As you know, Zingiberis Rhizoma recens *(shēng jiāng)* has an extraordinary ability to calm nausea and vomiting. Although I used a large dose (30g), it was not decocted with the other herbs. It was crushed and soaked to extract the juice. Then just 5ml of the juice were added to each dose of the cooked decoction. This method will not exacerbate the heat.

Chen Xiu-Yuan recommended this formula for "all types of barricades," and I would say that he had excellent insight. He wrote that, according to his experience, "if the patient cannot ingest the decoction, remove Zingiberis Rhizoma *(gān jiāng)*, add a small amount of Zingiberis Rhizomatis Succus *(jiāng zhī)*, and then have them sip it slowly. This small modification, which is an ancient method, has worked repeatedly." I have used the formula over the years to treat stubborn cases of vomiting. I do not remove the Zingiberis Rhizoma *(gān jiāng)*, but simply add Zingiberis Rhizomatis Succus *(jiāng zhī)*. I have found this to be very effective.

PHYSICIAN B   If what Chen Xiu-Yuan writes is correct, can we think of this formula as a main prescription for stubborn vomiting?

DR. YU   No, you should not think of it like that. If, for example, the vomiting is the result of Stomach yin deficiency and the tongue is red with a scanty coating, this formula would not be appropriate. If, however, the problem is due to heat being trapped within cold, this is a very useful approach. For example, in reference to Ginger, Scutellaria, Coptis, and Ginseng Decoction *(gān jiāng huáng qín huáng lián rén shēn tāng)*, Ke Yun-Bo wrote, "In cases of chronic vomiting with heat that is trapped [by the cold], [where] it has been unbeneficial to use Aucklandiae Radix *(mù xiāng)*, Amomi Fructus *(shā rén)*, Citri reticulatae Pericarpium *(chén pí)*, and Pinelliae Rhizoma preparatum *(zhì bàn xià)*, administer [Ginger, Scutellaria, Coptis, and Ginseng Decoction *(gān jiāng huáng qín huáng lián rén shēn tāng)*] and all will be peaceful and easy." I would encourage you all to ponder Ke Yun-Bo's words, as it makes it clear that the cold trapping in the heat is the focus of the problem. He clearly has something to teach us.

PHYSICIAN C   In the past, I have seen you use Inula and Haematite Decoction *(xuán fù dài zhě tāng)* with Zingiberis Rhizomatis Succus *(jiāng zhī)* to treat a few cases of recalcitrant vomiting. Why did you not use that formula in this case?

DR. YU   In this case, not only did the patient vomit food quickly after eating, but she also regurgitated the decocted formulas that she was prescribed. I also knew that a previous physician had tried to use Inula and Haematite Decoction *(xuán fù dài zhě tāng)* with no success. Further, it seemed unlikely that the addition of Zingiberis Rhizomatis Succus *(jiāng zhī)* would be sufficient to overcome the bad taste of Inulae Flos *(xuán fù huā)*. Ultimately, I was afraid that using that formula, even with the addition of Zingiberis Rhizomatis Succus *(jiāng zhī)*, would simply be walking over ground that had already been covered.

3.6 **Constipation**

Constipation for three years

With a well-conceived strategy, what need is there for conforming to convention?

胸有成竹, 何須從俗

■ CASE HISTORY

Patient: *38-year-old woman*

INTAKE EXAMINATION
DATE: December 5, 1987

For three years, the patient had suffered from constipation, only having a bowel movement once every six-to-seven days. The stool was hard, and when the patient passed stools, her anus was extremely painful. She had frequently used enemas and oral medicines, such as phenolpthalein tablets, Hemp Seed Pill *(má zǐ rén wán),* and Sennae Folium *(fān xiè yè),* but the effects had been minimal. Her tongue lacked moisture and the sides were red. It had a thin, yellow coating with scant fluids. The patient's pulse was wiry and rough.

Differentiation of Patterns and Discussion of Treatment

PHYSICIAN A   This pattern of long-term constipation seems to be due to deficiency. In the Chinese medicine textbooks, there are only two patterns for deficiency constipation: qi deficiency and blood deficiency.

In cases of qi deficiency, there are symptoms such as shortness of breath, lack of strength, defecation that does not move smoothly, and stools that are neither dry nor hard. The tongue is pale and tender and the pulse is deficient and weak. Appropriate treatment consists of augmenting the qi and moistening the Intestines with a formula such as Astragalus Decoction *(huáng qí tāng)* from the late 18th-century work *Appendices to the Golden Cabinet (Jīn guì yì)*, which consists of Astragali Radix *(huáng qí)*, Citri reticulatae Pericarpium *(chén pí)*, Cannabis Semen *(huǒ má rén)*, and honey.

In cases of blood deficiency, there are symptoms such as lusterless complexion, dizziness, and palpitations. The tongue is very pale and the pulse is fine and rough. Appropriate treatment consists of nourishing blood and moistening dryness with a formula such as Master Shen's Moisten the Intestines Pill *(rùn cháng wán)*, which consists of Angelicae sinensis Radix *(dāng guī)*, Rehmanniae Radix *(shēng dì huáng)*, Cannabis Semen *(huǒ má rén)*, Persicae Semen *(táo rén)*, and Aurantii Fructus *(zhǐ ké)*.

Does this case fit into one of these patterns?

DR. YU The blood-deficiency constipation pattern described in the textbooks is not seen very commonly in the clinic. Furthermore, blood-deficiency patients don't usually list constipation as their chief complaint. Put another way, in terms of the symptoms described for this pattern, constipation is rarely the patient's main issue. It is only in books that it appears this way.

Qi-deficiency constipation, however, is worth discussing. What is qi-deficiency constipation? It seems to be a pattern in which the patient strains in the bathroom, sweats, has shortness of breath, and has difficulty passing stool, even though the stool itself is neither dry nor hard. This clearly describes a middle burner qi deficiency with a lack of sufficient force to push out the stool. Not only are purgatives contraindicated in these cases, but even intestine-moistening substances such as Cannabis Semen *(huǒ má rén)* and honey, which are used in Astragalus Decoction *(huáng qí tāng)*, should be used with extreme caution, because enriching-moistening herbs can harm the yang qi of the middle burner.

For this type of constipation I generally use a large packet of Tonify the Middle to Augment the Qi Decoction *(bǔ zhōng yì qì tāng)* to tonify the Spleen and cause the clear to ascend. I combine that with Calm the Stomach Powder *(píng wèi sǎn)* to harmonize the Stomach and to cause turbidity to descend. I add Armeniacae Semen *(xìng rén)* and Eriobotryae Folium *(pí pá yè)* to disseminate and to clarify the Lung qi. When Spleen qi rises, Stomach qi descends, and Lung qi disseminates, the pivot mechanism then functions properly and this leads to smooth bowel movements.

Finally, when I write about these cases, I usually avoid the use of the term 'constipation,' but instead use terms such as 'stools that fail to move smoothly,' 'impeded defecation,' or 'difficult defecation.' Furthermore, I will add a note to specify that the stool is not dry. Although using this language is long-winded, it helps me to avoid falling into a fixed pattern and reminds me about the importance of correctly identifying the cause of the symptoms before determining the appropriate treatment.

PHYSICIAN B The symptom of constipation has too many different names. Modern books on the subject usually divide constipation into four distinct types: heat, excess, qi, and deficiency. The influential Ming-dynasty physician Zhang Jing-Yue wanted to avoid this annoyance and so simply divided constipation into two types: yin knotting and yang knotting. In your experience, which type of constipation is most commonly seen in the clinic?

DR. YU   Deficiency constipation is the most common type that I have treated. The most important pathodynamic is insufficiency of Spleen yin with Intestinal dryness. This type is referred to as 'habitual' constipation in biomedicine.

PHYSICIAN A   How is it that the type of constipation you say you treat most frequently is not even mentioned in standard textbooks?

DR. YU   The Spleen is the ultimate yin (至陰 *zhì yīn*) of yin. 'Ultimate' means 'large' and we can say that its fluid permeates the entire body. However, the character 至 *zhì* also means far-reaching, and so we can also say that the Spleen distributes essence throughout the body. When Spleen yin is insufficient, the fluids of the whole body become depleted and the Stomach and Intestines are the first to be affected by this. Why? Because, as it says in Chapter 45 of *Basic Questions (Sū wèn)*, "the Spleen manages the proper movement of fluids on behalf of the Stomach."

Patients with constipation from insufficiency of Spleen yin are commonly seen with symptoms such as hunger without a desire to eat, thirst without a desire to drink, dry lips, emaciation, fatigue, lack of strength, a pale tongue that lacks moisture, and a thin, dry tongue coating. The patient above fits this pattern.

In terms of well-known classical formulas that are used to enrich Spleen yin, one of the first to know is Peony and Licorice Decoction *(sháo yào gān cǎo tāng)*. The early modern physician Zhang Xi-Chun praised this formula for its ability to transform yin with sour and sweet flavors, and he would add Ginseng Radix *(rén shēn)* for its strong ability to nourish Spleen yin. When I treat habitual constipation caused by insufficiency of Spleen yin and Intestinal dryness, I generally use Peony and Licorice Decoction *(sháo yào gān cǎo tāng)* as follows:

Paeoniae Radix alba *(bái sháo)*	30-50g
Glycyrrhizae Radix *(gān cǎo)*	5-10g
Glycyrrhizae Radix preparata *(zhì gān cǎo)*	5-10g

These herbs greatly enrich Spleen yin. To this I add Cassiae Semen *(jué míng zǐ)* 30g and wine-prepared Cistanches Herba *(jiǔ ròu cōng róng)* 30g for their ability to moisten the Intestines and to unblock the bowels. Generally, the treatment is quite effective.

However, there are some stubborn cases in which there is distinct abdominal distention. For these cases, I add dry-fried Raphani Semen *(chǎo lái fú zǐ)* 30-50g to unblock the bowels and to cause the qi to descend, which accelerates the effect of the formula. The case above is an example of this usage. The rationale for using Raphani Semen *(lái fú zǐ)* in these cases is that its ability to eliminate distention and to cause the qi to descend is similar to Aurantii Fructus immaturus *(zhǐ shí)* and Magnoliae officinalis Cortex *(hòu pò)*, but its effect in unblocking the bowels is even stronger. Thus, the use of Raphani Semen *(lái fú zǐ)* can be expanded into cases of excess, heat, and wind constipation. Furthermore, because its nature is moistening, it causes qi to descend and also unblocks the bowels without injuring the yin. Thus, it is suitable for deficiency constipation due to Intestinal dryness. If abdominal distention is absent, replace Raphani Semen *(lái fú zǐ)* with Armeniacae Semen *(xìng rén)* 15g and Eriobotryae Folium *(pí pá yè)* 30g, as noted above, to disseminate and to clarify the Lung qi, thereby "removing the lid in order to open the teapot." These strategies will yield quick results.

PHYSICIAN A   According to Chinese medical literature, substances that enrich Spleen yin should be sweet, bland, and neutral, or sweet, cool, and moistening. Why do you use Cistanches Herba *(ròu cōng róng)*, which is a warm substance that supplements Kidney yang?

DR. YU   There is no question that when the Spleen yin is insufficient, one should nourish the Spleen. Nonetheless, according to Chapter 1 of *Basic Questions,* "The Kidneys govern water. It receives the essence of the five yin organs and six yang organs and then stores it." Once the Kidney yin is ample, it will be easier to enrich the Spleen yin. To enrich the Spleen yin without supplementing the Kidney is incorrect. Unfortunately, most substances that enrich Kidney yin are gentle, yin-type substances that are lacking in the power to create movement. This has led to difficulties for later generations of physicians who enthusiastically invoke the principle of "increasing water to move the boat."

Cistanches Herba *(ròu cōng róng)* enters the Kidney and Bladder channels. It is traditionally used to warm and tonify the Kidney yang. However, as noted in the *Treasury of Words on the Materia Medica (Běn cǎo huì yán)*, this warming tonification is special in that it is "warm, but not hot; tonifying, but not overpowering; warming, but not drying; slippery, but not draining; thus, it is referred to as *cōng róng*, which means 'unhurried' and 'leisurely.'" Although it is a yang herb, its nature is moistening, fluid, and gentle. It enriches the Kidney and replenishes essence. In a larger dosage, it also creates movement; thus, Cistanches Herba *(ròu cōng róng)* moistens the Intestines and unblocks the bowels. Within this one naturally-occurring substance is the ability to tonify yang, replenish essence, moisten the Intestines, and unblock the bowels. This is truly rare.

If you consider the formula that I generally use, there is a large dose of gentle, yin-natured herbs such as Paeoniae Radix alba *(bái sháo)*, Glycyrrhizae Radix *(gān cǎo)*, and Cassiae Semen *(jué míng zǐ)*. These substances must be accompanied by something like Cistanches Herba *(ròu cōng róng)*, which has the ability to generate yang qi. Only then will the formula be able to stimulate peristalsis and to achieve the effect of moistening the Intestines and unblocking the bowels. In fact, Cistanches Herba *(ròu cōng róng)* is the only herb in the formula for which there is no substitute.

The diagnosis in this case was insufficiency of Spleen yin with Intestinal dryness. I used Peony and Licorice Decoction *(sháo yào gān cǎo tāng)* with a large dosage of Paeoniae Radix alba *(bái sháo)* and additional herbs.

Treatment and Outcome

Paeoniae Radix alba *(bái sháo)* 30g

Glycyrrhizae Radix *(gān cǎo)* 5g

Glycyrrhizae Radix preparata *(zhì gān cǎo)* 5g

Cassiae Semen *(jué míng zǐ)* 30g

wine-prepared Cistanches Herba *(jiǔ ròu cōng róng)* 30g

After three packets, the patient was still unable to pass stool and her abdominal distention was unbearable. I therefore added 50g of dry-fried Raphani Semen *(chǎo lái fú zǐ)*.

After one packet, the patient's bowels had opened and her abdominal distention had decreased markedly. In order to secure the treatment effect, I removed the Raphani Semen *(lái fú zǐ)* and gave her 12 more packets of the original prescription. Three months later the symptoms had not recurred.

Follow-up Intake Examination

One year later, however, the patient returned. After a period of fatigue and stress during which she neither ate nor slept well, her constipation had returned. Although she tried taking the same formula again, it did not work this time. Furthermore, taking it seemed to intensify feelings of drooping distention in her lower abdomen.

The results of the second intake examination were as follows: a bowel movement every 2-3 days, unformed stool, straining to pass stool, spontaneous sweating, shortness of breath, and mild abdominal distention with a sinking sensation. Shortly after having a bowel movement, she would again have the sensation of needing to defecate and would then return to the bathroom. It was quite upsetting. Her tongue was tender and red with a thin, white coating. Her pulse was wiry and weak.

I considered this to be sinking of the middle qi and weakness of the transportive functions of the Spleen; thus, I chose a modification of Tonify the Middle to Augment the Qi Decoction *(bǔ zhōng yì qì tāng)*:

Astragali Radix *(huáng qí)*	30g
Codonopsis Radix *(dǎng shēn)*	30g
Atractylodis macrocephalae Rhizoma *(bái zhú)*	60g
Cimicifugae Rhizoma *(shēng má)*	6g
Bupleuri Radix *(chái hú)*	6g
Platycodi Radix *(jié gěng)*	6g
Zingiberis Rhizoma *(gān jiāng)*	10g
Angelicae dahuricae Radix *(bái zhǐ)*	10g
Glycyrrhizae Radix preparata *(zhì gān cǎo)*	6g

After eight packets, the patient's bowel movements were much smoother and the stool was well formed. Her sweating and shortness of breath had also decreased. Her tongue and pulse were unchanged. Because of the fact that she was busy with work, she was unable to continue taking the herbs in decoction form. I advised her to frequently take both Tonify the Middle to Augment the Qi Decoction *(bǔ zhōng yì qì tāng)* and Restore the Spleen Decoction *(guī pí tāng)* in pill form.

Disease	Main Symptoms	Pattern Identification	Treatment Method	Formula
HABITUAL CONSTIPATION	Stubborn constipation and abdominal distention	Spleen yin deficiency and Intestinal dryness	Enrich the Spleen and moisten the Intestines	Peony and Licorice Decoction *(sháo yào gān cǎo tāng)*
HABITUAL CONSTIPATION	Unformed stool and straining	Sinking of middle qi and weakness of Splenic movement	Augment the Spleen qi	Tonify the Middle to Augment the Qi Decoction *(bǔ zhōng yì qì tāng)*

REFLECTIONS AND CLARIFICATIONS

PHYSICIAN A   The famous formula for treating insufficiency of Spleen yin with Intestinal dryness is Hemp Seed Pill *(má zǐ rén wán),* and yet, it seems as though you never use this formula. Why not?

DR. YU   The ability of Hemp Seed Pill *(má zǐ rén wán)* to enrich Spleen yin is quite limited. In fact, although the use of the formula has been expanded to include habitual constipation from Spleen yin deficiency, the formula does not match this pattern.

Today, constipation that occurs after surgery is often treated with Hemp Seed Pill *(má zǐ rén wán),* and although it unblocks the bowels at the beginning, typically, after a while, the constipation recurs. The longer the patient takes the formula, the less effective it becomes. Eventually, when the formula ceases to work at all, many of these patients will resort to harsh draining substances such as Sennae Folium *(fān xiè yè)* in order to temporarily unblock the bowels. Given this situation, my feeling is that physicians do not truly understand when to use Hemp Seed Pill *(má zǐ rén wán).*

Line 247 of the *yáng míng* section in the *Discussion of Cold Damage (Shāng hán lùn)* states: "When the dorsal pedis pulse is floating and rough, floating means that the Stomach qi is strong [from a pathogen] and rough means that urination is frequent. As the floating and the rough grapple with each other, bowel movements will be hard and the Spleen will be bound. Hemp Seed Pill *(má zǐ rén wán)* governs."

The essential pathodynamic of this pattern is Stomach heat damaging the Spleen. The Spleen is restrained by the Stomach heat and is thereby unable to move the fluids of the Stomach. The fluids thus do not moisten the Intestines properly, leading to hard stool. Zhang Zhong-Jing composed Hemp Seed Pill *(má zǐ rén wán)* by starting with Minor Order the Qi Decoction *(xiǎo chéng qì tāng),* which drains heat, unblocks the bowels, and eliminates distention, and Rhei Radix et Rhizoma *(dà huáng),* Magnoliae officinalis Cortex *(hòu pò),* and Aurantii Fructus immaturus *(zhǐ shí).* To this base, he added Cannabis Semen *(huǒ má rén),* Armeniacae Semen *(xìng rén),* and Paeoniae Radix alba *(bái sháo).*

Given that he started with Minor Order the Qi Decoction *(xiǎo chéng qì tāng),* we can conclude that this pattern belongs within the classification of *yáng míng* bowel excess. Because the bound heat damages the fluids, leading to dryness, he added Cannabis Semen *(huǒ má rén),* Armeniacae Semen *(xìng rén),* and Paeoniae Radix alba *(bái sháo)* to moisten Intestinal dryness. Later physicians have used this formula to treat heat-type constipation, which manifests with symptoms such as constipation, scanty yellow urine, fever, abdominal distention, abdominal pain, dry mouth, thirst, a red tongue with a yellow coating, and a rapid pulse; these are all signs of heat. In this case, the formula matches the pattern and good results are reliable.

However, when considering habitual constipation from Spleen yin insufficiency with Intestinal dryness, the fact that it is called 'habitual' indicates that it usually develops slowly and lasts over a long period of time. Further, it is not generally accompanied by a whole set of heat symptoms. Why then would someone recommend using Hemp Seed Pill *(má zǐ rén wán)* over a long period of time?

PHYSICIAN C   Although Minor Order the Qi Decoction *(xiǎo chéng qì tāng)* is the base of the formula, historical commentators have noted that the formula is named after Cannabis Semen *(huǒ má rén)* and that it should be considered the chief ingredient, given its ability to moisten Intestinal dryness and to unblock the bowels. Further, Armeniacae Semen *(xìng rén)* also moistens the Intestines and unblocks the bowels. Finally, Paeoniae Radix alba *(bái sháo)* harmonizes the nutritive aspect and relaxes tension. The combination of Rhei Radix et Rhizoma *(dà huáng)*, Aurantii Fructus immaturus *(zhǐ shí)*, and Magnoliae officinalis Cortex *(hòu pò)* drains heat, discharges excess, moves qi, and guides out stagnation. In the notes following the formula in the source text, it states, "Take the above six ingredients and make into pills. ...Take three times a day. Increase the dosage until the desired affect is achieved." The fact that the formula is made into pills highlights that the formula is a moderate, moistening formula that directs downward. Would it not be fair to say that it is from this suggestion that the origin of the use of Hemp Seed Pill *(má zǐ rén wán)* for habitual constipation arises?

DR. YU   It is not as simple as that. Just because the name of the formula is Hemp Seed Pill *(má zǐ rén wán)*, the chief ingredient is Cannabis Semen *(huǒ má rén)*? According to the traditional dosages of the pill version of the formula, Rhei Radix et Rhizoma *(dà huáng)* is 500g, whereas Cannabis Semen *(huǒ má rén)* is just 2 *shēng*, which is around 30-60g. From that perspective, Rhei Radix et Rhizoma *(dà huáng)* in a large dosage is given primacy to emphasize its ability to drain heat and to unblock the bowels.

In this pattern, the knotted heat is relatively mild compared to the pattern for which Minor Order the Qi Decoction *(xiǎo chéng qì tāng)* is intended, and the damage to fluids is relatively severe. Thus, we can say that Hemp Seed Pill *(má zǐ rén wán)* is built on the functional foundation of Minor Order the Qi Decoction *(xiǎo chéng qì tāng)* to drain heat, unblock the bowels, and eliminate fullness. The addition of Cannabis Semen *(huǒ má rén)*, Armeniacae Semen *(xìng rén)*, and Paeoniae Radix alba *(bái sháo)* works to moisten Intestinal dryness. The change from decoction to pill creates a moderate downward-draining formula, but even so, once the stool moves, the formula should no longer be taken. The formula is not named after the primary ingredient, Rhei Radix et Rhizoma *(dà huáng)*, but is instead named after the assistant, Cannabis Semen *(huǒ má rén)*, as a way of highlighting the secondary pathodynamic of fluid damage and Intestinal dryness. In this way, Zhang Zhong-Jing was calling attention to the fact that this pattern is fundamentally different than the basic Order the Qi Decoction *(chéng qì tāng)* patterns.

To return to the original point, this formula treats the basic pathodynamic of knotted heat. There is no avoiding this point, regardless of what the name of the formula might highlight with regards to fluid damage or Intestinal dryness. Modern textbooks classify this formula as one of the primary formulas for heat constipation and this classification makes a great deal of sense.

If the formula is instead used for deficiency constipation, or for a long period of time, it is difficult to avoid damaging yin because of the bitter, drying natures of Rhei Radix et Rhizoma *(dà huáng)*, Aurantii Fructus immaturus *(zhǐ shí)*, and Magnoliae officinalis Cortex *(hòu pò)*. The common notion that Hemp Seed Pill *(má zǐ rén wán)* nourishes Spleen yin and that it can be used for a long period of time without ill effects is actually quite far from the truth.

PHYSICIAN A   Presently, many physicians consider treating habitual constipation with a large dose of Atractylodis macrocephalae Rhizoma *(bái zhú)*. Why did you not consider this approach?

DR. YU   Actually, I was one of the first physicians to use that approach, as you can readily find in the case records. Everyone knows that using a large dose (~60g) of Atractylodis macrocephalae Rhizoma *(bái zhú)* to unblock the bowels was first introduced by the famous physician from Beijing, Wei Long-Ji, in the 1970s. This idea caused quite a stir in Chinese medicine circles at the time and my colleagues and I began to use it in the clinic and to develop this application. Why is it that Atractylodis macrocephalae Rhizoma *(bái zhú)*, which is traditionally used to strengthen the Spleen and to stop diarrhea, can also be used to unblock the bowels? In a publication[12] on this topic, we stated that in moderate dosages, Atractylodis macrocephalae Rhizoma *(bái zhú)* strengthens the Spleen and stops diarrhea, yet in large dosages, it improves the transportive function of the Spleen and unblocks the bowels, thus revealing its regulatory action on bowel function.

In recent years, I have only used this method very rarely. For one thing, I have seldom encountered a case of chronic constipation that did not respond to the other formulas that I normally use, and for another, it is necessary to use unprocessed Atractylodis macrocephalae Rhizoma *(shēng bái zhú)*. In my local herb markets, this is difficult to procure. In any case, large dosages of Atractylodis macrocephalae Rhizoma *(bái zhú)* are used to treat stool that is not clearly formed, but is still difficult to pass. It is not to be used for constipation when the stool is dry.

PHYSICIAN D   You have said that most of the constipation patients that you treat exhibit a deficiency cold pattern. Why do you think that is the case?

DR. YU   I would speculate that the pressures of modern life have contributed to this. Nowadays, the common lifestyle involves overeating, poor sleeping habits, bad dietary choices, insufficient exercise, and mental stress. How could this not deplete the body's qi and fluids? Add to this the frequent use of antibiotics, air conditioning, and pollution and one can see how modern life is deleterious to the qi and fluids and can give rise to deficiency cold patterns.

....

12. Du Guang-Hua, Yu Guo-Jun, "The Revelation of Using Atractylodis macrocephalae Rhizoma *(bái zhú)* to Unblock the Bowels." Journal of Chinese Medicine, Vol. 11, 1982.

CHAPTER 4

Liver and Gallbladder System Disorders

4.1 Costal pain

Costal pain for three years

A physician discovers a miraculous formula by treating himself

醫者自療悟妙方

■ CASE HISTORY

Patient: *35-year-old woman*

The patient had chronic hepatitis for three years. She frequently experienced pain when she moved along with a stabbing pain in the lateral costal regions. The pain was accompanied by a stifling sensation in the chest, abdominal distention, belching, nausea, and vomiting. She had tried both Chinese and Western medicines and obtained no marked improvement.

INTAKE EXAMINATION

Her tongue was slightly red. The tip and the sides were filled with small, dark purple dots. The coating was thin, yellow, and slightly greasy. Her pulse was wiry and fine. Her liver descended below the costal margin by 3cm. Her GPT[1] was 60 U/L and her TTT[2] was 9U/L.

....

1. GPT = Alanine Aminotransferase (ALT) (GPT): normal value is 7-56U/L.
2. TTT= Thymol Turbidity Test: normal should be <6U/L. Note that this test is no longer used.

Differentiation of Patterns and Discussion of Treatment

PHYSICIAN A   In this case of chronic hepatitis with lateral costal pain, physicians had tried many different treatment strategies over a long period of time. These included dredging the Liver and regulating the qi, clearing heat and resolving dampness, invigorating the blood and transforming stasis, and nourishing yin and softening the Liver. None of these strategies yielded significant results. Did you have some other strategy to try?

DR. YU   The liver resides in the costal region and the Liver channel spreads throughout this area; thus, lateral costal pain is closely associated with Liver disease. It seemed to me that since so many strategies had been tried and yielded no results, we should consider whether the specific and unique circumstance that led to the pain had been overlooked. I believed that specific circumstance to be suspended thin-mucus obstructing the Liver collaterals.

Chapter 20 of the *Divine Pivot (Líng shū)* states that "If there is a pathogen in the Liver, there will be pain in both lateral costal regions." Here, 'pathogen' certainly includes thin-mucus, as is explained in many ancient references. For example, Chapter 12 of the *Essentials from the Golden Cabinet (Jīn guì yào lüè)* states that, "After consumption of liquids, fluid flows into the area below the lateral costal regions, causing coughing, spitting of saliva, and pain with movement. This pattern is called suspended thin-mucus." At line 41 of the *Systematic Differentiation of Warm Pathogen Diseases (Wēn bìng tiáo biàn),* Wu Ju-Tong observes:

> When there is pain in the lateral costal regions associated with lurking summerheat or damp-warmth, whether or not there is coughing, no chills but only tidal fevers, or actually chills and fever like a malarial condition, one should not mistake this for a Bupleuri Radix *(chái hú)* pattern. Cyperus and Inula Decoction *(xiāng fù xuán fù huā tāng)* governs.

Wu Ju-Tong considered this type of lateral costal pain to be caused by fluid in the Liver, as was originally suggested in *Essentials from the Golden Cabinet (Jīn guì yào lüè),* and treated it with Ten-Jujube Decoction *(shí zǎo tāng).* Because this pattern was relatively mild, I felt I could use a milder formula, Cyperus and Inula Decoction *(xiāng fù xuán fù huā tāng),* to flush away thin-mucus and to unblock the collaterals.

Treatment and Outcome

The pattern was suspended thin-mucus obstructing the Liver collaterals. The formula was a modification of Cyperus and Inula Decoction *(xiāng fù xuán fù huā tāng):*

vinegar-prepared Cyperi Rhizoma *(cù zhì xiāng fù)*	10g
Inulae Flos *(xuán fù huā)* [wrapped separately]	10g
standard Pinelliae Rhizoma praeparatum *(fǎ bàn xià)*	10g
Poria *(fú líng)*	15g
Citri reticulatae Pericarpium *(chén pí)*	10g
Armeniacae Semen *(xìng rén)*	10g
Coicis Semen *(yì yǐ rén)*	20g
Trichosanthis Semen *(guā lóu rén)*	10g
Dalbergiae odoriferae Lignum *(jiàng xiāng)*	15g
Platycodi Radix *(jié gěng)*	10g

Instructions: one packet every two days

After 15 packets, there was no more pain upon movement. The stabbing pain and other symptoms were reduced in severity.

I continued the original formula with the following modifications:

REMOVED:

> standard Pinelliae Rhizoma praeparatum *(fǎ bàn xià)*
> Citri reticulatae Pericarpium *(chén pí)*

ADDED:

> Salviae miltiorrhizae Radix *(dān shēn)* 15g
> Moutan Cortex *(mǔ dān pí)* 10g
> Rubiae Radix *(qiàn cǎo gēn)* 15g
> Paeoniae Radix rubra *(chì sháo)* 10g
> Eupolyphaga/Stelophaga *(tǔ biē chóng)* [honey-fried, ground to
>   powder, and mixed into the hot decoction] 3g
> Chinese scallions *(cōng jīng)* . . . . 9 stalks

After 15 more packets, the stabbing pain had completely resolved. The tongue had become pale-red with a thin, white coating and there were no longer dark purple spots on the sides and tip of the tongue. The pulse was wiry and moderate.

I then proceeded with Six-Gentlemen Decoction with Bupleurum and Peony *(chái sháo liù jūn zǐ tāng)* in order to achieve the best long-term outcome.

The patient took this formula for about three months and, with the exception of occasional feelings of poor appetite, weakness, and being easily fatigued, she was completely normal. On re-examination her liver was only 1.5cm below the costal margin and liver function tests were normal.[3]

Disease	Primary Symptoms	Differentiation	Treatment Method	Formula
Lateral costal area and hypochondriac pain	Pain with movement and a stabbing pain in the hypochondria and lateral costal areas	Suspended thin-mucus obstructing the Liver collaterals	Flush thin-mucus and unblock collaterals	Cyperus and Inula Decoction *(xiāng fù xuán fù huā tāng)*

REFLECTIONS AND CLARIFICATIONS

PHYSICIAN B   In thinking about clinical approaches to lateral costal pain, I would say that we often forget about the treatment method of flushing away thin-mucus and unblocking the collaterals. The fact that you were able to cure this case with a modified version of Cyperus and Inula Decoction *(xiāng fù xuán fù huā tāng)* suggests that this formula could perhaps be used more broadly. Is this a secret formula?

. . . .

3. This case was published in a 1987 volume entitled *Selected Papers by Young Chinese and Japanese Doctors of Traditional Medicine (Zhōng Rì qīng nián zhōng yī lùn wén xuǎn).* Although at first glance the case seems quite ordinary, the response in the medical community after its publication that led to it being included in this book demonstrates that it generated a certain amount of interest.

DR. YU   What do you mean by "secret formula"? It is right there clearly in the *Systematic Discussion of Warm Pathogen Diseases (Wēn bìng tiáo biàn)*.[4]

PHYSICIAN A   The ancient texts refer to lateral costal pain secondary to thin-mucus, lurking summerheat, damp-warmth, etc., but in this case the pain was caused by hepatitis!

DR. YU   It is clear in the clinic that there are many factors that can give rise to lateral costal pain from pathogenic thin-mucus, besides thin-mucus, lurking summerheat, or damp-warmth. Nonetheless, one of the primary pathodynamics involved in this pattern is thin-mucus obstructing the Liver collaterals. When there is lack of free flow, there is pain.

Recently this pattern is regarded by many to be similar to biomedically-defined conditions such as exudative pleurisy or pleural effusion. In the recent past, I have treated cases of acute hepatitis, chronic hepatitis, chronic cholecystitis, and asthma that had similarities to this pattern.

Nonetheless, to effectively use this formula, it is critical to understand the most important point: the lateral costal pain only occurs when the patient moves. This is what the term 'pain upon movement' (引痛 *yǐn tòng*, literally 'pulling pain') means in these classics. You must pay attention that the pain is primarily a pain upon movement or dragging pain, and not distention pain, stabbing pain, or dull pain. Further, when the patient is still, there is typically little or no pain; but as soon as the patient moves—changing positions, turning to one side or the other, lifting the head, or walking—then the pain is constant.

This information will only come from taking a good medical history, so let that be a warning to those who would neglect this part of the exam! Because many physicians do not understand the specific nature of this symptom, in the early stages of this condition, it is often mistaken for a Bupleuri Radix *(chái hú)* pattern.

PHYSICIAN A   How is it that you discovered the special nature of this symptom and this specific treatment strategy?

DR. YU   There is a traditional saying that only an experienced physician is a good one. When I was younger, how could I possibly have had that degree of perception and insight? I learned all of this from my teacher, Dr. Jiang. As a young man, he was sick and needed to treat himself. Then, during that difficult time, he had the good fortune to study with the famous master physician Chen Ding-San, who taught him a great deal.

When Dr. Jiang was 20 he contracted a cold during mid-autumn. He had a cough, alternating fever and chills, as if he had malaria, and pain upon movement in the lateral costal regions. He decided to use a modification of Minor Bupleurum Decoction *(xiǎo chái hú tāng)*, and when this was unsuccessful, he went to his teacher for help. Dr. Chen laughed and said, "This is not a Bupleuri Radix *(chái hú)* pattern, but a Cyperus and Inula Decoction *(xiāng fù xuán fù huā tāng)* pattern." He then used the original formula:

Cyperi Rhizoma *(xiāng fù)* 9g

---

4. This material is found in the text at line 41 of the Lower Burner Section. In fact, the connection with Ten-Jujube Decoction *(shí zǎo tāng)* and the suggestion to use Cyperus and Inula Decoction *(xiāng fù xuán fù huā tāng)* for milder cases is made in the source text by Wu Ju-Tong.

Inulae Flos *(xuán fù huā)* 9g
Perillae Fructus *(zǐ sū zǐ)* 9g
Citri reticulatae Pericarpium *(chén pí)* 9g
Poria *(fú líng)* 9g
standard Pinelliae Rhizoma praeparatum *(fǎ bàn xià)* 15g
Coicis Semen *(yì yǐ rén)* 15g

The decoction made Dr. Jiang very nauseous and he felt that the bitter herbs were very difficult to swallow. As soon as he swallowed them he would begin to retch. He continued to retch and after about a half day he spit up a small bowlful of sticky mucus. After that, surprisingly, the lateral costal pain and the fever and chills completely resolved.

Dr. Jiang was happy with the efficacy of the formula and so went to his teacher to ask about it. Dr. Chen showed him the passage from the *Systematic Discussion of Warm Pathogen Diseases (Wēn bìng tiáo biàn)*. At that point, he understood that he had misdiagnosed himself as having a Bupleuri Radix *(chái hú)* pattern, just as his teacher had said. However, if it was not a Bupleuri Radix *(chái hú)* pattern, even though it had lateral costal pain and alternating chills and fever, how should one understand it? According to Wu Ju-Tong's note on the formula, "This pattern is due to a seasonal pathogen becoming newly intertwined with internal fluids." That made the situation abundantly clear.

After a period of time, Dr. Jiang accumulated more and more experience. He was able to compare Bupleuri Radix *(chái hú)* patterns with those of Cyperus and Inula Decoction *(xiāng fù xuán fù huā tāng)* and he noticed that although the chills and fever in both patterns were similar, the chest and lateral costal symptoms were markedly different.

Bupleuri Radix *(chái hú)* patterns are characterized by the presence of an unpleasant fullness in the chest and lateral costal region, perhaps accompanied by pain, but definitely not pain upon movement. The pattern is from a formless pathogenic qi constrained in the *sháo yáng,* and it tends toward the half exterior portion of a half exterior-half interior pattern. Cyperus and Inula Decoction *(xiāng fù xuán fù huā tāng)* patterns are characterized by the presence of pain upon movement in the chest and lateral costal regions, but no unpleasant fullness. The pattern is the result of a pathogen with form comprised of pathogenic water and thin-mucus collected in the chest and lateral costal regions. It tends toward the half interior portion of a half exterior-half interior pattern. This is the crux of the differential diagnosis of these two patterns.

PHYSICIAN C   Your explanation seems unable to completely avoid an issue that has not been settled by either ancient or modern physicians—where exactly is the location of *sháo yáng* disease?

DR. YU   While we may not be able to completely avoid that issue from an intellectual perspective, we can still focus on clinical observation. From Dr. Jiang's perspective, the two most commonly occurring patterns of *sháo yáng* disease seen in the clinic are Bupleuri Radix *(chái hú)* patterns and Cyperus and Inula Decoction *(xiāng fù xuán fù huā tāng)* patterns.

Furthermore, establishing the precise location of *sháo yáng* disease, in the final analysis, will bump up against the problem of establishing exactly what organs are associated with the interstices and the pores, as well as the chest and lateral costal region. Chapter 1 of the *Essentials from the Golden Cabinet* states that "The interstices are the places where the Triple Burner connects and communicates with the genuine base [of qi] and it is the place where blood and qi pour out. The pores are the textured grain of the skin and organs." Thus we can say that the interstices and pores belong to the Triple Burner. Further, while the chest and lateral costal region, which includes aspects of the chest, abdomen, and body cavity, is within the outer form of the body, at the same time it is outside of the organs. This is also a location of the Triple Burner. As the mid-Qing physician Chen Xiu-Yuan wrote, "In the interior, the *sháo yáng* governs the Triple Burner; in the exterior, it governs the interstices and the pores." So these are all locations of *sháo yáng* disease.

PHYSICIAN B   It seems to me that the main issue that should be addressed is the absence of alternating fever and chills in this case of lateral costal pain secondary to chronic hepatitis. If we strictly adhere to the principle of matching the symptom presentation to the formula, it is then inappropriate to use Cyperus and Inula Decoction *(xiāng fù xuán fù huā tāng)* in this case.

DR. YU   Exterior symptoms do not necessarily need to be present in order to use this formula. This insight is also from Dr. Jiang's experience. He said that he learned this through a direct experience of his own, which he illustrated with the saying, "When a fish drinks water he knows if it is hot or cold simply by drinking it." When he was in his 60s, Dr. Jiang contracted neuritis of the facial nerves, which quickly resolved. It was during mid-autumn and he then contracted a cold, but had no clear exterior symptoms, only pain upon movement in the right lateral costal region, which was not initially significant. The same night, the pain became more severe and started to extend back to the area around the kidneys. In the middle of the night, the pain became so severe that he was unable to roll over or to take a deep breath. He needed to be supported by family members in order to sit up.

The next morning he was diagnosed with lobar pneumonia and the Western doctor recommended antibiotics. Dr. Jiang instead wrote this formula for himself with the addition of Dalbergiae odoriferae Lignum *(jiàng xiāng)*, Sinapis Semen *(bái jiè zǐ)*, and Trichosanthis Semen *(guā lóu rén)*. He took one packet, and by nightfall, the pain was significantly reduced. He took one more packet and the pain was gone.

Over many years, Dr. Jiang used this formula to treat a large number of patients with pleurisy or pleural effusion and most of them had no exterior symptoms. Generally, after taking 2-4 packets, the lateral costal pain would be controlled. When a thin-mucus pathogen obstructs the Liver collaterals, in disorders such as chronic hepatitis, chronic cholecystitis, and asthma, exterior symptoms are also often absent. By modifying the base formula according to the presenting symptoms, excellent results will be achieved if the patient takes the formula consistently.

So when Dr. Jiang advocated studying ancient books, first he emphasized that we "should not allow the words to get in the way of the sentence, nor the sentence to get in the way of the sense." Secondly, we should always link the classical material as closely as possible to its clinical applications.

PHYSICIAN B   When I consider the herbs in this formula, they seem very ordinary, and yet the results are quite outstanding. It seems likely to me that there must be some secret with regard to modifying the formula to transform such an ordinary formula into one that is so extraordinary. Is that correct?

DR. YU   In fact, many classical formulas, as well as well-known contemporary formulas, are constructed of ordinary ingredients. My view is that this is a matter of accurately addressing the etiology and pathodynamic. If the clinical efficacy is distinct and re-peatable, why not use ordinary substances? In his own explanation of the formula, Wu Ju-Tong wrote:

> Cyperi Rhizoma *(xiāng fù)* and Inulae Flos *(xuán fù huā)* effectively unblock the Liver collaterals and drive out thin-mucus below the ribs. Perillae Fructus *(zǐ sū zǐ)* and Armeniacae Semen *(xìng rén)*[5] direct the Lung qi downward and trans-form thin-mucus. This is known as building up metal in order to calm wood. Citri reticulatae Pericarpium *(chén pí)* and standard Pinelliae Rhizoma praepa-ratum *(fǎ bàn xià)* truly eliminate thin-mucus. Poria *(fú líng)* and Coicis Semen *(yì yǐ rén)* open the *tài yīn* and close the *yáng míng*, which follows the adage that to treat water, one must bolster earth. When the water in the main channel of the river rises up, one should open the side branches of the river.

From the perspective of clinical efficacy, I would say that Wu's words do not overstate the matter.

PHYSICIAN B   Although Wu Ju-Tong writes that "Cyperi Rhizoma *(xiāng fù)* and Inulae Flos *(xuán fù huā)* effectively unblock the Liver collaterals and drive out thin-mucus below the ribs", Inulae Flos *(xuán fù huā)* does not enter the Liver channel.

DR. YU   Cyperi Rhizoma *(xiāng fù)* enters the Liver channel and it can guide Inulae Flos *(xuán fù huā)* to enter the Liver and unblock the collaterals.

- If there are accompanying symptoms of a pathogen obstructing the interstices and pores, such as alternating fever and chills, one can also add Artemisiae annuae Herba *(qīng hāo)* and Bupleuri Radix *(chái hú)* to open the interstices and to drive out the pathogen.

- For dizziness owing to upward counterflow of thin-mucus, one can add Poria, Cinna-mon Twig, Atractylodes, and Licorice Decoction *(líng guì zhú gān tāng)* to transform thin-mucus and direct counterflow downward.

- For Spleen deficiency and a failure of transportation, causing epigastric focal disten-tion and abdominal distention, one can add Six-Gentlemen Decoction with Auck-landia and Amomum *(xiāng shā liù jūn zǐ tāng)* to strengthen the Spleen and assist transportation.

- If damp turbidity encumbers the Spleen, causing a thick, greasy tongue coating and a poor appetite, one can add a large dose of Acori tatarinowii Rhizoma *(shí chāng pǔ)*,

....

5. *Translators' note:* While the original formula does not contain Armeniacae Semen *(xìng rén)*, it is mentioned in the commentary for the formula in the *Systematic Differentiation of Warm Patho-gen Diseases (Wēn bìng tiáo biàn)*.

Eupatorii Herba *(pèi lán)*, and Pogostemonis Herba *(guǎng huò xiāng)* to transform turbidity and to awaken the Spleen.

- Where there is static blood congealing in the collaterals, causing stabbing pain in the lateral costal region, one can add Dalbergiae odoriferae Lignum *(jiàng xiāng)*, Salviae miltiorrhizae Radix *(dān shēn)*, Rubiae Radix *(qiàn cǎo gēn)*, Eupolyphaga/Stelophaga *(tǔ biē chóng)* and other substances to dispel stasis and to unblock the collaterals.

This is not a secret method of modification. One simply must observe the clinical presentation and modify the formula accordingly.

4.1.1 Costal pain

A multi-year case of chronic cholecystitis

Confusion born from an intractable, recurrent illness

為病之易反易復,纏綿難愈所困惑

■ CASE HISTORY

Patient: *56-year-old woman*

After moving south to Sichuan from the northern part of China, the patient developed shoulder and back pain, reduced appetite, and fatigue, all of which she attributed to difficulty acclimating to her new environment. A physician that she consulted said that the rain and dampness in Sichuan had mixed with wind-cold to produce painful obstruction, leading to the shoulder and back pain. He attributed her fatigue and poor appetite to dampness encumbering the Spleen. The physician first prescribed formulas such as Notopterygium Decoction to Overcome Dampness *(qiāng huó shèng shī tāng)* and Five-Accumulation Powder *(wǔ jī sǎn)*, but there was no change in the patient's shoulder and back pain. He then switched to Patchouli/Agastache Powder to Rectify the Qi *(huò xiāng zhèng qì sǎn)*, Five-Ingredient Powder with Poria *(wǔ líng sǎn)*, Qi-Pushing Powder *(tuī qì sǎn)*,[6] and Minor Decoction [for Pathogens] Stuck in the Chest *(xiǎo xiàn xiōng tāng)* with the addition of Curcumae Radix *(yù jīn)* and Dalbergiae odoriferae Lignum *(jiàng xiāng)*, but the patient's poor appetite and fatigue remained unchanged. Having taken hundreds of packets of herbs over the past few years, and seeing no change in her condition, she had completely lost confidence in the possibility that treatment could help her.

....

6. *Translators' note:* Qi-Pushing Powder *(tuī qì sǎn)*: bran-fried Aurantii Fructus *(fū chǎo zhǐ ké)*, Cinnamomi Cortex *(ròu guì)*, Curcumae longae Rhizoma *(jiāng huáng)*, Glycyrrhizae Radix praeparata *(zhì gān cǎo)*. This formula comes from the 13th-century work by Yan Yong-He, *Formulas to Aid the Living*.

INTAKE EXAMINATION
DATE: March, 18, 1990

Her complexion was greenish, yellow, and slightly dark. The darkness was particularly distinct around the bridge of the nose. She was fatigued, short of breath, and her speech was sluggish. She had pain in her shoulder and back, especially on the right side. The patient complained of dull pain in the right lateral costal region, a stifling sensation of fullness in the epigastrium, and distention in the lower abdomen. Her appetite was poor and she had an aversion to rich, greasy foods. Her mouth was dry and she reported having a bitter taste. The patient's bowel movements were somewhat loose. Her tongue was a bit red with a thin, yellow, and slightly greasy coating, and her pulse was wiry and soggy.

Differentiation of Patterns and Discussion of Treatment

PHYSICIAN A   Ultimately, this patient received a Western medical diagnosis of chronic cholecystitis, scleroatrophic gallbladder, and gallbladder polyps. Because the subjective symptoms were so varied, it was difficult to determine the priority of these conditions. This made decisions about diagnosis and treatment quite difficult.

  The previous physician first considered the patient's shoulder and back pain, which he diagnosed as wind-damp-cold painful obstruction, to be the primary disorder, and therefore he prescribed a formula that dispersed wind, scattered cold, and eliminated dampness. Subsequently, he made a diagnosis of Spleen encumbered by dampness to account for the patient's poor appetite and fatigue, and thus he chose formulas to awaken the Spleen, resolve dampness, properly move qi, and transform phlegm. However, after two years of these formulas, there was no improvement.

DR. YU   The patient's complexion, which was greenish, yellow, and slightly dark, is clear evidence that there was a disharmony of wood and earth. The symptoms of dull right-sided lateral costal pain, lower abdominal distention, aversion to rich greasy foods, and dry mouth with bitter taste are all evidence of Liver constraint with Gallbladder heat. Finally, fatigue, shortness of breath, sluggish speech, poor appetite, fullness with a stifling sensation in the epigastrium, and slightly loose stools clearly indicate Spleen deficiency, Stomach cold, qi stagnation, and damp obstruction. Thus, the complete diagnosis is Liver constraint, Gallbladder heat, Spleen deficiency, Stomach cold, qi stagnation, and damp obstruction.

PHYSICIAN B   What explains the shoulder and back pain?

DR. YU   This is diseased wood overwhelming earth. When earth is deficient, pooling thin fluids convert into phlegm. Phlegm-dampness flows into the channels and collaterals of the shoulder and the back, obstructing qi transformation and the qi dynamic. This causes blockage, which in turn produces pain.

PHYSICIAN B   It appears that your ability to clearly understand the pathodynamic of this case is related to the fact that you inquired thoroughly about the patient's subjective symptoms and then put them all together. This suggests that the more thorough the four examinations, the better. This is especially true of the history or questioning examination. It is only through this type of thorough investigation that we can avoid the bias of "treating only the head for headache and treating only the foot for foot pain."

DR. YU   However, I would suggest that *thorough* is not the same as *holistic*. Modern Western medicine certainly stresses being thorough and would not suggest "treating only the head for headache and treating only the foot for foot pain." Chinese medicine also stresses being thorough, but its unique strength lies in its holism. The *Yellow Emperor's Inner Classic (Huáng Dì nèi jīng)* states that "if you understand the essentials, then one word can represent the whole; if you do not, endless [words] will never do so." This phrase profoundly expresses the idea of one versus many in relation to pattern identification. The basic idea is to emphasize the importance of striving to understand the pathodynamic from a broad, holistic perspective.

In the case presented here, the description of subjective symptoms seems chaotic and confusing. However, viewing them through the lens of wood-earth disharmony, a broad, holistic perspective, allowed me to make sense of the symptoms. One is then able to avoid the situation described in Chapter 1 of the *Divine Pivot (Líng shū)*: "Not knowing what is important, one squanders words endlessly."

PHYSICIAN A   I have heard that you spent many years researching chronic cholecystitis. Could you tell us something about what you learned?

DR. YU   In my early years of practice, chronic cholecystitis was quite common where I worked. Because I was a new physician without much experience, and because the descriptions of this disorder in books rarely seemed to match clinical reality, I had no choice but to gradually develop my own understanding.

After many years of experience, I did begin to have a sense of these patients. Chronic cholecystitis patients, regardless of whether or not they have gallstones, generally report many subjective symptoms. During the interview process, these patients will describe a seemingly jumbled set of disparate symptoms, which can be extremely confusing. If the physician is not adept at putting these symptoms together in a meaningful way, it can be very difficult to understand the primary complaint and to deal with the apparent contradictions. Thus, it is not easy to avoid using a symptomatic herbal formula, a strategy which rarely yields satisfying results.

My clinical investigations determined that this disease primarily affects the Liver, Gallbladder, Spleen, and Stomach. Recurrent right-sided upper abdominal pain that may or may not radiate to the shoulder and back, and a chronic bitter taste in the mouth, are suggestive of Liver constraint, Gallbladder heat, and a loss of the management of dredging and draining. Fullness and a stifling sensation in the epigastric region, poor appetite, reduced food intake, belching, indefinable epigastric discomfort, shortness of breath, and weakness indicate Spleen-Stomach deficiency and loss of adjustment of the middle burner's function of directing the pure upward and the turbid downward. Other possible symptoms include worry, anger, and an exacerbation of symptoms following ingestion of rich and oily or cold and raw foods. The sides of the tongue are often red and the coating is thin and white or thin, slightly yellow, and greasy. The pulse is often wiry, frail, and slightly slippery.

Appropriate treatment is to dredge the Liver, clear the Gallbladder, strengthen the Spleen, and harmonize the Stomach. I often combine two formulas to get quick results: Bupleurum, Gentian, and Oyster Shell Decoction *(chái dǎn mǔ lì tāng)* from the contemporary Sichuanese physician Jian Yu-Guang, and Nurture the Spleen and Sooth the Liver Decoction *(péi pí shū gān tāng)* from Zhang Xi-Chun:

Bupleuri Radix *(chái hú)* 10g
Ostreae Concha *(mǔ lì)* 30g
Gentianae Radix *(lóng dǎn cǎo)* 3-6g
Atractylodis macrocephalae Rhizoma *(bái zhú)* 10g
Astragali Radix *(huáng qí)* 10g
Citri reticulatae Pericarpium *(chén pí)* 10g
ginger Magnoliae officinalis Cortex *(jiāng hòu pò)* 6g
Hordei Fructus germinatus *(mài yá)* 10g
dry-fried Setariae (Oryzae) Fructus germinatus *(chǎo gǔ yá)* 10g
Gigeriae galli Endothelium corneum *(jī nèi jīn)* 6g
Paeoniae Radix alba *(bái sháo)* 12g
Zingiberis Rhizoma recens *(shēng jiāng)* 6g
Glycyrrhizae Radix *(gān cǎo)* 6g

In this formula, Bupleuri Radix *(chái hú)* and Hordei Fructus germinatus *(mài yá)* dredge the Liver and spread out areas that are constrained; Gentianae Radix *(lóng dǎn cǎo)*, Ostreae Concha *(mǔ lì)*, and Paeoniae Radix alba *(bái sháo)* clear and restrain Gallbladder fire; Astragali Radix *(huáng qí)*, Atractylodis macrocephalae Rhizoma *(bái zhú)*, and Glycyrrhizae Radix *(gān cǎo)* strengthen the Spleen and direct the clear upward; and Citri reticulatae Pericarpium *(chén pí)*, ginger Magnoliae officinalis Cortex *(jiāng hòu pò)*, dry-fried Setariae (Oryzae) Fructus germinatus *(chǎo gǔ yá)*, and Zingiberis Rhizoma recens *(shēng jiāng)* harmonize the Stomach and direct turbidity downward.

MODIFICATIONS:

• If the bitter taste in the mouth is severe, increase Gentianae Radix *(lóng dǎn cǎo)* to 10g.

• If fullness and a stifling sensation in the chest and diaphragm is severe, remove Atractylodis macrocephalae Rhizoma *(bái zhú)* and Paeoniae Radix alba *(bái sháo)*, and add Allii macrostemi Bulbus *(xiè bái)* 10g.

• For chronic tendency toward watery stool, add Coptidis Rhizoma *(huáng lián)* 3g, Dioscoreae Rhizoma *(shān yào)* 15g, and Agrimoniae Herba *(xiān hè cǎo)* 30g. This is because a small dose of Coptidis Rhizoma *(huáng lián)* clears heat associated with failed movement and transformation (this is why it is said to fortify the Stomach in small doses); Dioscoreae Rhizoma *(shān yào)* tonifies the Spleen and binds up diarrhea; and Agrimoniae Herba *(xiān hè cǎo)* is a tonifying herb that is also astringent and can treat diarrhea.

• When there is stiffness and pain upon movement in the shoulder and back, add Curcumae longae Rhizoma *(jiāng huáng)* 10g.

In 1972, I saw a 32-year-old woman with an eight-year history of cholecystitis without gallstones. Her symptoms included poor appetite, bitter taste, dull right-sided lateral costal pain, aching pain in the shoulders and back, fullness and a stifling sensation in the epigastric area, and slightly loose stools. Her tongue coating was white and greasy. Her pulse was soggy and slippery.

I chose to give her Bupleurum, Gentian, and Oyster Shell Decoction *(chái dǎn mǔ lì tāng)* plus Three-Seed Decoction *(sān rén tāng)* with the addition of Pogostemonis Herba *(guǎng huò xiāng)*, Eupatorii Herba *(pèi lán)*, Platycodi Radix *(jié gěng)*, and Agrimoniae Herba *(xiān hè cǎo)*. After taking ten packets, the bitter taste had resolved, the lateral costal pain and epigastric fullness had greatly reduced, and the stool was formed. I then changed her to the combination of Bupleurum, Gentian, and Oyster Shell Decoction *(chái dǎn mǔ lì tāng)* and Nurture the Spleen and Sooth the Liver Decoction *(péi pí shū gān tāng)*, and she took 16 packets. At that point, all her symptoms had resolved. After that time, when she occasionally had a recurrence of the symptoms, she took 3-4 packets of the latter formula and the symptoms would resolve.

In recent years, I have been using more classical formulas. As I reviewed this case, it appeared to me that a combination of Bupleurum and Cinnamon Twig Decoction *(chái hú guì zhī tāng)* and Bupleurum, Cinnamon Twig, and Ginger Decoction *(chái hú guì jiāng tāng)* might have yielded even better results.

In the case described at the beginning of this chapter, I diagnosed the patient with Liver constraint, Gallbladder heat, Spleen deficiency, and Stomach cold, accompanied by qi stagnation and damp obstruction.

Appropriate treatment consisted of dredging the Liver, clearing the Gallbladder, strengthening the Spleen, warming the Stomach, moving the qi, and transforming dampness.

The formula was a modification of Bupleurum and Cinnamon Twig Decoction *(chái hú guì zhī tāng)* combined with Bupleurum, Cinnamon Twig, and Ginger Decoction *(chái hú guì jiāng tāng)*:

Bupleuri Radix *(chái hú)* 15g
Scutellariae Radix *(huáng qín)* 6g
standard Pinelliae Rhizoma praeparatum *(fǎ bàn xià)* 10g
Codonopsis Radix *(dǎng shēn)* 12g
Glycyrrhizae Radix *(gān cǎo)* 3g
Zingiberis Rhizoma recens *(shēng jiāng)* 5g
Cinnamomi Ramulus *(guì zhī)* 10g
Paeoniae Radix alba *(bái sháo)* 12g
Zingiberis Rhizoma *(gān jiāng)* 5g
Ostreae Concha *(mǔ lì)* 30g
Trichosanthis Radix *(tiān huā fěn)* 12g
Curcumae longae Rhizoma *(jiāng huáng)* 10g

Instructions: two packets

I encouraged the patient to reduce her worry and anger, and to avoid both oily, rich and cold, raw foods. I also told her that from a Western medical perspective, the locus of her problem was in the gallbladder. As such, I encouraged her to have imaging done in order to confirm that diagnosis.

SECOND VISIT: After taking the formula, she noticed a reduction in right-sided lateral costal pain, fullness and the stifling sensation in the epigastric region, lower abdominal distention, and poor appetite. She also reported that the imaging studies confirmed that she had chronic cholecystitis, gallbladder atrophy, and gallbladder polyps. Because this confirmed my diagnosis, it gave her additional confidence in the treatment.

To the above formula, I added Mume Fructus *(wū méi)* 20g, Clematidis Radix *(wēi líng xiān)* 10g, Bombyx batryticatus *(bái jiāng cán)* 6g, and Pheretima *(dì lóng)* 6g. (The last two ingredients were baked, ground to a fine powder, and washed down with the drained liquid from the decoction.)

THIRD VISIT: After taking six packets of the formula, the patient's right-side lateral costal pain, fullness and stifling sensation in the epigastric region, and lower abdominal distention had essentially resolved. The aching and pain in her shoulder and back had markedly diminished. Her appetite had improved and her bowels were formed. Her tongue was normal and her pulse was wiry and moderate.

From the above formula, we removed Cinnamomi Ramulus *(guì zhī)*, Zingiberis Rhizoma *(gān jiāng)*, Ostreae Concha *(mǔ lì)*, and Trichosanthis Radix *(tiān huā fěn)*, and added Astragali Radix *(huáng qí)* 30g and Citri reticulatae Pericarpium *(chén pí)* 10g.

RESULTS: After 45 packets of the formula given in the third visit, all of the symptoms completely resolved. Her complexion was comparatively rosy and moist without a trace of illness. At a one-year follow-up, she reported that she was still doing very well.

Disease	Primary Symptoms	Differentiation	Treatment Method	Formula
Chronic cholecystitis	Dull right-sided lateral costal pain, shoulder and back pain, poor appetite, bitter taste	Liver constraint, Gallbladder heat, Spleen deficiency, Stomach cold	Soothe the Liver, clear the Gallbladder, strengthen the Spleen, warm the Stomach	Bupleurum and Cinnamon Twig Decoction *(chái hú guì zhī tāng)* plus Bupleurum, Cinnamon Twig, and Ginger Decoction *(chái hú guì jiāng tāng)*

Reflections and Clarifications

PHYSICIAN A   Dr. Yu, do you feel that this patient was completely cured? Was there a complete reversal of the chronic cholecystitis, gallbladder atrophy, and gallbladder polyps?

DR. YU   From the perspective of Western medicine, I do not know. The patient was unwilling to do further testing, so I have no way to answer that question. Nonetheless, all of the symptoms had completely resolved, her complexion was comparatively rosy and moist without a trace of illness, and upon follow-up after one year, she reported that she was still doing very well. So from the perspective of Chinese medicine, can we not consider that a clinical cure?

PHYSICIAN C   According to your diagnostic process, the holistic treatment principle involved regulating the Liver, Gallbladder, Spleen, and Stomach. However, you chose two formulas: Bupleurum and Cinnamon Twig Decoction *(chái hú guì zhī tāng)* and Bupleurum, Cinnamon Twig, and Ginger Decoction *(chái hú guì jiāng tāng)*, both from the *tài yáng* section of the *Discussion of Cold Damage (Shāng hán lùn)*. The former is a mild formula to simultaneously resolve the *tài yáng* and the *sháo yáng*, whereas the latter is a formula that harmonizes the *sháo yáng* and warms and transforms cold thin-mucus. It seems as though neither formula has much to do with the Spleen and Stomach and yet the effect was excellent. What is the rationale behind the formula's success?

DR. YU   It is true that Bupleurum and Cinnamon Twig Decoction *(chái hú guì zhī tāng)* is, as you say, a mild formula to simultaneously resolve the *tài yáng* and the *sháo yáng*. Its source is line 146 of the *Discussion of Cold Damage (Shāng hán lùn)*: "Cold damage for six or seven days with feverishness, slight chills, annoyingly painful joints of the limbs, mild vomiting, and knots of the supports below the Heart,[7] [means] that the external pattern has not yet gone: Bupleurum and Cinnamon Twig Decoction *(chái hú guì zhī tāng)* governs." If you take a mechanistic view of the formula which says that there must be an exact match between the symptoms in the line and the use of the formula, you have a shallow and limited view of the formula.

This formula is a combination of Minor Bupleurum Decoction *(xiǎo chái hú tāng)* and Cinnamon Twig Decoction *(guì zhī tāng)*. From a six-channel perspective, Minor Bupleurum Decoction *(xiǎo chái hú tāng)* can push a pathogen out of the body by using the *sháo yáng* pivot in order to thrust out *tài yáng* qi. It unblocks and treats the symptoms, as described at line 97 of the *Discussion of Cold Damage (Shāng hán lùn)*, that are produced when "the blood is weak, the qi expended, and the pores and interstices open, pathogenic qi can enter and contend with the normal qi."

If we consider the same formula from the perspective of the yin and yang organs, Bupleuri Radix *(chái hú)* and Scutellariae Radix *(huáng qín)* dredge the Liver and clear the Gallbladder; Ginseng Radix *(rén shēn)*, Glycyrrhizae Radix *(gān cǎo)*, standard Pinelliae Rhizoma praeparatum *(fǎ bàn xià)*, Zingiberis Rhizoma recens *(shēng jiāng)*, and Jujubae Fructus *(dà zǎo)* strengthen the Spleen and harmonize the Stomach. In fact, from a holistic perspective, Minor Bupleurum Decoction *(xiǎo chái hú tāng)* is an excellent formula for regulating the Liver, Gallbladder, Spleen, and Stomach.

With regards to Cinnamon Twig Decoction *(guì zhī tāng)*, esteemed physicians have extolled its virtues. For example, the 17th-century writer Xu Bin stated that "for external presentations it resolves the flesh and harmonizes the nutritive and protective; for internal presentations, it transforms qi and regulates yin and yang."

In my opinion, in this context the phrase *qi transformation* refers to the formula's ability to transform and to generate essence qi from food and drink. In this way it helps to restore and strengthen the functions of the Spleen and Stomach. In doing so, it encourages the continual production of qi and blood, which then spreads throughout the five yin organs, the six yang organs, and the limbs and bones. Thus, we can say that its connection to the Spleen and the Stomach is significant.

As for Bupleurum, Cinnamon Twig, and Ginger Decoction *(chái hú guì jiāng tāng)*, it originates from line 147 of the *Discussion of Cold Damage (Shāng hán lùn)*:

----

7. *Translators' note:* "Knots of the supports" (支結 *zhī jié*) refers to a feeling of something inside the upper abdomen, which feels both as if it is propping up the abdomen and inducing the feeling of being all knotted up.

When there has been cold damage for five or six days that had already been
sweated and was then purged, with fullness and slight knotting in the chest and
ribs, impeded urination, thirst without vomiting, sweating only from the head,
alternating chills and fever, and irritability in the chest, it means that [the exte-
rior] has not yet been released, and Bupleurum, Cinnamon Twig, and Ginger
Decoction (chái hú guì jiāng tāng) governs.

This passage is an example of a shào yáng disease accompanied by internal knotting
of thin-mucus. The formula harmonizes the shào yáng, drives out thin-mucus, and
disperses knots. In the case described here, the formula is used in the following ways:
Bupleuri Radix (chái hú) and Scutellariae Radix (huáng qín) dredge the Liver and clear
the Gallbladder; Cinnamomi Ramulus (guì zhī), Glycyrrhizae Radix (gān cǎo), and
Zingiberis Rhizoma (gān jiāng) warm and transform the cold thin-mucus affecting
the Spleen and Stomach; and Ostreae Concha (mǔ lì) and Trichosanthis Radix (tiān
huā fěn) drive out thin-mucus and disperse knots. Thus, we can see that the formula
simultaneously treats the Liver, Gallbladder, Spleen, and Stomach. The combination
of Bupleurum, Cinnamon Twig, and Ginger Decoction (chái hú guì jiāng tāng) and
Bupleurum and Cinnamon Twig Decoction (chái hú guì zhī tāng) fully maximizes the
effect of both formulas as they dredge the Liver, clear the Gallbladder, strengthen the
Spleen, harmonize the Stomach, move the qi, and transform dampness.

PHYSICIAN C   After the patient went in for imaging, you added Mume Fructus (wū méi),
Clematidis Radix (wēi líng xiān), Bombyx batryticatus (bái jiāng cán), and Pheretima
(dì lóng). Can you explain the rationale for these additions?

DR. YU   These substances were added to eliminate the patient's gallbladder polyps. In
Chinese medicine, we view polyps as static, congealed phlegm. Surprisingly, as it is
astringent, many contemporary physicians still use Mume Fructus (wū méi). This is
worth pondering.

   I think that the source of this may be from a version of Mume Pill (wū méi wán)
(consisting of only Mume Fructus (wū méi) and vinegar) that appears in Formulas to
Aid the Living (Jì shēng fāng). In recent years, physicians have used this formula in
conjunction with substances such as Manitis Squama (chuān shān jiǎ),[8] Notoginseng
Radix (sān qī), and Bombyx batryticatus (bái jiāng cán) to transform stasis, unblock
the collaterals, grind away hardness, and disperse knots. This combination has been
used to effectively treat polyps affecting areas such as the rectum, duodenum, vocal
cords, and the cervix.

   Last year, I treated a woman in her 50s for cervical spine hyperplasia. During the
course of treatment, she developed a corn-kernel sized polyp beneath her tongue. The
Western physicians wanted to operate on the polyp, but the patient was afraid to have
surgery and asked if it could be treated with Chinese medicine. To her formula, I added
Mume Fructus (wū méi) 20g and Bombyx batryticatus (bái jiāng cán) 6g (ground into
a fine powder and swallowed with the decoction liquid). After eight packets, the polyp
had disappeared without any problems.

   In recent years, whenever I treat gallbladder polyps, I always use the combination

8. *Translators' note:* Due to its endangered species designation, this substance is no longer available.

of Mume Fructus *(wū méi)*, Clematidis Radix *(wēi líng xiān)*, Bombyx batryticatus *(bái jiāng cán)*, and Pheretima *(dì lóng)*. The Confucian classic *Book of Documents (Shū jīng)* states that the sour flavor promotes the bending and straightening power of wood. Mume Fructus *(wū méi)* is extremely sour. In the presence of the extremely thick qi of wood, then within restraining, there is a great force of unblocking and dredging. Clematidis Radix *(wēi líng xiān)* is acrid, aromatic, and mobilizing. It has a special ability to attack and to dissipate. Further, from pharmacological studies, we know that these two medicinal substances have a relatively strong ability to enable the functions of the gallbladder. Bombyx batryticatus *(bái jiāng cán)* and Pheretima *(dì lóng)* excel at transforming phlegm, unblocking the collaterals, grinding away hardness, and dispersing knots. Sadly, written case studies of this type of usage are not numerous. I hope that this is an area that people are motivated to expand upon in the future.

PHYSICIAN C   From what I have seen clinically, this disease easily recurs and it is difficult to treat the root. What have you observed?

DR. YU   I have treated chronic cholecystitis for many years and I have frequently encountered this problem of the disease recurring. It is difficult to treat the root, even if you are meticulous in your application of matching the treatment principle, treatment method, formula, and herbs.

However, I have found three important points that can assist in the process of quickly reducing the symptoms and improving the patient's constitution.

The first is that the dredging and clearing should be done to an appropriate degree. Patients suffering from this disorder are generally constitutionally weak, the disease course is often long, and deficiency and excess are intermixed: deficiency of the Spleen and Stomach mixed with excess of the Liver and Gallbladder. Liver constraint and Gallbladder heat require dredging and clearing. But if all you do is dredge and clear, or do so excessively, this will eventually injure the source qi of the Spleen and Stomach, aggravating the poor appetite, shortness of breath, and lack of strength. Thus, we should dredge and clear to the appropriate degree, and optimally, this should be done simultaneously with strengthening the Spleen and harmonizing the Stomach throughout the treatment.

The second point is that we should be cautious when using bitter, cold herbs. In these patients, the Spleen and Stomach are already weak, intake and assimilation of food is poor, and in general, cold, bitter herbs are poorly tolerated. Given that Gallbladder heat is present in these patterns and that using bitter, cold herbs is critical, we are faced with a conundrum.

Through years of experience I have developed quite a deep knowledge of the substances that clear and direct Gallbladder fire downward. These herbs are able to increase the function of the Gallbladder, but are hard on the Spleen and Stomach, so we must use small doses. In cases where the stools are loose, we must be even more cautious. Only small doses of Gentianae Radix *(lóng dǎn cǎo)* and Coptidis Rhizoma *(huáng lián)* can be used, perhaps 1.5-3g. These herbs effectively clear Gallbladder heat, but also firm up the Stomach and Intestines, so they can be used in cases with loose stools. However, if the loose stools are chronic, then only Coptidis Rhizoma *(huáng lián)* should be used because, as noted in the 6th-century work *Miscellaneous Records of Famous Physicians (Míng yī bié lù)*, it can firm up the Intestines and regulate the Stomach.

The third point has to do with additional advice that should be given to the patient. They must be encouraged to cultivate a good emotional outlook and to be optimistic and cheerful. Further, they must avoid oily, rich foods, as well as raw and cold foods. More than a few patients who have not responded well to the formula, or who have had recurrences, have not heeded this advice; thus, it is important to emphasize these points to the patient.

4.2 Liver abscess

High fever with shivering for one month (liver abscess)

Unexpected, simultaneous appearance of mutually incompatible disease dynamics

互相矛盾的病機竟然同時並存

■ CASE HISTORY

Patient: *39-year-old man*

About two weeks before he became sick, the patient went through a period of emotional difficulty and attempted to alleviate his worries with alcohol. His sleep and food intake during that time were poor and he was also listless. One day, he realized that he was feeling increasingly chilled and his whole body was aching. His temperature was 38.5°C (101.3°F). As the day progressed into night, he developed a high fever with shivering. His temperature reached 39.5°C (103.1°F).

The first physician he saw viewed the situation as intruding cold enwrapping heat and prescribed Bupleurum and Kudzu Decoction to Release the Muscle Layer *(chái gé jiě jī tāng)*. After two packets of the formula the patient sweated profusely and his fever fell to 38°C (100.4°F). However, a few hours later, it shot back up.

A second physician felt that the sweating had not resolved the illness, and noting that the tongue coating was yellow, thick, and greasy, diagnosed damp-warmth. He prescribed Sweet Dew Special Pill to Eliminate Toxin *(gān lù xiāo dú dān)* plus Artemisiae annuae Herba *(qīng hāo)* and Eupatorii Herba *(pèi lán)*. After four packets, not only had the patient's tongue coating not waned, but his fever had increased to between 39°C–39.5°C (102.2°F–103.1°F) and was accompanied by severe chills, sweating, and feeling flustered and alarmed.

The third physician consulted by the patient diagnosed a cold contraction owing to yang deficiency and thus prescribed Ephedra, Asarum, and Aconite Accessory Root Decoction *(má huáng xì xīn fù zǐ tāng)* plus Ginseng Radix rubra *(hóng shēn)*. After one packet, the chills, sweating, and alarm ceased and the fever dropped to 38°C (100.4°F). However, the next day, the high fever and shivering returned with the temperature increasing to 40°C (104°F).

The fourth physician palpated the patient's abdomen and found epigastric fullness and a stifling sensation. He also noted that the tongue coating was gray-yellow, moldy, and greasy. He diagnosed a pathogen lurking in the membrane source and prescribed two packets of a modification of Reach the Source Drink *(dá yuán yǐn)*. There was no alleviation in the symptoms.

Given that he had not been out of bed for 12 days and that his blood tests appeared abnormal, there was fear of a severe malady. He was therefore admitted to the hospital where he planned to treat his symptoms with Western medicine.

On ultrasound, the left lobe of the liver was found to have a 5.5cm x 9.5cm area of inflammatory changes.

He was diagnosed with a liver abscess and treated with ampicillin, gentamycin, and metronidazole intravenously for seven days. This medication was combined with seven packets of Chinese herbs to clear heat, resolve toxicity, drain the Liver, unblock the collaterals, flush phlegm, and promote urination. However, the fever remained unchanged. At that point, the doctors began using hydrocortisone and the fever quickly declined to 37°C (98.6°F) or below. However, within days of stopping the hydrocortisone, the fever returned to 38.5°C–39.5°C (101.3°F–103.1°F) and the blood tests remained abnormally high.

The Western physicians explained to the patient that the abscess was already purulent and that they wanted to perform a percutaneous drainage of the purulent fluid. The patient was fearful and thus refused and asked that he be treated with Chinese medicine.

Intake Examination
DATE: November 15, 1992

The patient's temperature was 39°C (102.2°F). His complexion was sallow and dark. He was emaciated, having lost 7 kg (15.4 lb), and exhausted. In the morning, he began to feel chills, but in the afternoon and into the evening, he experienced tidal fevers and copious sweating. He reported epigastric focal distention with fullness and a stifling sensation that worsened with pressure. He had a foul taste in his mouth and his food intake was reduced. The patient's bowel movements were loose and his urine was scanty and dark yellow. The body of his tongue was pale and dark with stasis spots on the left side and the coating was gray-yellow, thick, moldy, and greasy. His pulse was soggy and rapid.

Differentiation of Patterns and Discussion of Treatment

PHYSICIAN A   Liver abscess in Western medicine is similar to that described in Chinese medicine. Is this case truly an example of Liver abscess? The *Concise Dictionary of Chinese Medicine (Jiǎn míng zhōng yī cí diǎn)* describes the pathodynamic of liver abscess as follows:

> In many cases, Liver constraint transforms into fire, the qi stagnates, and the blood becomes static; this accumulates and produces an abscess. It can also be the result of accumulated dampness producing phlegm, which collects and steams, giving rise to an abscess. In the early stages, there is dull pain in the area around LV-14, which gradually evolves into distending pain in the right lateral costal region that worsens with pressure. The patient cannot lie on the right side. The discomfort is frequently accompanied by chills and fever with a wiry, rapid pulse. If the condition lingers, the distending pain in the local area may become severe and be accompanied by fullness, distention, and unrelenting fever. If left untreated over a long period, this situation may lead to a bursting of the abscess, resulting in diarrhea with pus and blood or spitting up of pus and blood.

In the present case, with the exception of high fever and severe chills, the symptoms are quite different from this presentation. As a result, the use of typical treatment strategies for liver abscess such as clearing heat and resolving toxicity, draining the Liver and unblocking the collaterals, and flushing phlegm and promoting urination were all quite useless.

You have emphasized the need to synthesize disease identification and pattern identification, as well as the importance of taking into account both the larger picture and the details. Further, you often remind us to "observe the pulse and the signs to understand what has gone wrong and then to use the appropriate strategy to treat." And you have admonished us to never proceed in a rigid, inflexible, 'paint-by-numbers' way. This case appears to be an excellent illustration of these challenges.

The patient does not seem to clearly match the Chinese medicine definition of liver abscess, nor the Western medicine definition. Was the Western medical diagnosis incorrect?

DR. YU The Western diagnosis was correct. It was determined through ultrasound, which is quite a sensitive tool for determining the presence of liver abscess. The incidence of liver abscess is relatively low and the incidence of misdiagnosis is relatively high, particularly in the early stage of the disorder. Prior to the time when ultrasound was routinely used in the clinic, the rate of misdiagnosis was even higher. In fact, there have been some cases in which the presence of a liver abscess was only found on autopsy.

The majority of liver abscesses occur in the right lobe of the liver. This clinical presentation is quite similar to the description of liver abscess in Chinese medicine. However, in the current case, the abscess occurred in the left lobe of the liver. The specific location of the symptoms was below the xiphoid process, what in Chinese medicine is referred to as the area "below the heart" (the epigastric region.) Thus, the patient complained of focal distention, fullness, stifling sensation, and distention in the epigastrium, which worsened with pressure.

If we just consider this one symptom, it would seem that this presentation is very similar to minor knotting in the chest (also translated into English as minor chest bind), as described at line 138 of the *Discussion of Cold Damage (Shāng hán lùn)*: "A minor knotting in the chest disease is right in the area below the heart. On pressure it is painful and the pulse is floating and slippery. Minor Decoction [for Pathogens] Stuck in the Chest *(xiǎo xiàn xiōng tāng)* governs."

PHYSICIAN A So why did you choose not to use that formula?

DR. YU If you consider the presentation just in the local area, this pattern seems very similar to that for which Minor Decoction [for Pathogens] Stuck in the Chest *(xiǎo xiàn xiōng tāng)* is used: phlegm-heat stuck in the chest. However, if you consider this patient from a more systemic perspective, the similarity disappears.

The patient experienced a month-long high fever and shivering which were unresolved with sweating. He then had severe chills, tidal fevers, copious sweating, foul taste in the mouth, loose stools, and scanty, dark yellow urine. His tongue coating was grey-yellow, thick, moldy, and greasy, and his pulse was soggy and rapid. Clearly, this was a damp-warmth pattern.

However, because multiple ineffective treatment strategies were pursued, such as dispersing and unblocking, transforming with aromatic herbs, and leaching out with bland herbs, it resulted in a pathodynamic that was hidden deeply in the body. It was clear from the patient's sallow-dark complexion and his dark-pale tongue with stasis spots that there was stasis in the collaterals. Also, not only did the use of Ephedra, Asarum, and Aconite Accessory Root Decoction *(má huáng xì xīn fù zǐ tāng)* plus Ginseng Radix rubra *(hóng shēn)* not exacerbate the symptoms, it actually lowered the patient's body temperature. Thus, it is clear that a veiled constitutional yang deficiency was one factor in the disorder.

From this it can be seen that the pattern is one of yang deficiency and damp-warmth.

PHYSICIAN B   In the textbooks discussing warm disease, there is no pattern of yang deficiency and damp-warmth. Does this presentation appear in the classical literature?

DR. YU   Although this specific pattern is not mentioned by name, similar patterns do appear in case records. This pattern is not uncommon in modern practice, and this case is a good example.

My thought was that this case involved yang deficiency, qi stagnation, knotting of damp-heat, and stasis in the Stomach collaterals.

The treatment therefore was to warm the yang, guide out stagnation, clear heat, resolve dampness, dispel stasis, and unblock the collaterals.

The formula selected was a combination of Ginger and Aconite Accessory Root Decoction *(gān jiāng fù zǐ tāng)*, Calm the Stomach Powder *(píng wèi sǎn)*, and Three-Seed Decoction *(sān rén tāng)* with modifications.

Aconiti Radix lateralis praeparata *(zhì fù zǐ)* [precook for 30 minutes]	30g
Zingiberis Rhizoma *(gān jiāng)*...	15g
Atractylodis Rhizoma *(cāng zhú)*...	15g
Ginger Magnoliae officinalis Cortex *(jiāng hòu pò)*.........................	20g
Citri reticulatae Pericarpium *(chén pí)*	15g
Armeniacae Semen *(xìng rén)*	15g
Coicis Semen *(yì yǐ rén)*..	30g
Platycodi Radix *(jié gěng)*	30g
standard Pinelliae Rhizoma praeparatum *(fǎ bàn xià)*	20g
Sargentodoxae Caulis *(hóng téng)*..	15g
Vaccariae Semen *(wáng bù liú xíng)*	15g
Manitis Squama *(chuān shān jiǎ)*[9].......................................	
[powder and take with strained decoction].............................	5g
Notoginseng Radix *(sān qī)*	
[powder and take with strained decoction].............................	5g

Instructions: Three packets. This was taken in conjunction with previously prescribed Western medications.

SECOND VISIT: The body temperature had decreased to between 37.5–38.5°C (99.5–101.3°F). The symptoms of chills, tidal fever, and epigastric focal distention had all lessened. The patient still complained of copious sweating, reduced food intake, and unformed stools.

....

9. *Translators' note:* This substance is not available in the West, nor any longer in China. For this reason, as a substitute, the author recommends increasing the dosage of Vaccariae Semen *(wáng bù liú xíng)* to 30g.

His tongue coating was slightly less yellow, greasy, thick, and moldy.

To the above formula, we added:

> Ginseng Radix rubra (*hóng shēn*) [cooked separately] 15g
> Astragali Radix (*huáng qí*)... 30g
> Agrimoniae Herba (*xiān hè cǎo*).. 60g

Instructions: Three packets. The patient continued with his previously-prescribed Western medications.

THIRD VISIT: The lab values of his blood tests were within normal range. His temperature had decreased to a range of 37.2–37.6°C (98.9–99.6°F). His chills, tidal fever, and epigastric focal distention had all resolved and his sweating was noticeably less. All that remained was the sensation of being roasted and then sweating when he drank or ate. His appetite was good, his stool was formed, and his urination was clear and smooth. His tongue was pale-red and the stasis spots on the left side of the tongue had resolved. The patient's moldy, greasy tongue coating was reduced by about half.

We then prescribed a modified version of Six-Gentlemen Decoction with Aucklandia and Amomum *(xiāng shā liù jūn zǐ tāng)* with Poria, Cinnamon Twig, Atractylodes, and Licorice Decoction *(líng guì zhú gān tāng).*

> Codonopsis Radix (*dǎng shēn*).. 15g
> Atractylodis macrocephalae Rhizoma (*bái zhú*) 15g
> Poria (*fú líng*)... 30g
> Glycyrrhizae Radix (*gān cǎo*).. 5g
> standard Pinelliae Rhizoma praeparatum (*fǎ bàn xià*) 15g
> Citri reticulatae Pericarpium (*chén pí*) 10g
> Amomi Fructus (*shā rén*)... 5g
> Aucklandiae Radix (*mù xiāng*) 10g
> Cinnamomi Ramulus (*guì zhī*)... 10g
> Astragali Radix (*huáng qí*)... 30g
> Notoginseng Radix (*sān qī*) [powder and take with strained decoction] ... 5g
> Platycodi Radix (*jié gěng*) 15g
> Sargentodoxae Caulis (*hóng téng*)... 15g

Instructions: Discontinue all Western medications, with the exception of vitamins.

After the patient had taken 12 packets of the formula over 12 days, all of his symptoms resolved. A follow-up ultrasound showed that in the left lobe of the liver there was a liquefaction zone[10] of 1.5cm x 1cm. He was discharged from the hospital to recuperate further at home.

We sent him home with the following post-treatment instructions:

1. Preparation of Notoginseng Radix *(sān qī)* as follows: Take 100g Notoginseng Radix *(sān qī)* and fry in chicken fat for two minutes. After this, its nature becomes warming and acrid, and, from a pharmacological perspective, it contains even more helpful saponins

10. In the early stage, a liver abscess is generally more solid. Later, a liquefaction zone may develop following cell death. As the abscess heals, this zone becomes smaller until, with complete healing, it disappears.

than Ginseng Radix *(rén shēn)*. After cooling, grind to a fine powder. Each morning and evening take 5g of the powder mixed in egg drop soup made with two eggs. Then add white sugar to taste and ingest.

2. Alternate between Aconite Accessory Root Pill to Regulate the Middle *(fù zǐ lǐ zhōng wán)* and Tonify the Middle to Augment the Qi Pill *(bǔ zhōng yì qì wán)*, taking each one every other day for a month.

On follow-up at six months, the patient had completely recuperated.

Disease	Primary Symptoms	Differentiation	Treatment Method	Formula
Liver abscess	High fever and shivering	Yang deficiency, qi stagnation, knotting of damp-heat, stasis in the Stomach collaterals	Warm the yang, guide out stagnation, clear heat, resolve dampness, dispel stasis, unblock the collaterals	Ginger and Aconite Accessory Root Decoction *(gān jiāng fù zǐ tāng)*, Calm the Stomach Powder *(píng wèi sǎn)*, and Three-Seed Decoction *(sān rén tāng)* with modifications

REFLECTIONS AND CLARIFICATIONS

PHYSICIAN A   The way that I understand yang deficiency with damp-heat is that the yang deficiency represents the constitution and the damp-heat represents the pathogen. If this is the case, is it not true that this pattern contradicts traditional theories in Chinese medicine?

PHYSICIAN B   I had the same thought. In the traditional theories of externally-contracted heat diseases, there is the objective rule of transformations: yin patterns transform into cold and yang patterns transform into heat. For example, there is the following explanation in the *Golden Mirror of the Medical Tradition (Yī zōng jīn jiàn)*:

> Diseases of the six channels always involve transformations related to cold damage. While the qi is the same, the diseases are different. How could it be otherwise? The form of the organs are variable and the transformations occur based on type, so they are varied. As it is clear that the various types of water and fire can overcome each other, how is it difficult to understand the principle of cold changing into heat? One could go on and on about the thousands of transformations, but all are contained inside yin/yang and exterior/interior.

This passage means that when a patient with a yang deficiency constitution contracts an external pathogen, it can only transform from yin and thus become a pattern of yang deficiency with cold and dampness. There is no way for this to transform into a yang deficiency with warmth and dampness. Dr. Yu, what are your thoughts on this?

DR. YU   The tenet that pathogens will transform from yin into cold and from yang into heat has a certain utility to it. Nonetheless, when we are discussing the myriad changes of actual diseases, it is extremely difficult to restrict oneself to a limited framework. We have to make general categorizations, as best we can, while recognizing that these cannot capture every incidence.

With regard to this type of disparity, not only do we see patients with yang deficiency and damp-warmth, we also see patients with yin deficiency and cold-dampness.
In severe cases, we may even come across more complicated sets of symptoms. We
may encounter patients simultaneously displaying symptoms that indicate multiple,
seemingly disconnected pathodynamics, or even multiple contradictory pathodynamics.

If we only consider the standard rules and methods, it will be very difficult for us to
reach a seamless match between the diagnosis, treatment principle, formula, and specific herbs. Lacking that, we can easily imagine what the therapeutic outcome will be.
In these cases, we must break out of our ruts, look for a new way forward, and boldly
use more complex formulations.

The modern physician Qiu Pei-Ran had a very deep insight into this situation.
He worked with many dysentery patients who were in critical condition. After these
patients had failed to respond to various treatments, he ultimately used large complex
formulas with Codonopsis Radix *(dǎng shēn)*, Rehmanniae Radix praeparata *(shú dì
huáng)*, Angelicae sinensis Radix *(dāng guī)*, Atractylodis macrocephalae Rhizoma *(bái
zhú)*, Coptidis Rhizoma *(huáng lián)*, Plantaginis Semen *(chē qián zǐ)*, Alismatis Rhizoma *(zé xiè)*, Scutellariae Radix *(huáng qín)*, Zingiberis Rhizoma *(gān jiāng)*, Aconiti
Radix lateralis praeparata *(zhì fù zǐ)*, Natrii Sulfas *(máng xiāo)*, Rhei Radix et Rhizoma
(dà huáng), Astragali Radix *(huáng qí)*, Saposhnikoviae Radix *(fáng fēng)*, Notopterygii
Rhizoma seu Radix *(qiāng huó)*, Mume Fructus *(wū méi)*, and Chebulae Fructus *(hē
zǐ)*. After just two days of herbs, these patients were cured.

When treating stubborn cases of chronic nephritis, he would sometimes combine
up to seven different treatment principles into one large formula: clear heat and resolve
toxicity, warm and tonify Kidney yang, augment Spleen qi, enrich yin and tonify blood,
dispel dampness and promote urination, release the exterior with acrid-warm herbs,
and bind up the lower burner. Often, blood-tonifying would be mixed with stasis-dispelling, qi-tonifying with dispersing knots, tonifying with purging, warming yang with
clearing heat, and binding with unblocking.

Dr. Qiu expressed his thinking about this by saying, "I fully comprehend that these
[prescriptions] seem to be a sundry mess of substances and a chaotic set of treatment
principles. Yet, in critical cases of severe disease, this synergistic strategy is highly effective."

PHYSICIAN A   In the case above, the patient had high fever and shivering for a month. He
was diagnosed by Western medicine with a liver abscess and treated with a combination
of antibiotics and Chinese herbs (clear heat and resolve toxicity, drain the Liver and
unblock the collaterals, flush phlegm and promote urination), with poor results.

After receiving the patient, you had a breakthrough in thinking about the case and
prescribed a large formula that focused primarily on warming yang and guiding out
stagnation, assisted by clearing heat and resolving dampness, while also dispelling stasis and unblocking the collaterals. This method produced excellent results. I have seen
no clinical reports of using warm and hot herbs to treat liver abscess. It would be very
useful if you could summarize this for me.

DR. YU   The critical point here is making the correct pattern identification, not what specific medicinal substances were used. Once I had made the diagnosis of yang deficiency

with damp-warmth, I then resolved to use a large, complex formula that combined Ginger and Aconite Accessory Root Decoction *(gān jiāng fù zǐ tāng)* with Calm the Stomach Powder *(píng wèi sǎn)* to warm the yang and to guide out stagnation, as the basis for the primary formula. To this, I added Three-Seed Decoction *(sān rén tāng)* to disseminate and facilitate the Triple Burner and to clear heat and resolve dampness. Finally, I added Manitis Squama *(chuān shān jiǎ)*,[11] Notoginseng Radix *(sān qī)*, and Vaccariae Semen *(wáng bù liú xíng)* to dispel stasis and to unblock the collaterals.

PHYSICIAN C   I still have a question. In Chapters 7 and 18 of the *Essentials from the Golden Cabinet (Jīn guì yào lüè)*, Zhang Zhong-Jing discusses Lung abscess and Intestinal abscess. His discussion is thorough and the suggested treatments are effective. We think of these texts as a primary source of information for these conditions. Given that liver abscess is certainly no less serious than lung or intestinal abscess, how is it that Zhang Zhong-Jing never addressed it in his writings?

DR. YU   It is true that liver abscess is not mentioned in the books of Zhang Zhong-Jing. In fact, liver abscess is not often mentioned in the whole of traditional literature. In the late Qing-dynasty text *Record of Surgical Cases of Ma Pei-Zhi (Mǎ Péi-Zhī wài kē yi àn)*, liver abscess is treated with Liver-Soothing Phlegm-Scouring Decoction *(shū gān dí tán tāng)*,[12] but I have never read a case report of someone successfully treating liver abscess with just this formula.

I wonder if the lack of written records regarding liver abscess in the traditional literature reflects the fact that physicians in the past rarely had success treating this condition? In fact, in contemporary case literature, there is no lack of examples of cases in which physicians failed when treating liver abscess solely using Chinese medicine. They then had no choice but to refer the patients for Western medical treatment, and, in some severe cases, for surgery.

In the case of liver abscess described above, the abscess had not become fully purulent. Even so, I did not rely solely on Chinese medicine, but proceeded with combined Chinese-Western treatment. As such, the question that I would like to ask to the Chinese medicine community is, how do we elevate the therapeutic efficacy of Chinese medical treatment of liver abscess so that there may come a day when we can rely solely on Chinese medicine to treat even severe cases of this problem? This example of treating a pattern of high fever and shivering should remind us all that in the clinic, we must be aware of non-standard presentations of liver abscess or transmutations of liver abscess patterns.

----

11. *Translators' note:* Due to its endangered status, this substance is no longer available. When we discussed this with Dr. Yu, he suggested that increasing the dose of Vaccariae Semen *(wáng bù liú xíng)* would be a reasonable substitution in this case.

12. Liver-Soothing Phlegm-Scouring Decoction *(shū gān dí tán tāng)*: Cyperi Rhizoma *(xiāng fù)*, Angelicae sinensis Radix *(dāng guī)*, Citri sarcodactylis Fructus *(fó shǒu)*, Citri reticulatae Exocarpium rubrum *(jú hóng)*, Trichosanthis Semen *(guā lóu rén)*, Curcumae Radix *(yù jīn)*, Poria *(fú líng)*, Perillae Caulis *(zǐ sū gěng)*, bran-fried Aurantii Fructus *(fū chǎo zhǐ ké)*, Notoginseng Radix *(sān qī)*, Pinelliae Rhizoma praeparatum *(zhì bàn xià)*, Bambusae Caulis in taeniam *(zhú rú)*.

4.3 **Headaches**

Distending orbital and periorbital pain for two months

Finding the simplicity in a complex situation to realize an easy solution

大有執簡馭繁，駕輕就熟之妙

■ CASE HISTORY

Patient: *16-year-old man*

Six months ago, the patient began to experience dizziness and headaches. Two months ago, the headaches became more severe following a cold and fever (39°C/102.2°F). The headaches were accompanied by lethargy, vomiting, dilated pupils, lack of visual clarity, swollen and painful throat, and difficulty swallowing, so he was admitted to the hospital for emergency treatment.

The Western medical diagnosis was viral meningitis and there was a question of intracranial pathology, but this was ruled out by CT scan in two different Western medical facilities. The patient stayed in the hospital for two weeks and during that time was sent to the ICU twice. He was treated effectively for the critical symptoms, but his headaches persisted. At that point, he left the hospital and began taking Chinese herbs.

The patient's primary symptom was distending pain in the orbit, supraorbital ridge, and temple. The pain was occurring three times in a 24-hour period and lasting for about two hours each time. The headache was frequently accompanied by throat pain and vomiting of watery mucus.

He first took Rambling Powder *(xiāo yáo sǎn)* plus Honeysuckle and Forsythia Powder *(yín qiáo sǎn)* modified, but after 17 packets with no effect, the prescription was changed to a combination of Xanthium Powder *(cāng ěr zǐ sǎn)*, Cimicifuga and Kudzu Decoction *(shēng má gé gēn tāng)*, Minor Bupleurum Decoction *(xiǎo chái hú tāng)*, and Evodia Decoction *(wú zhū yú tāng)* modified. (The combined formula contained more than 19 ingredients, including Evodiae Fructus *(wú zhū yú)* and Zingiberis Rhizoma recens *(shēng jiāng)*, each at 3g, as well as Codonopsis Radix *(dǎng shēn)* and Jujubae Fructus *(dà zǎo)*, each at 10g.) There was no observable improvement after 20 packets.

INTAKE EXAMINATION
DATE: January 2, 1988

The symptoms were as described above. In addition, he had recently begun to experience irritability, dry mouth, unquenchable thirst, poor appetite, and stools that tended to be loose. His tongue was red and there were densely clustered red spots on the tip and sides. The coating was white, slightly yellow, thick, and greasy. His pulse was wiry, slippery, and slightly rapid.

Differentiation of Patterns and Discussion of Treatment

DR. YU　　Line 378 of the *Discussion of Cold Damage (Shāng hán lùn)* states, "For dry retching, vomiting of frothy mucus, Evodia Decoction *(wú zhū yú tāng)* governs."

Because this line is found in the *jué yīn* section, the location of the headache is at the vertex (the *jué yīn* Liver channel and the Governing vessel intersect at the vertex). Also, inferring the pattern from the formula, this clearly pertains to cold. According to the principle that "all interior [conditions] must manifest on the outside," there should be a group of generalized symptoms, including the tongue and the pulse, that indicate cold. According to clinical experience, this is indeed a general rule.

However, it is worth pointing out that this general principle cannot cover all situations. In recent years, I have used Evodia Decoction *(wú zhū yú tāng)* to treat quite a few headache patients with accompanying symptoms of nausea and vomiting of clear fluids or frothy mucus. Not all of them had symptoms of deficiency cold in the Liver and Stomach with ascending counterflow of turbid yin, or a tongue and pulse that would match that diagnosis. In fact, some of them had heat signs. Also, the location of the headache was not always the vertex.

Adhering rigidly to the standard patterns will significantly restrict your usage of the formula and you will never be confident to use Evodia Decoction *(wú zhū yú tāng)* by itself in a flexible way or in a large dosage. This reminds us that we must not allow our clinical reasoning to become set in fixed patterns.

After repeatedly reviewing this pattern, it seemed to me that the headache and vomiting in this case were objective indicators of the Evodia Decoction *(wú zhū yú tāng)* presentation. It is a shame that the previous physician did not trust this formula enough and therefore added a huge number of additional ingredients, thereby reducing the efficacy of the treatment due to his own lack of confidence. Perhaps it would be worthwhile to simply let the full force of the formula come through in order to address this illness.

However, after examining the patient, I determined that a significant number of heat signs were present and so I had to consider how best to use this formula. If I decided not to use it, then what formula should I use? This forced me to ask the patient more questions, and I thus discovered that he had, over the last few years, begun the habit of swimming in the river every day from March through October. Furthermore, he frequently ate fruit and iced foods. Finally, he reported that because his schoolwork was very demanding, he frequently consumed very concentrated tea in order to stay awake.

Treatment and Outcome

At that point, my mind was made up and I went ahead with Evodia Decoction *(wú zhū yú tāng)*:

```
Evodiae Fructus (wú zhū yú) ............................................. 15g
Zingiberis Rhizoma recens (shēng jiāng) ............................. 15g
Codonopsis Radix (dǎng shēn) ......................................... 30g
Jujubae Fructus (dà zǎo) ................................................. 30g
```

I told him that he should first try two packets, and that even if the dry mouth and sore throat got worse, he should nonetheless finish both packets of herbs.

SECOND VISIT (1/4): (Dr. Jiang Er-Xun saw the patient for this visit, because Dr. Yu was out of town.) After taking the first packet, the orbital and periorbital pain decreased substantially, as did the sore throat, and the patient's vomiting had ceased. His dry mouth and irritability had also decreased. After finishing the second packet, the pain was essentially gone. The only remaining symptoms were mild abdominal fullness along with a slight stifling sensation.

Three more packets of the original formula were prescribed, with the dosage of both Codonopsis Radix *(dǎng shēn)* and Jujubae Fructus *(dà zǎo)* reduced to 15g, and with the addition of ginger Magnoliae officinalis Cortex *(jiāng hòu pò)* 15g and standard Pinelliae Rhizoma praeparatum *(fǎ bàn xià)* 10g.

THIRD VISIT (1/8): The pain was completely gone, the patient's appetite had returned, his abdomen felt comfortable, and his bowel movements had returned to normal. His tongue body was basically unchanged with a thin, white, faintly-yellow coating. His pulse was no longer rapid, but was still wiry and slightly slippery. At that point, we prescribed Six-Gentlemen Decoction *(liù jūn zǐ tāng)* plus Cinnamomi Ramulus *(guì zhī)* (which is similar to Poria, Cinnamon Twig, Atractylodes, and Licorice Decoction *[líng guì zhú gān tāng]*) and advised him to take this for a while to secure the treatment effect. On his three-year follow-up he had had no recurrences.

Disease	Primary Symptoms	Differentiation	Treatment Method	Formula
Headache	Vomiting of frothy mucus and headache	Cold congealed in the Liver and Stomach, upward counterflow of turbid yin	Warm the Liver and the Stomach, raise the clear, direct the turbid downward	Evodia Decoction *(wú zhū yú tāng)*

Reflections and Clarifications

PHYSICIAN A   I agree that it is correct to avoid inflexible thinking, but I still would have worried about all the heat signs that were present in this case. Is it really possible that Evodia Decoction *(wú zhū yú tāng)* can be used for headaches in a heat pattern? This patient clearly displayed many heat signs such as dry mouth, unquenchable thirst, a red tongue with red spots on the tip and sides, a white, slightly-yellow tongue coating that was also thick and greasy, and a wiry, slippery, slightly rapid pulse. Why is it that you still used Evodia Decoction *(wú zhū yú tāng)*, which is very acrid and hot?

PHYSICIAN B   I have the same impression! There have been many articles written about the use of Evodia Decoction *(wú zhū yú tāng)* for headaches. The pathodynamic in these headache cases is Liver-Stomach deficiency cold with counterflow of turbid yin. Evodia Decoction *(wú zhū yú tāng)* warms the Liver and Stomach, directs the clear upward, and turbidity downward. Since it directly addresses the pathodynamic, the clinical effects are excellent. However, as my colleague already stated, this patient did not clearly show signs of this pathodynamic, such as cold limbs, aversion to cold in the abdomen and stomach, cold-type abdominal pain, a pale tongue with a white slippery coating, and a wiry, sunken pulse or a wiry, slow pulse. In fact, this patient displayed just the opposite: a number of distinct heat signs. Still, quite unexpectedly to me, you chose to use an unmodified Evodia Decoction *(wú zhū yú tāng)* and the dosages were large. Your decision is hard to understand.

DR. YU   If I had not had my own misgivings about this group of heat signs, I would not have persisted in asking the patient about his lifestyle and history. For the last few years, between March and October, this patient had consistently gone swimming in the river, had frequently eaten fruit and iced food, and had consumed concentrated tea. This lifestyle history was very enlightening to me.

   If we consider the lifestyle history and the efficacy of the formula, we can infer that congealed and knotted cold had been retained in his abdomen for a long period of time. This hindered the smooth movement of yang qi. Over time this led to constraint, which in turn produced heat. Another possibility is that the haze of cold qi forced the yang qi upward, producing symptoms that give the appearance of flushing ascent of heat.

   This case highlights the keys to properly utilizing Evodia Decoction *(wú zhū yú tāng)*. The first is to fully grasp the characteristic signs and symptoms of this pattern: headache accompanied by vomiting of watery mucus. The second key is the need to incorporate the patient's lifestyle and treatment history into your analysis. In this way, you can see through the façade of floating heat signs to discern the patient's underlying yin-cold nature.

PHYSICIAN A   It seems that you are using a formula-pattern correspondence. My understanding of this formula-pattern correspondence is that if one sees dry retching, vomiting of watery mucus, and headache, one can then freely use Evodia Decoction *(wú zhū yú tāng)*. You do not need to fuss over whether or not all the signs and symptoms correspond to a pattern of Liver-Stomach deficiency cold with counterflow of turbid yin. Furthermore, one need not consider if the pattern is exterior or interior, channel or organ, recent or chronic, or any of these factors. Is that correct?

DR. YU   That is correct. You see, Zhang Zhong-Jing, by describing the unique symptoms of "dry retching, vomiting of watery mucus, and headache," has already amply captured the unique nature of this disorder.

   The 12th-century writer Cheng Wu-Ji, in *Annotation and Explanation of the Discussion of Cold Damage (Zhù Jiě Shāng Hán Lùn)*, explains that "Dry retching and vomiting of watery mucus results from interior cold; headache results from cold qi attacking upward. Give Evodia Decoction *(wú zhū yú tāng)* to warm the interior and to disperse cold." To put it another way, Zhang Zhong-Jing's pattern analysis was quite precise and he provided an extremely effective remedy. In the clinic, as long as the symptoms correspond, you can use the formula freely. The rapid clinical effect seen in this case is an illustration of the principle of "finding the simplicity in a complex situation to realize an easy solution."

   It is also worth rethinking a trend of the last few years, which is to stress the flexibility of differentiating patterns to determine treatment (which I agree is important) and to ignore the basic principle of formula-pattern correspondence. This trend is detrimental

PHYSICIAN B   So in this case, the patient had contracted viral meningitis and was treated with Western medicine. When the critical phase had passed, he was left with pain in and around the eyes. He was originally treated with 17 packets of a combined Rambling Powder *(xiāo yáo sǎn)* and Honeysuckle and Forsythia Powder *(yín qiáo sǎn)*, which was ineffective. Then he was given 20 packets of a combination of Xanthium Powder *(cāng ěr zǐ sǎn)*, Cimicifuga and Kudzu Decoction *(shēng má gé gēn tāng)*, Minor Bupleurum Decoction *(xiǎo chái hú tāng)*, and Evodia Decoction *(wú zhū yú tāng)*, also without effect. This process lasted two months. You gave him a large dosage of Evodia Decoction *(wú zhū yú tāng)* and achieved very quick results. This really opened my eyes! However, it has also left me with a question. The patient had previously taken a large combined formula that included Evodia Decoction *(wú zhū yú tāng)* but the clinical results were disappointing. Why was that the case?

DR. YU   That formula combined Xanthium Powder *(cāng ěr zǐ sǎn)*, Cimicifuga and Kudzu Decoction *(shēng má gé gēn tāng)*, Minor Bupleurum Decoction *(xiǎo chái hú tāng)*, and Evodia Decoction *(wú zhū yú tāng)* and had a total of 19 herbs. Furthermore, the dosages were small. It is possible that there was a conflict within the formula that prevented better results.

As everyone knows, Zhang Zhong-Jing wrote in his preface to the *Discussion of Cold Damage (Shāng hán lùn)* that he "diligently sought the guidance of the ancients and widely gathered various remedies." Through clinical application, he sifted through these formulas, testing and verifying their efficacy, and passed down to us a group of highly effective formulas based on his experiences. For example, Evodia Decoction *(wú zhū yú tāng)* only contains four herbs and seems very unremarkable. In reality, its usage is full of possibilities. If you decide to make your own additions because you suspect that the formula has too few herbs to be effective, or you are afraid that the patient will be skeptical of the effects of a small formula, you will often negatively affect the outcome. If, through observing formula-pattern correspondence and using the original formula you can achieve outstanding clinical results, why is there any need to add superfluous ingredients? Is this not like adding legs to a drawing of a snake?

Of course, sometimes there is a need to make some modifications according to the patient's clinical presentation. Nonetheless, if you add too many ingredients, they may eclipse the original formula or make the original formula unrecognizable. Further, if you make so many changes that the original formula is unrecognizable, yet still say, "this is a modified classical formula," well, you cannot be taken seriously. We would all do well to think deeply about the words of the early 20th-century master, Chen Xun-Zhai: "Classical formulas are most valuable when unmodified."

PHYSICIAN D   When you use Evodia Decoction *(wú zhū yú tāng)* to treat headaches, what is the standard dosage of the ingredients?

DR. YU   I generally start with Evodiae Fructus *(wú zhū yú)* and Zingiberis Rhizoma recens *(shēng jiāng)* at no less than 15g, and Codonopsis Radix *(dǎng shēn)* and Jujubae Fructus *(dà zǎo)* at no less than 30g. After the clinical effects are clear, one can consider reducing the dosage.

4.4 **Dizziness**

Dizziness for 17 years

Chinese medicine need not be slow-acting

中醫不是"慢郎中"

■ CASE HISTORY

Patient: *Ms. Xu, 28-year-old woman, cadre*

When she was 8-years old, after accidentally falling into water, the patient became both frightened and cold. This shock and exposure to cold led her to be bedridden for more than a month, and after that her general condition gradually deteriorated. At age 11, she started to experience dizziness. The attacks were marked by lightheadedness, vertigo, tinnitus, and nausea. These episodes occurred 5–6 times per year.

When she was 20, Ms. Xu was treated by an itinerant physician and was prescribed the lead-containing mineral, processed galenite (鉛粉 *qiān fěn*), to treat her dizziness. She took 6g each day for three days. As a result, she developed lead poisoning. She was treated for four months at the West China Hospital of Sichuan Medical University, and at the end of that time, the patient's main lead-poisoning symptoms had disappeared, but her dizziness was significantly worse. She frequently experienced lightheadedness and vertigo, and when it was severe she felt like the earth and sky were both spinning, which left her reluctant to open her eyes. She also suffered from distending pain in her eyeballs, as well as visual disturbances, tinnitus, blocked ears, trembling of the arms and legs, dry heaves, and irritability.

She was diagnosed with inner-ear dizziness, and over the last eight years has been treated in many different hospitals, with both Western medicine and Chinese medicine. She has taken substances that calm the Liver and subdue yang, extinguish wind and relieve spasms, nourish the Liver and Kidneys, fortify the Spleen and transform phlegm. Treatment also included bug substances to search and to dig out stagnation in the channels and collaterals. After taking hundreds of packets, there was no significant improvement, and she was unable to consistently attend work.

INTAKE EXAMINATION
DATE: February 17, 1986

The symptoms were as described above. Her tongue was red with a thin, white coating. Her pulse was sunken and fine.

Differentiation of Patterns and Discussion of Treatment

PHYSICIAN A   In general, patients experiencing dizziness respond quickly to Western medicine and many cases resolve spontaneously.

DR. YU   It is true that some cases resolve spontaneously, but actually this is uncommon. In cases of severe, acute dizziness, commonly-used Western drugs such as sedatives, antiemetics, and anticholinergic drugs are often ineffective. Frequently, these patients are referred to the Chinese medicine department.

PHYSICIAN B   But isn't it true that we cannot draw an equivalence between dizziness in Western medicine and Chinese medicine?

DR. YU   What do we mean by dizziness? The term is made up of two characters: 眩暈 *xuàn yùn*. The first refers to visual disturbances and blurred vision, the second to a spinning sensation in the head. Nonetheless, when you carefully investigate both classical texts and modern textbooks, you find that the broad category labeled 'dizziness' includes not only lightheadedness, but also symptoms such as a heavy feeling in the head with instability of the legs and no spinning sensation.

In Western medicine, one can make a clear differentiation between 'true vertigo', also known as 'true dizziness', and other types of dizziness. True vertigo, which is also referred to as rotational vertigo, is the result of vestibular nerve disease or labyrinthine disease. True vertigo is characterized by such symptoms as dizziness with a feeling that the person himself is spinning or that the room is spinning, nausea, vomiting, tinnitus, hearing loss, nystagmus, headache, and ataxia.

Dr. Jiang thought that, in order to insure correct pattern identification, simple light-headedness or symptoms such as a feeling that the head is heavy and the legs light without a spinning sensation should not be included under the rubric of 眩暈 *xuàn yùn* or dizziness. Dr. Jiang strongly believed in using knowledge from Western medicine in the service of Chinese medicine. He frequently said that "stones from other mountains may be used to polish jade."

PHYSICIAN C   Dr. Jiang's clarification of the definition of dizziness is original and thought-provoking. How can we use the theories of Chinese medicine to correctly identify and distinguish true vertigo?

DR. YU   First, we should explore historical literature that discusses dizziness and carefully analyze what we find. While we can delight in the joys of the literature, we must avoid simply reading whatever comes to hand and accepting what we read without critical thought.

For example, it is written that "there is no dizziness without wind," "there is no diz-ziness without fire," "there is no dizziness without phlegm," and "there is no dizziness without deficiency." While there is truth in each of these statements, each is incomplete. Further, because these statements relate to the broad category of dizziness, were we to use these ideas to explain the etiology and pathodynamic of the narrower category of true vertigo, it would necessarily be overly general and abstract.

Dr. Jiang believed that we should pay special attention to the writings of Zhang Zhong-Jing who primarily approached dizziness from the perspective of *sháo yáng* ministerial fire flaring upward and upward counterflow of phlegm and thin-mucus. Zhang Zhong-Jing used formulas such as Minor Bupleurum Decoction *(xiǎo chái hú tāng)*, Poria, Cinnamon Twig, Atractylodes, and Licorice Decoction *(líng guì zhú gān tāng)*, Alismatis Decoction *(zé xiè tāng)*, and Minor Pinellia plus Poria Decoction *(xiǎo bàn xià jiā fú líng tāng)*. These seem to match up well with the special symptoms of true vertigo.

From this idea of *sháo yáng* ministerial fire flaring upward and upward counterflow of phlegm and thin-mucus, we can determine the overarching etiology and pathodynamic of true vertigo: wind, fire, phlegm, and deficiency.

On the basis of Dr. Jiang's teaching, I diagnosed this patient as having Spleen and Kidney deficiency with ascendant disturbance by wind, fire, and phlegm.

Treatment and Outcome

We dispensed a modified formula that was devised by my teacher, Jiang Er-Xun: Bupleurum, Dried Tangerine Peel, and Alismatis Decoction *(chái chén zé xiè tāng)*:[13]

Bupleuri Radix *(chái hú)*	10g
Scutellariae Radix *(huáng qín)*	6g
standard Pinelliae Rhizoma praeparatum *(fǎ bàn xià)*	10g
Codonopsis Radix *(dǎng shēn)*	15g
Poria *(fú líng)*	12g
Citri reticulatae Pericarpium *(chén pí)*	10g
Glycyrrhizae Radix *(gān cǎo)*	3g
Atractylodis macrocephalae Rhizoma *(bái zhú)*	10g
Alismatis Rhizoma *(zé xiè)*	30g
Uncariae Ramulus cum Uncis *(gōu téng)* [add 10–15 minutes from end]	12g
Chrysanthemi Flos *(jú huā)*	10g
Gastrodiae Rhizoma *(tiān má)* [grind to a fine powder and mix into strained decoction]	10g
Zingiberis Rhizoma recens *(shēng jiāng)*	10g
Paeoniae Radix alba *(bái sháo)*	12g
Ostreae Concha *(mǔ lì)*	30g

RESULTS: After three packets the patient's dizziness was significantly reduced, as was her distending eyeball pain, dry heaves, and irritability. After 25 packets, all symptoms had resolved.

I followed up with the patient two years later and she reported that occasionally, when she encountered emotional problems, she would sometimes have a sensation of lightheadedness or mild dizziness. These episodes were quickly addressed with 2–3 packets of the original formula.

Disease	Main Symptoms	Pattern Identification	Treatment Method	Formula
Dizziness	Lightheadedness, vertigo, tinnitus, nausea, and vomiting	Upward flaring of ministerial fire, counterflow ascent of phlegm and thin-mucus, and Spleen and Kidney deficiency	Dispel wind, clear fire, dislodge phlegm, tonify the Spleen	Bupleurum, Dried Tangerine Peel, and Alismatis Decoction *(chái chén zé xiè tāng)*

....

13. *Translators' note:* This formula is a modified combination of Minor Bupleurum Decoction *(xiǎo chái hú tāng)*, Two-Aged [Herb] Decoction *(èr chén tāng)*, Six-Gentlemen Decoction *(liù jūn zǐ tāng)*, and Alismatis Decoction *(zé xiè tāng)*.

Reflections and Clarifications

PHYSICIAN C   There is something that I don't completely understand. Is there really any difference between "*sháo yáng* ministerial fire flaring upward and upward counterflow of phlegm and thin-mucus" and "there is no dizziness without phlegm"?

DR. YU   From the idea of "*sháo yáng* ministerial fire flaring upward and upward counterflow of phlegm and thin-mucus" we can derive the entire etiology and pathodynamic of true vertigo: wind, fire, phlegm, and deficiency. That in no way equates with the extremely narrow idea of "there is no dizziness without phlegm."

PHYSICIAN B   You said that "*sháo yáng* ministerial fire flaring upward and upward counterflow of phlegm and thin-mucus" describes the entire etiology and pathodynamic of true vertigo: wind, fire, phlegm, and deficiency. I have never heard this idea before. Where does it come from?

DR. YU   *Shào yáng* ministerial fire and *jué yīn* wind-wood have an exterior-interior relationship. The presence of wind increases the momentum of fire. The presence of fire increases the danger of wind. This epitomizes mutual causality. Upward counterflow of phlegm and thin-mucus generally has Spleen and Kidney deficiency at its root. Would you agree that this explains the derivation of the concept of wind, fire, phlegm, and deficiency?

Of the people who have pondered this issue over the ages, I hold in high esteem the early 19th-century physician Chen Xiu-Yuan (also known as Chen Nian-Zu).

- While in his discussion of dizziness, he considers wind as the primary factor, he explains it together with the presence of fire, phlegm, and deficiency. His work reveals some subtle ideas and contains critical information. He states in his *Collection of Medical Writings Following the Work of Others (Yī xué cóng zhòng lù)*, "This type of wind does not come from the exterior, but is from *jué yīn* wind-wood." When wood is exuberant, it generates wind.

- Furthermore, because *jué yīn* wind-wood "shares a common location with *sháo yáng* ministerial fire, qi counterflow of *jué yīn* creates wind, which then gives rise to fire."

- When discussing deficiency, he writes that, "The creation of wind influences the dynamic of wood, such that wood overcomes earth." Further, "The Kidneys are the mother of the Liver and they govern the storage of essence. When essence is deficient, the brain becomes empty, resulting in heaviness of the head." This is the child pilfering the mother's qi.

- Speaking of phlegm, he states that "When earth is diseased, pooling thin-mucus becomes phlegm."

To summarize, wind, fire, and phlegm are the branches of dizziness, while Spleen and Kidney deficiency is its root. Chen Xiu-Yuan ends by saying, "When one speaks of deficiency, one is speaking of the root cause of the disease; when one speaks of excess, one is talking of the manifestations of the disease. Together they form the core for best practice."

Dr. Jiang felt that these ideas of Chen Xiu-Yuan were incredibly perceptive and that the application of them to understanding the cause of true vertigo was quite accurate. He emphasized, though, that the onset of vertigo was not the product of wind, fire, phlegm, and deficiency as individual factors, but when they combined as a group.

For this reason, he did not agree with Zhang Jing-Yue's statement that "For patients with dizziness, deficiency accounts for 80–90%, while fire and phlegm are only implicated in 10–20%." In the clinic, patients with dizziness generally present with a whole set of symptoms indicating upward disturbance by wind, fire, and phlegm. How is it possible that we can use deficiency alone to explain this?

PHYSICIAN C   But Dr. Jiang did not deny the importance of deficiency, correct?

DR. YU   Of course he did not deny its importance. Without deficiency, it becomes very difficult to satisfactorily explain the genesis of upward disturbance by wind, fire, and phlegm. As I said, Chen Xiu-Yun considered deficiency to be the root of dizziness. We can consider deficiency as either a latent or constitutional disease cause.

No matter how we understand it, we should remember that vertigo comes about from a combination of wind, fire, phlegm, and deficiency. Fundamentally, it is a pattern of root deficiency with branch excess. And we must treat it by simultaneously addressing both root and branch.

PHYSICIAN C   There is one thing that confounds me about this case. If this pattern involves phlegm and thin-mucus, shouldn't we expect to see evidence of this in the pulse and on the tongue? I would expect to see a greasy tongue coating and a wiry or slippery pulse, but in this case, the tongue is red with a thin, white coating and the pulse is sunken and fine.

DR. YU   In the clinic there are no fixed tongue and pulse signs associated with true vertigo caused by *sháo yáng* ministerial fire rising and counterflow of phlegm and thin-mucus. Although it is true that a greasy tongue coating is common in phlegm and thin-mucus patterns, the absence of a greasy coating or even a complete absence of tongue coating does not mean that phlegm and thin-mucus are also absent.

Many of the patients that Dr. Jiang treated for dizziness had tongues that were pale-red with a thin white coating or no coating at all. Tonifying qi and blood or enriching yin and settling yang in these patients was ineffective. Switching to a strategy of scouring phlegm, driving out thin-mucus, dispelling wind, and clearing fire produced effective results. That the pulse is also not fixed goes without saying. Further study of the mechanisms involved in this pattern is certainly worthwhile and may reveal additional information.

PHYSICIAN C   You mentioned simultaneous root and branch treatment. I have to say that when considering opinions from both ancient and modern physicians about exactly what this means, the opinions are distinct, varied, and often conflicting. It has left me feeling unsure of what to do. Could you comment on this a bit?

DR. YU   Well, that is a long story! Chen Xiu-Yuan offered the critique that "He Jian [an honorific name for the 12th-century writer Liu Wan-Su] and his followers would clear fire, dispel wind, and flush phlegm in their treatments, but they did not understand the etiology of these things." He also said, "I have taken a look at the works of Zhang Jing-Yue and his idea about primarily tonifying deficiency in these cases. His method does not work. Having sought the answers in the works of antiquity, it seems that Zhang Jing-Yue's notion of deficiency and excess is static and inflexible and he lacks a thorough understanding of the workings of wind and fire."

However, it should be noted that when treating dizziness, Chen Xiu-Yuan did not always employ simultaneous root and branch treatment, and the same could be said of Zhu Dan-Xi. Sometimes they would use a single-herb formula, Rhei Radix et Rhizoma *(dà huáng),* in order to drain fire. Sometimes they would use Restore the Left [Kidney] Drink *(zuǒ guī yǐn),* modified with the addition of Cervi Cornu pantotrichum *(lù róng)* wine, Six-Ingredient Pill with Rehmannia *(liù wèi dì huáng wán),* or Kidney Qi Pill *(shèn qì wán),* in order to tonify the Kidneys. And sometimes they would use Tonify the Middle to Augment the Qi Decoction *(bǔ zhōng yì qì tāng)* in order to tonify the Spleen.

The famous and influential early Qing-dynasty physicians Cheng Guo-Peng and Ye Tian-Shi proposed the use of simultaneous root and branch treatments, such as strengthening the Spleen and augmenting the qi in combination with transforming phlegm and directing counterflow downward; or enriching the Liver and Kidneys in combination with calming the Liver and anchoring yang. While these seem like well-considered and excellent treatment methods, I would say that these approaches may be insufficient to the task of effectively reducing the symptoms during an acute episode of vertigo.

In modern discussions of the treatment of dizziness, there has been a tendency to emphasize the branch treatment. For example, using Inula and Haematite Decoction *(xuán fù dài zhě tāng)* for upward counterflow of Liver qi caused by phlegm congestion. Another example is the use of Alismatis Decoction *(zé xiè tāng)* to treat prodding thin-mucus. Also, some people propose the strategy of using Warm Gallbladder Decoction *(wēn dǎn tāng)* for the acute phase of the illness and Two-Aged [Herb] Decoction plus Ginseng and Astragalus *(shēn qí èr chén tāng)* once the illness has abated. These different strategies each demonstrate something worthwhile and should be considered.

PHYSICIAN C   Which method did Dr. Jiang choose to follow?

DR. YU   Dr. Jiang's methodology differs somewhat from the previously described methods. In the acute phase, he emphasized simultaneous root and branch treatment, focusing on dispelling wind, clearing fire, dislodging phlegm, and tonifying the Spleen. After the dizziness has abated, he would then slowly treat the root.

PHYSICIAN A   In the previous discussion about the root deficiency of this disorder you mentioned both the Spleen and the Kidneys. However, in the root-branch treatment that you suggested, there is only treatment of the Spleen, not the Kidneys. Why is that?

DR. YU   In Dr. Jiang's opinion, during the acute phase of dizziness, the ascendant counterflow of phlegm and thin-mucus is a very important aspect of the pathology. Medicinal substances that tonify the Kidneys would not only be relatively slow acting in this situation, but they would also tend to impede progress due to their cloying nature, thereby making it difficult to achieve a quick resolution of the branch symptoms. Thus, it is best to wait for the dizziness to abate before tonifying the Kidneys.

Dr. Jiang has told me about using a variety of formulas such as Six-Ingredient Pill with Rehmannia *(liù wèi dì huáng wán)*, Eight-Ingredient Pill with Rehmannia *(bā wèi dì huáng wán)*, Restore the Left [Kidney] Drink *(zuǒ guī yǐn)*, and Restore the Right [Kidney] Pill *(yòu guī wán)* in his efforts to resolve dizziness. However, the effects were minimal or even completely absent. The problem was not with the formulas, but with the timing of their usage.

Thus, Dr. Jiang places the emphasis on the Spleen when treating the root in these cases. This must be done with some skill so as to emphasize improving the Spleen's transportive function and harmonizing the Stomach. By improving the Spleen's transportive function, one can transform phlegm, and by harmonizing the Stomach, one can arrest retching. When the Spleen effectively transports, it is better able to ward off encroachment by the Liver. As a result, the wanton movement of wind-wood is reduced. As wind-wood is calmed, ministerial fire becomes tranquil. Once this has occurred, the branch manifestations of wind, fire, and phlegm quickly dissipate. This method illustrates the principle of directly treating the root so as to indirectly treat the branch.

PHYSICIAN A   In this case, the patient not only experienceed dizziness for 17 years, but also had lead poisoning. Further, her constitution was rather weak. Given that she had undergone Western and Chinese medical treatment without any improvement, this seems to qualify as 'stubborn' dizziness. Although your treatment was not extremely rapid—it took 25 packets before she was cured—the treatment and the formula were consistent from start to finish. This outcome seems to me relatively good.

I understand that Dr. Jiang's formula, Bupleurum, Dried Tangerine Peel, and Alismatis Decoction *(chái chén zé xiè tāng)*, has been used on hundreds of patients and generally has an excellent clinical effect, often resolving the dizziness within two to four packets. It seems that this method should be more widely known.

I would like to know the basic ingredients of the formula, the typical dosage range, the formula dynamics, and the typical usage.

DR. YU   Bupleurum, Dried Tangerine Peel, and Alismatis Decoction *(chái chén zé xiè tāng)* is composed of Minor Bupleurum Decoction *(xiǎo chái hú tāng)*, Two-Aged [Herb] Decoction *(èr chén tāng)*, Six-Gentlemen Decoction *(liù jūn zǐ tāng)*, and Alismatis Decoction *(zé xiè tāng)*. To this base, we add Gastrodiae Rhizoma *(tiān má)*, Uncariae Ramulus cum Uncis *(gōu téng)*, and Chrysanthemi Flos *(jú huā)*. The typical prescription would be:

Bupleuri Radix *(chái hú)*	10g
Scutellariae Radix *(huáng qín)*	6-10g
standard Pinelliae Rhizoma praeparatum *(fǎ bàn xià)*	10g
Codonopsis Radix *(dǎng shēn)*	12-15g
Glycyrrhizae Radix *(gān cǎo)*	3-5g
Jujubae Fructus *(dà zǎo)*	10-12g
Zingiberis Rhizoma recens *(shēng jiāng)*	6-10g
Citri reticulatae Pericarpium *(chén pí)*	10g
Poria *(fú líng)*	15g
Atractylodis macrocephalae Rhizoma *(bái zhú)*	10-15g

Alismatis Rhizoma *(zé xiè)*... 10-15g
Gastrodiae Rhizoma *(tiān má)*
      [powdered and mixed into hot decoction]............................... 10g
Uncariae Ramulus cum Uncis *(gōu téng)*
      [added 10-15 minutes before end] 12g
Chrysanthemi Flos *(jú huā)* 10g

Minor Bupleurum Decoction *(xiǎo chái hú tāng)* acts on the *sháo yáng* pivot dynamic to vent constrained fire, raise the clear, and direct the turbid downward. Two-Aged [Herb] Decoction *(èr chén tāng)* transforms phlegm and resolves counterflow. Alismatis Decoction *(zé xiè tāng)* flushes away thin-mucus and promotes water metabolism.

Minor Pinellia plus Poria Decoction *(xiǎo bàn xià jiā fú líng tāng)* is also part of this formula. The formula resolves counterflow, transforms phlegm, flushes away thin-mucus, and arrests retching. Dr. Jiang's formula also contains Six-Gentlemen Decoction *(liù jūn zǐ tāng)*, which treats the root by improving the transportive function of the Spleen and by harmonizing the Stomach. Gastrodiae Rhizoma *(tiān má)*, Uncariae Ramulus cum Uncis *(gōu téng)*, and Chrysanthemi Flos *(jú huā)* are included to soften and moisten in order to extinguish Liver wind.

According to the principle of "treating different diseases with the same treatment," we can expand the range of suitable conditions for which the formula is prescribed. It can be used for dizziness from hypertension or from cerebral arterial insufficiency, as long as the presenting symptoms match the clinical presentation of true vertigo.

Recently, I used this formula to treat dizziness associated with disease of the cervical vertebrae. Because of the etiology of this disorder I removed Citri reticulatae Pericarpium *(chén pí)*, Chrysanthemi Flos *(jú huā)*, Poria *(fú líng)*, Glycyrrhizae Radix *(gān cǎo)*, and Uncariae Ramulus cum Uncis *(gōu téng)* and added a large dosage (30-60g) of Puerariae Radix *(gé gēn)*. This herb guides fluids to the head and neck so as to soothe the sinews and to alleviate spasms. I also added a large dosage (30-60g) of Chuanxiong Rhizoma *(chuān xiōng)* in order to invigorate blood, transform stasis, unblock the collaterals, and relieve pain. I have used this strategy with more than ten patients and achieved satisfactory results.

ADDENDUM: ONE FURTHER QUESTION

PHYSICIAN D As you discussed earlier, once the symptoms have subsided the proper procedure would be to then tonify the Kidneys. However, in this case the patient was never given a follow-up Kidney-tonifying formula and yet her symptoms did not resurface. Please explain.

DR. YU It has now been many years since we treated that patient and she has not had any relapses. Although she is no longer young, she does not look her years. I recently treated her father and he related that in the time since her treatment she has been taking good care of her body and paying special attention to various techniques that nourish health. She has had no major illnesses and has not taken tonifying herbs.

Dizziness has its root in Kidney deficiency, but this aspect of the etiology may be hidden behind the disease dynamic or the constitution. In theory, one should tonify the Kidneys, but if there are no typical Kidney-deficiency symptoms, it is difficult to select herbs. Thus, it is said that "tonifying with herbs is not as good as tonifying with food, and even that is not as good as tonification of the spirit."

A small number of patients suffering from dizziness display Kidney-deficiency symptoms. For these patients, when the dizziness ceases one can suggest dietary therapy, spiritual therapies such as meditation, and health-nourishing practices as the principal treatment methods. If desired, this can be accompanied by herbs that tonify Kidney qi (not Kidney yin or Kidney yang) such as Cuscutae Semen *(tù sī zǐ)*, Eucommiae Cortex *(dù zhòng)*, Taxilli Herba *(sāng jì shēng)*, Dipsaci Radix *(xù duàn)*, Psoraleae Fructus *(bǔ gǔ zhī)*, Epimedii Herba *(yín yáng huò)*, Morindae officinalis Radix *(bā jǐ tiān)*, Dioscoreae Rhizoma *(shān yào)*, and Astragali complanati Semen *(shā yuàn zǐ)*.

Historically, there is an ongoing debate in Chinese medicine about whether Spleen tonification is inferior to Kidney tonification or Kidney tonification is inferior to Spleen tonification. This debate has no clinical value, as the proper treatment strategy depends on the precise circumstances. As Goethe wrote, "Grey, dear friend, is all theory, And green the golden tree of life."

For cases like this I often employ dietary therapy with the goal of tonifying the Liver, Spleen, and Kidneys simultaneously with the four black ingredients and walnuts.

Recipe: Mix together and grind into a powder equal parts walnuts, dry-fried black beans, dry-fried black rice, dry-fried black sesame seeds. Take 50-100 grams of this powder and mix it with water to make a thin paste and then bring that to a boil and simmer for 15 minutes (or cook in a microwave for three minutes). Eat this every morning. I have prescribed this treatment many times, and if the patient is consistent in taking it, the results are excellent. To achieve even better results, add one part each of Poria *(fú líng)* and Dioscoreae Rhizoma *(shān yào)* and 0.5 parts of Gigeriae galli Endothelium corneum *(jī nèi jīn)* to the above ingredients before grinding.

In summary, qi gong, taijiquan, and other health-promoting exercises, combined with dietary therapy as in the recipe I mentioned, should form the basis of post-dizziness treatment. Also, when faced with a case where dizziness has ceased and one's goal is to prevent recurrence, it is best to carefully analyze the patient's current situation and treat what is found instead of reflexively tonifying the Kidneys.

4.4.1 Dizziness

Vertigo for many years

Seeking a long-term treatment that results in two years without relapse

追求2年不復發的遠期治療

■ CASE HISTORY

Patient #1: *42-year-old woman*

The patient reported having attacks of vertigo for more than ten years. Episodes were brought on by any number of factors, such as catching a cold, exhaustion, insomnia, or a bout of anger. When the symptom occurred, she felt that everything in her visual field was spinning and she was afraid to open her eyes. The vertigo was accompanied by tinnitus, hearing loss, and nausea, which when severe, could result in retching and vomiting.

She was diagnosed by Western medicine with Ménière's syndrome. When the vertigo occurred, she would take an assortment of Western and Chinese medicines, which would generally take a week or even longer to start to control the symptoms. While she had gone as long as six months between episodes, they could recur as frequently as twice within a month, and there was no doubt that they would recur. She also experienced significant hearing loss in her right ear.

Five years ago, my teacher Dr. Jiang Er-Xun treated her and prescribed Bupleurum, Dried Tangerine Peel, and Alismatis Decoction *(chái chén zé xiè tāng)*, as described on page 122: Bupleuri Radix *(chái hú)*, Scutellariae Radix *(huáng qín)*, standard Pinelliae Rhizoma praeparatum *(fǎ bàn xià)*, Codonopsis Radix *(dǎng shēn)*, Atractylodis macro-cephalae Rhizoma *(bái zhú)*, Alismatis Rhizoma *(zé xiè)*, Poria *(fú líng)*, Citri reticulatae Pericarpium *(chén pí)*, Gastrodiae Rhizoma *(tiān má)*, Uncariae Ramulus cum Uncis *(gōu téng)*, Chrysanthemi Flos *(jú huā)*, Zingiberis Rhizoma recens *(shēng jiāng)*, and Jujubae Fructus *(dà zǎo)*.

After taking two packets, her vertigo stopped as did the rest of the symptoms. The patient was very happy with the result and she requested the formula so that she could prepare some of it to address any future recurrences. From that time on, when the vertigo recurred, she would quickly take a packet or two of this formula and the symptoms would quickly abate, without taking any Western medication. When she was asymptomatic, she followed Dr. Jiang's advice and took Six-Gentlemen Pill with Aucklandia and Amomum *(xiāng shā liù jūn zǐ wán)* and Rambling Pill *(xiāo yáo wán)*. But the vertigo still occasion-ally reappeared and the hearing in her right ear was still reduced, which worried her. She came to the clinic to ask if there was something more that could be done.

Patient #2: *47-year-old woman*

The patient had experienced vertigo off and on for 18 years. The first occurrence was three months after the delivery of her child via cesarean section. Her visual fields became dark and everything began to spin. This symptom was accompanied by nausea, vomiting, and tinnitus in the right ear with a feeling of blockage. After the first episode, she generally had recurrences about 1-3 times per year. The hearing in her right ear gradually decreased. She has been diagnosed with Ménière's syndrome.

For the last eight years, she had been seen in Dr. Jiang's clinic and each time she was given modifications of Bupleurum, Dried Tangerine Peel, and Alismatis Decoction *(chái chén zé xiè tāng)*, which would resolve the vertigo after 2-4 packets. She had also gone to another hospital clinic where the vertigo was diagnosed as being the result of unresolved blood stasis. She took more than 40 packets of Drive out Stasis from the Mansion of Blood Decoction *(xuè fǔ zhú yū tāng)* and Tonify the Yang to Restore Five-tenths Decoction *(bǔ yáng huán wǔ tāng)*, but these did nothing to control the recurrences.

INTAKE EXAMINATION

Patient #1

The patient's complexion was slightly greenish-yellow. Her sleep was poor and she has had significant hearing loss in her right ear. The tongue was pale-red with a thin white coating. The pulse was wiry and fine.

Patient #2

The patient's complexion was slightly dark. The hearing in her right ear was reduced. Her tongue was pale red. The right side of the central area of the patient's tongue was purplish. Her pulse was wiry, fine, and rough.

Differentiation of Patterns and Discussion of Treatment

DR. YU   Vertigo is seen frequently, easily recurs, and is difficult to cure completely. Physicians over the years have offered ideas, such as "there is no vertigo without wind," "there is no vertigo without fire," "there is no vertigo without phlegm," and "there is no vertigo without deficiency." All of these ideas have merit, but they are all limited.

My teacher, Jiang Er-Xun, combined these ideas in developing a treatment strategy for vertigo. He suggests that the fundamental pathodynamic of vertigo involves wind, fire, phlegm, and deficiency. His treatment strategy is to dispel wind, clear heat, dislodge phlegm, and tonify deficiency. He created a formula for this purpose, called Bupleurum, Dried Tangerine Peel, and Alismatis Decoction *(chái chén zé xiè tāng)*.

This formula is actually a combination of four formulas: Minor Bupleurum Decoction *(xiǎo chái hú tāng)*, Two-Aged [Herb] Decoction *(èr chén tāng)*, Alismatis Decoction *(zé xiè tāng)*, and Six-Gentlemen Decoction *(liù jūn zǐ tāng)*. On the basis of a wealth of clinical experience, I can tell you that this formula generally reduces the acute symptoms of vertigo within 2-4 packets. It is fast-acting and effective.

Even though this formula is very effective, there are some cases that are particularly recalcitrant and in which long-term efficacy is elusive. What qualifies as long-term efficacy? I would say that at the least, the patient should be without a recurrence for two years.

In recent years, I have treated a few of these recalcitrant cases. I have created a modification of Bupleurum, Dried Tangerine Peel, and Alismatis Decoction *(chái chén zé xiè tāng)* that includes herbs to invigorate blood and dispel stasis. I now have a few cases in which patients have not had a recurrence in more than two years.

Treatment and Outcome

CASE #1

In this case, because the patient's symptoms responded quickly to Bupleurum, Dried Tangerine Peel, and Alismatis Decoction *(chái chén zé xiè tāng)*, there seemed to be no need to change the basic formula. I added some substances to invigorate blood and dispel stasis. I also changed the formula from a decoction to a powder, so that it would be milder and appropriate for long-term use.

Bupleuri Radix (chái hú).. 100g
Scutellariae Radix (huáng qín)... 100g
standard Pinelliae Rhizoma praeparatum (fǎ bàn xià) 150g
Pseudostellariae Radix (tài zǐ shēn) 150g
Atractylodis macrocephalae Rhizoma (bái zhú)......................... 100g
Alismatis Rhizoma (zé xiè)... 200g
Poria (fú líng)... 150g
Citri reticulatae Pericarpium (chén pí) 100g
Puerariae Radix (gé gēn) 500g
vinegar-fried Cyperi Rhizoma (cù chǎo xiāng fù)...................... 100g
Moutan Cortex (mǔ dān pí)... 100g
Gastrodiae Rhizoma (tiān má).. 100g
Uncariae Ramulus cum Uncis (gōu téng) 100g
Acori tatarinowii Rhizoma (shí chāng pǔ)............................... 100g
Chrysanthemi Flos (jú huā) 100g
Notoginseng Radix (sān qī)... 100g

Instructions: All of the ingredients except Notoginseng Radix (*sān qī*) were cooked until brittle. Then the Notoginseng Radix (*sān qī*) was mixed in and the entire formula was ground to a fine powder. The patient was instructed to mix 10g in water and add enough sugar to make it palatable. One dose was to be taken three times each day with meals.

After two months, the patient reported that she was sleeping peacefully and that her head was quite clear.

I gave her another round of the same formula, with the dosage of Notoginseng Radix (*sān qī*) increased to 200g. Afterward, she reported positive changes in her hearing. Over a two-year period, although she had caught a cold about four times, and had periods of fatigue, anger, and insomnia, there had been no recurrence of the vertigo.

CASE #2

Given the pulse, tongue, and complexion, it was clear that blood stasis was present in this case. Furthermore, over ten years' time, phlegm and stasis had entered the collaterals and the root of the disease was deeply set. Plant substances were insufficient for this type of case, so I turned to a creature-based substance in order to attack and to drive out the stasis from every corner.

Bupleurum, Dried Tangerine Peel, and Alismatis Decoction
(*chái chén zé xiè tāng*), modified

Bupleuri Radix (chái hú).. 100g
Scutellariae Radix (huáng qín)... 100g
standard Pinelliae Rhizoma praeparatum (fǎ bàn xià) 100g
Pseudostellariae Radix (tài zǐ shēn) 150g
Atractylodis macrocephalae Rhizoma (bái zhú)......................... 100g
Alismatis Rhizoma (zé xiè)... 200g
Citri reticulatae Pericarpium (chén pí) 150g
Puerariae Radix (gé gēn) 500g
Acori tatarinowii Rhizoma (shí chāng pǔ)............................... 200g
Notoginseng Radix (sān qī)... 200g
Hirudo (shuǐ zhì)... 100g

Instructions: All of the ingredients, except Notoginseng Radix *(sān qī)* and Hirudo *(shuǐ zhì)*, were cooked until brittle. Then the Notoginseng Radix *(sān qī)* and Hirudo *(shuǐ zhì)* were mixed in and the entire formula was ground to a fine powder. The patient was instructed to mix 10g in water and add enough sugar to make it palatable. One dose was to be taken three times each day with meals.

During the time that she was taking this formula, the patient had one episode of acute vertigo. Two packets of Bupleurum, Dried Tangerine Peel, and Alismatis Decoction *(chái chén zé xiè tāng)*, unmodified, resolved it.

After finishing the powder, her tongue still appeared to be slightly dark, but the purplish area of the tongue looked more pale and her hearing had improved a bit.

At this point, as she had made substantial improvement, I decided to change my approach and simplify things. I had Notoginseng Radix *(sān qī)* 1200g and Hirudo *(shuǐ zhì)* 150g separately ground into fine powders. The Hirudo *(shuǐ zhì)* was placed in enteric capsules with each capsule containing 0.25g. *(Note:* this is the preferred method of administering this substance today.) While no symptoms remained that were clearly related to blood stasis, the tongue showed that this aspect of the problem had not fully resolved and I was concerned about blood stasis playing a role in a possible recurrence.

The patient was instructed to make a 200ml decoction from Acori tatarinowii Rhizoma *(shí chāng pǔ)* 15g and Astragali Radix *(huáng qí)* 30g, every day. The former herb is good at opening the orifices and removing filth, while the latter tonifies the qi in a way that increases the efficacy of the former. This decoction was divided in half and taken together with 4g of Notoginseng Radix *(sān qī)* powder and two capsules of Hirudo *(shuǐ zhì)*, twice a day.

The patient proceeded with this regimen for four months, after which time her tongue had become pale-red with no sign of purple. Her hearing had significantly improved. Over the course of the next three years, she had had no recurrences of vertigo.

Disease	Main Symptoms	Pattern Identification	Treatment Method	Formula
Vertigo	Recurrent vertigo	Wind, fire, phlegm, deficiency, and stasis	Dispel wind, clear fire, dislodge phlegm, tonify deficiency, invigorate blood, and dispel stasis	Bupleurum, Dried Tangerine Peel, and Alismatis Decoction *(chái chén zé xiè tāng)* modified with medicinal substances to invigorate blood and to dispel stasis

Reflections and Clarifications

PHYSICIAN A   Throughout history, physicians have been aware of the fact that static blood can cause vertigo. The Ming-dynasty physician Yu Tuan wrote in his *Correct Transmission of Medicine (Yī xué zhèng chuán)*, "Additionally, in patients who vomit blood and then are dizzy, there is dead blood in the chest, blocking the Heart orifice. It is appropriate to move the blood and to clear the Heart in order to restore health." Modern Western medicine also recognizes that traumatic injury can lead to static blood, which can cause localized ischemia and hypoxia in the head and result in vertigo.

Dr. Jiang had mastered a wide range of medical doctrines and he proposed the model of wind, fire, phlegm, and deficiency for these patients. Why do you think he did not include blood stasis?

DR. YU When we were organizing Dr. Jiang's medical writings, from what we could tell he had never even considered the relationship between blood stasis and vertigo. Although I could not believe that, in reviewing the case records of those he treated for vertigo, it appears that he never addressed blood stasis in any of these cases. Dr. Jiang had even lectured to an advanced class, pouring out his knowledge about the treatment of vertigo, but he did not even touch upon blood stasis.

PHYSICIAN B In the first case above, when we consider the signs and symptoms, there does not seem to be any evidence of blood stasis. It seems that your addition of blood-moving substances to the formula was done as a way of clarifying the diagnosis, what is termed in Western medicine "diagnosis by treatment." She took the powder for four months and then suffered no recurrence of the vertigo for more than two years. This result suggests that the formula matched the pattern, that there was in fact static blood present, and that "prolonged disease had entered the collaterals."

DR. YU We also need to remember the interrelationship of phlegm and stasis. Many years ago now, the modern master Dong Han-Liang wrote a treatise on this topic.[14] Dr. Dong describes a cycle in which phlegm gives rise to stasis and stasis brews phlegm. The two are interconnected in terms of cause and effect, and essentially the interrelationship can produce a vicious cycle. Thus, when treating phlegm, we should not forget stasis, and when treating stasis, we should not forget phlegm. One point that is worth mentioning is that although many intractable cases are the result of stasis, the stasis may be lodged so deeply that there are no obvious signs of static blood. As a result, when treating these cases of intractable disease, the adage that one should "observe the pulse, signs, and symptoms, and then treat accordingly" may be insufficient.

PHYSICIAN C When considering vertigo caused by stasis in the modern clinic, the most frequently seen and the easiest to understand are the cases of vertigo caused by trauma to the head or the neck. However, the two cases above appear to be related to the ear. From the perspective of Western medicine, aural vertigo is the result of excessive lymph fluid in the inner ear or a blockage in the absorption of fluid, such that there is a fluid buildup. From a Chinese medical perspective, this would relate to water and thin-mucus, which would be treated with formulas such as Poria, Cinnamon Twig, Atractylodes, and Licorice Decoction *(líng guì zhú gān tāng)* or Alismatis Decoction *(zé xiè tāng)*. These formulas unblock yang and transform water or strengthen the Spleen and move water. Do water and thin-mucus have any relationship with static blood?

DR. YU Yes, the relationship is quite close. In Chapter 14 of the *Essentials from the Golden Cabinet (Jīn Guì Yào Lüè)* it is said that "[When the movement of] blood is inhibited, pathogenic water develops." And if we turn this around, what happens when the movement of water is inhibited? It can influence the circulation of blood and fluids, which,

14. *Translators' note:* This refers to Dong Han-Liang, "Tentative Discussion on the Interrelationship between Phlegm and Stasis *(Shì tán tán yū xiāng guān lùn)*." Journal of Chinese Medicine *(Zhōng yì zá zhì)*. 21(9):7-10, 1980.

over time, can produce static blood. This phenomenon is referred to traditionally as "the mutual affliction of stasis and water."

It is worth noting that because the primary disease factor in aural vertigo is pathogenic water and thin-mucus, or phlegm and thin-mucus, signs of static blood may not be clear or may even be absent. As a result, we must employ a type of investigational methodology in diagnosis and treatment. This methodology is suggested by the following line in Chapter 74 of the *Basic Questions (Sū wèn)*: "If [the signs] are there, look for [the pathodynamic]. If [the signs] are missing, [also] look for them." In particular, when we are reviewing the patient's history of treatment, we should carefully consider the herbs and formulas that have been used before and then do a systematic consideration of how to proceed.

PHYSICIAN C   Thinking about a "systematic consideration of how to proceed" reminds me of a question. Given that aural vertigo relates directly to the ear, shouldn't we consider the connections to the ear? In Chapter 17 of the *Divine Pivot (Líng shū)*, it says that the "Kidney qi connects with the ears." Thus, when there is disease that affects the ear, its root is in the Kidneys. Furthermore, the Kidneys store essence, and as the same chapter states, "loss of essence results in deafness." In the clinic, patients with vertigo accompanied by tinnitus, a feeling of blockage in the ears, and even, in severe cases, decrease or loss of hearing, are considered to have essence deficiency, not blood stasis.

DR. YU   While it is true that *Divine Pivot (Líng shū)* states that the Kidney qi connects with the ears, Chapter 4 of the *Basic Questions (Sū wèn)* states that the Heart's "opening orifice is the ear." The Heart governs the blood, and thus, when the Heart vessels are impeded, it can result in stasis in the ear collaterals. This simply follows as a matter of course.

I think that it is important to remember that the *Inner Classic (Nèi jīng)* is an ancient book that was neither completed by one individual nor during one time period. As a result, although the information in the text is valuable and profound, it is incumbent on us as readers not to lose sight of the different perspectives represented within the text and of the potential for contradictions and bias.

PHYSICIAN A   In the first case, you chose to use Moutan Cortex *(mǔ dān pí)* and Notoginseng Radix *(sān qī)* as the substances to invigorate the blood and to dispel stasis. In modern materia medica, Moutan Cortex *(mǔ dān pí)* is categorized as an herb that clears heat and cools the blood. Notoginseng Radix *(sān qī)* is categorized as an herb that stops bleeding. Does this not imply that the main functions of these two herbs are not invigorating the blood and dispelling stasis?

DR. YU   In modern materia medica, the categorization scheme reflects the influence of Western pharmacology. However, most of the substances that we use in Chinese medicine are from the natural world; they are plants, animals, and minerals, with complicated ingredients. As such, their functions are multi-faceted. Any attempt at categorization is therefore primarily done in comparison to other medicinal substances. These categorizations should not be viewed mechanistically or simplistically; otherwise, they become useless.

For example, Moutan Cortex *(mǔ dān pí)* clears heat and cools the blood and also invigorates the blood and dispels stasis. Which functions are primary and which are secondary is actually worth contemplating. From my experience, I would say that Moutan Cortex *(mǔ dān pí)* dispels stasis, but is not strong enough to break up stasis. In thinking about appropriate usage, it can be used in a wide variety of patterns including those with heat, cold, deficiency, and/or excess. It is red and it enters the Heart and I consider it to be one of the more "authentic" blood-invigorating, stasis-dispelling herbs.

PHYSICIAN A   Considering the way of thinking that you have just expressed, it is easier for me to understand your usage of Notoginseng Radix *(sān qī)*. Although it is included in the category of substances that stop bleeding, it also effectively invigorates the blood and dispels stasis. In fact, its unique functionality is that it stops bleeding without causing stasis and that it dispels stasis without damaging the blood.

DR. YU   The early 20th-century physician Zhang Xi-Chun truly admired the ability of Notoginseng Radix *(sān qī)* to transform stasis and to generate new blood. He thought that it could "be used in place of Purge Static Blood Decoction *(xià yū xuè tāng)* from the *Essentials from the Golden Cabinet* and that it is safer and more reliable than Purge Static Blood Decoction *(xià yū xuè tāng)*." The famous modern physician from Chengdu, Shen Shao-Jiu, said regarding Notoginseng Radix *(sān qī)* that its functions could be greatly affected through different combinations: combining it with attacking herbs, it attacks; combining it with tonifying herbs, it tonifies.

PHYSICIAN A   The formula also contains Hirudo *(shuǐ zhì)*, which is slightly toxic. It breaks up and drives out blood stasis. Its fierceness and violence sets it apart from the relative moderation of Notoginseng Radix *(sān qī)* and Moutan Cortex *(mǔ dān pí)*. In the second case, the patient used it for more than four months. Was there not some concern about damaging the normal qi?

DR. YU   In my usage of Hirudo *(shuǐ zhì)*, I have also absorbed the influence of Zhang Xi-Chun. Dr. Zhang explained the effects of Hirudo *(shuǐ zhì)* as follows in his *Essays on Medicine Esteeming the Chinese and Respecting the Western (Yī xué zhōng zhōng cān xī lù)*:

> It is salty in taste, black in color, its qi is putrefied, and its nature is neutral. Because it is salty, it has an affinity for the blood level; because it comes from a blood-consuming animal, it is effective at breaking up blood [stasis]; because its qi is putrefied, it has a synergy with static blood, but not with new blood; thus, it breaks up blood stasis without damaging new blood. … Its ability to break up static blood is an innate ability of Hirudo *(shuǐ zhì)*, it is not the result of it being fierce and violent.

Dr. Zhang stressed many times that it was "most appropriate to use Hirudo *(shuǐ zhì)* untreated; absolutely do not roast it first."

If Hirudo *(shuǐ zhì)* is cooked in a decoction or a draft, the fishy smell and taste becomes quite extreme, and after ingesting it, patients readily vomit. So, when I use Hirudo *(shuǐ zhì)* in a prepared formula, I usually use it as a powder.

One more thing that everyone seems to have ignored is the fact that one other important herb was used in both formulas in a large dosage to invigorate the blood and to unblock the collaterals: Puerariae Radix *(gé gēn)*. In the *Discussion of Cold Damage (Shāng hán lùn)*, Kudzu Decoction *(gé gēn tāng)* is used to treat a "stiff and craned" nape and upper back. The formula discharges exterior conditions, disperses cold, soothes the sinews, releases spasms, and also invigorates the blood and unblocks the collaterals. In modern materia medica, Puerariae Radix *(gé gēn)* is placed in the category of acrid, cool, exterior-releasing substances; I believe that the placement overlooks important aspects of this herb's functionality. In the *Divine Husbandman's Classic of the Materia Medica (Shén Nóng běn cāo jīng)*, Puerariae Radix *(gé gēn)* is said to treat "all [types of] obstruction," which refers to conditions of blockage and lack of flow. After many years of clinical practice, I can state that not only does Puerariae Radix *(gé gēn)* invigorate the blood and unblock the collaterals, it also raises the clear. It guides other blood-invigorating, collateral-unblocking substances to the head, vertex, and face, including all the orifices. It is actually an irreplaceable primary ingredient in this formula.

4.5 Constraint

Biliary-cardiac syndrome

What is the best way to approach a case that is prone to misdiagnosis?

容易誤診怎麼辦?

■ CASE HISTORY

Patient: *56-year-old woman*

Over the past five years, the patient has experienced chest and lateral costal area pain and palpitations. She was diagnosed with coronary heart disease. She has frequently taken medications such as dipyridamole, Compounded Salvia tablets *(fù fāng dān shēn piàn)*[15] and Notoginseng tablets *(sān qī piàn)*. She interspersed this with Drive out Stasis from the Mansion of Blood Decoction *(xuè fǔ zhú yū tāng)* and Trichosanthes Fruit, Chinese Garlic, and Wine Decoction *(guā lóu xìe bái bái jiǔ tāng)*. While sometimes there seemed to be improvement, in the end no progress was made. She often eats greasy, rich food, which leads to episodes of lateral costal and hypochondriac pain that radiates to the shoulder and back. This pain is accompanied by chest pain, palpitations, and rapid fluctuations in body temperature.

Previously, an EKG revealed changes in the ST-T wave. After she was given medications to combat infection, as well as anti-spasmodics and pain relievers, her situation improved. Her EKG also returned to normal.

An ultrasound revealed two gallstones, each measuring about 0.5cm. She took more than ten packets of Decoction to Expel Stones from the Gallbladder Duct *(dǎn dào pái*

---

15. This consists of Salviae miltiorrhizae Radix *(dān shēn)*, Notoginseng Radix *(sān qī)*, and Borneolum *(bīng piàn)*.

shi tāng) without any improvement. She has done nothing else up to this point and her physical condition is less than optimal.

INTAKE EXAMINATION
DATE: October 30, 1995

Her appetite was poor. She experienced shortness of breath, dizziness, dull pain in the chest and ribs, palpitations, constipation, and dry mouth with a bitter taste. Her tongue was tender-red and her pulse was wiry and fine.

Differentiation of Patterns and Discussion of Treatment

DR. YU   Given the clinical presentation for this patient, we can consider biliary-cardiac syndrome.

PHYSICIAN A   I am not familiar with that syndrome.

DR. YU   Biliary-cardiac syndrome, also known as gall heart syndrome, is a biomedical disease name, which indicates a syndrome that is characterized by transient angina, cardiac arrhythmia, and abnormal EKG caused by biliary tract infection.

Just as in this case, when there is an active biliary tract infection, it causes changes in the ST-T wave in the EKG, and once the infection is controlled, the EKG returns to normal. This is completely in accord with the diagnosis of biliary-cardiac syndrome. This disease name was not formally established until 1977. Modern medicine's discovery of this syndrome was quite late.

In fact, biomedical research into the relationship between the gallbladder and the heart also started quite late. According to the literature, it was not until 1961 that anyone began to consider a relationship between gallstones and heart disease. In 1975, researchers pointed out a connection between biliary duct diseases and heart disease. And it was not until 1977 that the concept of biliary-cardiac syndrome was put forward.

PHYSICIAN B   The description of biliary-cardiac syndrome is clear, and thus it should be difficult to misdiagnose. Yet, in the literature, the rate of misdiagnosis is not low. What is the reason?

DR. YU   One reason is that this syndrome is rare, and in fact, some physicians may not have ever seen it. Another reason is that some physicians have a rigid way of thinking. If they see angina or chest pain, they immediately equate that with angina associated with coronary heart disease.

In order to avoid misdiagnosis or a missed diagnosis it is necessary to clearly grasp the three main factors associated with biliary-cardiac syndrome. The first is recurrent biliary tract infections. The second is that the biliary tract infections lead to transient angina, which, unlike coronary heart disease, is not associated with a sensation of pressure in the chest, or a feeling of fear and dread, or a feeling that one is about to die. The third is transient changes in the ST-T wave in the EKG, which returns to normal once the biliary tract infection is controlled. In cases of coronary heart disease with angina, there are generally persistent ST-T wave changes in the EKG. If you are clear about all of this, how can a misdiagnosis occur?

Given this situation, for patients with gallbladder disease who do not experience angina, chest pain, or palpitations, it is appropriate for physicians to have the concept of biliary-cardiac disease in mind and to have considered a plan of action in order to avoid a misdiagnosis or a missed diagnosis.

PHYSICIAN A   Why is it that biliary tract infections can lead to angina and arrhythmia?

DR. YU   According to modern medical research, biliary tract infection causes a dilation of the biliary tract, which increases the pressure in the bile duct. Then, as a result of a nervous system reflex response, the coronary artery begins to spasm. There is a decrease in blood flow to the heart muscle, which becomes ischemic, giving rise to angina and arrhythmia.

PHYSICIAN A   The biliary tract infection is the original cause of this syndrome; thus, Western medical treatment focuses on controlling the infection, while also using antispasmodics and analgesics. If there are gallstones, which can cause recurrent infections, this situation can cause great suffering for the patient and surgery may then be appropriate. Nonetheless, there are articles that report that even after surgery, some patients will only have a reduction in the angina or arrhythmia, not a complete resolution.

Therefore, we can say that Chinese medicine has an advantageous position with regard to the treatment of biliary-cardiac syndrome. Given that situation, how does Chinese medicine view differentiation and treatment of this syndrome?

DR. YU   On the basis of clinical observations, most biliary-cardiac syndrome patients who are in the acute phase (while the biliary tract infection is active) manifest a group of symptoms that can be categorized as Liver-Gallbladder constraint, internal collection of phlegm-heat, and obstruction in the Heart collaterals. Appropriate treatment involves a combination of Frigid Extremities Powder *(sì nì sǎn)*, Bupleurum Decoction [for Pathogens] Stuck in the Chest *(chái hú xiàn xiōng tāng)*, and Salvia Drink *(dān shēn yǐn)*. Optimally, a combination of Chinese and Western medicines is employed to address root and branch, in order to resolve this urgent situation.

During the stable stage (with no evidence of infection), it is necessary to carefully consider the state of the qi dynamic and qi transformation of the Liver, Gallbladder, and Heart. The correct determination of the disease factors underlying the symptoms will lead one to the proper treatment.

PHYSICIAN B   Biliary-cardiac syndrome naturally involves the Gallbladder and the Heart, but you suggested that we also consider the qi dynamic and qi transformation of the Liver. Why should we consider the Liver?

DR. YU   Western medicine emphasizes the physical substance of the viscera, while in Chinese medicine, we emphasize qi transformation, by which I mean the function. These two are completely different medical systems. In Chinese medicine, the Gallbladder is considered an accessory to the Liver. The surplus of the Liver qi pours into the Gallbladder and becomes the bile. Thus, diseases of one organ can easily affect the other. For example, when the Liver becomes constrained, the Gallbladder will also suffer from constraint, and vice versa. Most herbs and formulas that dredge the Liver also promote free flow in the Gallbladder, and Gallbladder-freeing herbs and formulas also dredge the Liver. Thus, classical formulas such as Frigid Extremities Powder *(sì nì sǎn)* and Minor Bupleurum Decoction *(xiǎo chái hú tāng)*, and other formulas in this family, are commonly used to treat both Liver and Gallbladder disease.

Liver constraint and Gallbladder constraint can both affect the Heart, forming a type of "triangular" disease dynamic.

PHYSICIAN A The intimate relationship between the Liver and Gallbladder is easy to understand. Is there also an intimate relationship between these organs and the Heart?

In the *Essentials from the Golden Cabinet (Jīn guì yào lüè)* there is a well-known section which states that when one "sees Liver disease, know that it will transmit to the Spleen," and it does not speak of the Heart. What is the basis of your statement that Liver and Gallbladder constraint can influence the Heart?

DR. YU The principles of medicine are very simple. According to five-phase theory, the Liver and Gallbladder are associated with wood and the Heart is associated with fire. Wood generates fire; thus, disease of the parent can affect the child.

PHYSICIAN B A moment ago you said that the relationship between the Gallbladder and the Heart is even more intimate than that shared by the Liver and Gallbladder. This information is both novel and striking. I would like more details.

DR. YU The Liver and the Gallbladder are both associated with wood. The Liver is yin wood and the Gallbladder is yang wood. The Heart is associated with fire, which is yang. Thus, both the Gallbladder and the Heart are associated with yang qi. According to the *Book of Changes (Yì jīng)*, "Sounds that are similar respond to each other and types of qi that are similar group together." Therefore, the relationship of the Gallbladder and the Heart is naturally even closer.

PHYSICIAN B During the discussion above, you frequently refer to Gallbladder constraint. Is this a new term?

DR. YU It is not a new term. In *Supplemented Collections on Patterns and Treatments (Zhèng zhì huì bǔ)* by the Qing-dynasty writer Li Yong-Cui, it is said that "When there is Gallbladder constraint, there is a bitter taste in the mouth, late afternoon fever, and continuous palpitations with a lack of tranquility." Bitter taste in the mouth is one of the primary symptoms. Late afternoon fever means a fever that occurs between 3 and 7 p.m. This time period is managed by the dry metal of *yáng míng*. Metal controls wood, which makes it so that wood has difficulty stretching out, thus there is a fever. Continuous palpitations with a lack of tranquility is clearly a disease of the Heart, and while these symptoms do not always occur in these patients, they can occur, especially in those with concurrent qi deficiency. This portion of the text is probably the earliest mention of Gallbladder constraint affecting the Heart.

As a starting point, we should consider that in this case, Gallbladder constraint affects the Heart and that qi and yin are both deficient. The treatment is to promote free flow in the Gallbladder, soothe the Heart, augment qi and nourish yin. The formula is a modification of combined Frigid Extremities Powder *(sì nì sǎn)* and Generate the Pulse Powder *(shēng mài sǎn)*.

Bupleuri Radix (*chái hú*) 10g

Paeoniae Radix alba (*bái sháo*) 30g

bran-fried Aurantii Fructus *(fū chǎo zhǐ ké)* 10g

Glycyrrhizae Radix praeparata *(zhì gān cǎo)* 10g

Panacis quinquefolii Radix *(xī yáng shēn)* [cook separately] 10g

Ophiopogonis Radix *(mài mén dōng)* 20g

Schisandrae Fructus *(wǔ wèi zǐ)* 10g

Cinnamomi Ramulus *(guì zhī)* 6g

Curcumae Radix *(yù jīn)* 10g

Tribuli Fructus (*cì jí lí*) 5g

Oroxyli Semen (*mù hú dié*) 10g

Mume Fructus *(wū méi)* 30g

After ten packets, there had been no episodes of chest and hypochondriac pain, nor had there been palpitations. The patient's appetite had increased and her bowels were moving smoothly. She no longer had dryness or a bitter taste in her mouth, and the shortness of breath she had been experiencing was significantly reduced.

She was then given ten more packets of the formula, to which was added Curcumae longae Rhizoma *(jiāng huáng)* 10g. During this period, the patient was advised to reduce intake of greasy, fatty foods, and to maintain a calm demeanor.

Upon ultrasound imaging, no stones were found. The only finding was that the wall of the gallbladder was not smooth.

Follow-up six months later revealed that there had been some occasional mild episodes of pain in the chest and ribs and palpitations. However, these symptoms were relieved with 3-5 packets of the original formula.

Disease	Primary Symptoms	Differentiation	Treatment Method	Formula
Gallbladder constraint (biliary-cardiac syndrome)	Chest and hypochondriac pain accompanied by heart palpitations	Gallbladder constraint affecting Heart and dual deficiency of qi and yin	Promote free flow in the Gallbladder, soothe the Heart, augment qi, and nourish yin	Frigid Extremities Powder *(sì nì sǎn)* plus Generate the Pulse Powder *(shēng mài sǎn)*

REFLECTIONS AND CLARIFICATIONS

PHYSICIAN B We recently reviewed your case records and it seems that in treating biliary-cardiac syndrome, you frequently use Frigid Extremities Powder *(sì nì sǎn)* plus Bupleurum Decoction [for Pathogens] Stuck in the Chest *(chái hú xiàn xiōng tāng)* and Salvia Drink *(dān shēn yǐn)*. Commonly-used herbs include Bupleuri Radix *(chái hú)*, Paeoniae Radix alba *(bái sháo)*, bran-fried Aurantii Fructus *(fū chǎo zhǐ ké)*, Glycyrrhizae Radix *(gān cǎo)*, Scutellariae Radix *(huáng qín)*, Pinelliae Rhizoma preparatum *(zhì bàn xià)*, Trichosanthis Semen *(guā lóu rén)*, Coptidis Rhizoma *(huáng lián)*, Platycodi Radix *(jié gěng)*, Salviae miltiorrhizae Radix *(dān shēn)*, Curcumae Radix *(yù jīn)*, Curcumae longae Rhizoma *(jiāng huáng),* and Mume Fructus *(wū méi)*.

DR. YU If you look at the formulas and herbs we have used to treat this condition, it is clear that the primary disease mechanism of biliary-cardiac syndrome is Liver-Gallbladder constraint, internal collection of phlegm-heat, and stasis in the Heart collaterals. Generally, these are patterns of excess.

However, in this case, we see a whole group of deficiency indicators, such as dull pain in the chest and ribs, palpitations, shortness of breath, dizziness, a tender, red tongue, and a wiry, fine pulse. The differentiation was Gallbladder constraint affecting the Heart with dual deficiency of qi and yin. The treatment principle was to promote free flow in the Gallbladder and soothe the Heart, augment qi and nourish yin. I used a modification of the combination of Frigid Extremities Powder *(sì nì sǎn)* and Generate the Pulse Powder *(shēng mài sǎn)*. The nature of these herbs is gentle and slowly they were able to be effective. This illustrates normal variation in treatment.

Most practitioners have a good understanding of the clinical application of Frigid Extremities Powder *(sì nì sǎn)* from the perspective of the *Discussion of Cold Damage (Shāng hán lùn),* and we have discussed many of its uses here. We can certainly say that it has a broad range of usage.

So why is it necessary at this point to discuss the usage of Frigid Extremities Powder *(sì nì sǎn)* for biliary-cardiac syndrome? On the one hand, misdiagnosis of this pattern is quite easy. On the other hand, this case illustrates normal variation in treatment and is what I frequently talk about with regards to "getting new ideas out of standard methods."

PHYSICIAN A   In this case, the pathodynamic is Gallbladder constraint affecting the Heart and dual deficiency of qi and yin. Cold signs are absent, yet the formula contains warm, acrid Cinnamomi Ramulus *(guì zhī).* Are these types of subtle points important?

DR. YU   Assisting with a small amount of warm, acrid Cinnamomi Ramulus *(guì zhī),* which enters the blood, when boosting the qi and nourishing yin, unblocks the Heart qi with warmth and facilitates the movement of the blood. In conjunction with Frigid Extremities Powder *(sì nì sǎn),* the combination more effectively promotes free flow in the Gallbladder and soothes the Heart.

If we look at the notes following Frigid Extremities Powder *(sì nì sǎn)* in the *Discussion of Cold Damage (Shāng hán lùn),* it states, "For palpitations, add Cinnamomi Ramulus *(guì zhī)* 5 *fēn.*" Palpitations are a disease of the Heart. Some people say that Frigid Extremities Powder *(sì nì sǎn)* has nothing to do with *shào yīn* disease; this indicates that they have not read the notes following the formula.

4.5.1 **Constraint**

Pain in the chest, ribs, and abdomen for half a year

When two different pathodynamics coexist side-by-side,
how do you decide which is primary and which is secondary?

兩組病機共存並列，分不清孰主孰次

■ CASE HISTORY

Patient: *Ms. Liu, 56-year-old woman*

Twelve years previously, the patient had contracted acute icteric hepatitis, which was treated successfully. Although she occasionally experienced dull pain in the liver area and fullness and a stifling sensation in the epigastrium, taking a few packets of Chinese herbs to dredge the Liver and to harmonize the Stomach would temporarily calm things down.

However, about six months ago, following a period of emotional upset and overwork, her minor symptoms of dull pain in the chest and ribs, fullness and a stifling sensation in the epigastrium, and scorching heat and bloating in the lower abdomen became much more severe. She took a total of more than 60 packets of various formulas, including modifications of Minor Bupleurum Decoction *(xiǎo chái hú tāng)*, Augmented Rambling Powder *(jiā wèi xiāo yáo sǎn)*, Pinellia and Poria Decoction *(bàn líng tāng)*, and Enrich Water and Clear the Liver Drink *(zī shuǐ qīng gān yǐn)*, with little improvement.

The patient worried constantly that her condition might be untreatable. Although she had many diagnostic tests performed, including x-rays, ultrasound, and endoscopy, no one could determine the nature of the problem.

INTAKE EXAMINATION
DATE: March 16, 1987

She presented with dull pain in the chest and ribs that occurred in the afternoon, fullness and a stifling sensation in the epigastrium, scorching heat and bloating in the lower abdomen, and frequent belching, all of which worsened in the evenings. She reported accompanying symptoms of dry and irritated eyes, chaotic dreams, dry mouth, bitter taste, and dry stool. Her tongue was pale-red with a thin, yellow coating that lacked moisture. Her pulse was wiry and fine.

Note: Although some of the complaints are labeled as "accompanying," which implies that they were secondary, it should be noted here that upon repeated questioning and discussion, the patient was unable to clearly label one group of the complaints as primary and another as secondary. All she could say was that she suffered from all of them.

Differentiation of Patterns and Discussion of Treatment

DR. YU   In this patient, the dull pain in the chest and ribs and scorching heat in the lower abdomen that was worse in the evening, accompanied by dry, irritated eyes, chaotic dreams, and a dry mouth and bitter taste, all clearly belong to Liver-Kidney yin deficiency.

The fullness and a stifling sensation in the epigastrium, bloating in the lower abdomen, and frequent belching all indicate Liver constraint with qi stagnation.

The patient indicated that all of these were equally worrisome and so treatment needed to consider both sets of symptoms. Thus, I viewed this case as a combination of Liver-Kidney yin deficiency and Liver constraint with qi stagnation.

Treatment and Outcome

The treatment was to enrich the Liver and Kidneys while dredging the Liver and moving the qi. The formula was a combination of Linking Decoction *(yī guàn jiān)* and Frigid Extremities Powder *(sì nì sǎn)*, with some additions.

Angelicae sinensis Radix *(dāng guī)*.. 10g
Rehmanniae Radix *(shēng dì huáng)*... 12g
Lycii Fructus *(gǒu qǐ zǐ)*.. 12g
Glehniae Radix *(běi shā shēn)*... 12g
Ophiopogonis Radix *(mài mén dōng)*... 15g
charred Toosendan Fructus *(chuān liàn zǐ tàn)*............................... 6g
Bupleuri Radix *(chái hú)*... 10g
Paeoniae Radix alba *(bái sháo)*.. 12g
bran-fried Aurantii Fructus *(fū chǎo zhǐ ké)*................................ 10g
Glycyrrhizae Radix *(gān cǎo)*... 5g
dry-fried Ziziphi spinosae Semen *(chǎo suān zǎo rén)*.................... 10g

Instructions: Three packets. I also reassured her that her condition was treatable and that it was vitally important that she work to change her attitude and adopt a more optimistic outlook.

SECOND VISIT: The dull pain in the ribs, fullness and stifling sensation in the epigastrium, and scorching heat and bloating in the lower abdomen had all decreased in severity. However, the dull pain in the patient's chest was unchanged and her stools remained dry.

To the previous formula I added:

Lilii Bulbus *(bǎi hé)*.. 30g
dry-fried Cassiae Semen *(chǎo jué míng zǐ)*................................. 20g
wine-prepared Cistanches Herba *(jiǔ cōng róng)*........................... 20g

I also changed Aurantii Fructus *(zhǐ ké)* to Aurantii Fructus immaturus *(zhǐ shí)*.

Instructions: three packets

THIRD VISIT: All of the symptoms had improved, including the chest pain, and her stools were less dry and her bowel movements smoother. Her tongue was pale-red with a thin, white coating. Her pulse was still wiry and fine. From the previous formula, I removed charred Toosendan Fructus *(chuān liàn zǐ tàn)* and added Tribuli Fructus *(cì jí lí)* 10g. I told her to take the formula until her symptoms completely resolved.

Three months later, the patient returned to my clinic with a cousin, who she was referring to me for treatment. At that time she reported that after taking eight packets of herbs, all of her symptoms had resolved.

Disease	Primary Symptoms	Differentiation	Treatment Method	Formula
Constraint pattern	Dull pain in the chest and ribs, fullness and a stifling sensation in the epigastrium, and scorching heat and bloating in the lower abdomen	Liver-Kidney yin deficiency, Liver constraint with qi stagnation	Enrich the Liver and Kidneys, dredge the Liver, move the qi	Linking Decoction *(yī guàn jiān)* plus Frigid Extremities Powder *(sì nì sǎn)*

Reflections and Clarifications

PHYSICIAN A   I have noticed that in treating Liver disease in which there is Liver-Kidney yin deficiency, you generally begin with Linking Decoction *(yī guàn jiān)*, then you add some Kidney-enriching herbs. You often get excellent results. More recently, I have also seen quite a few cases in which you combined Linking Decoction *(yī guàn jiān)* and Frigid Extremities Powder *(sì nì sǎn)*. It is impossible to deny the good results, but I would fear ridicule if I combined these two formulas because of how completely different the treatment principles and realm of treatment of the two formulas seem to be. From the perspective of basic theory, they seem incompatible.

To be specific, Linking Decoction *(yī guàn jiān)* combines a large group of moistening herbs that enrich Liver-Kidney yin with just one herb, Toosendan Fructus *(chuān liàn zǐ)*, to dredge the Liver and move the qi, so as to tonify without causing stagnation. Frigid Extremities Powder *(sì nì sǎn)*, on the other hand, is a strong formula that focuses specifically on dredging the Liver and moving the qi. I would have some misgivings about putting the two formulas together.

If the disorder being treated is primarily the result of Liver-Kidney yin deficiency, as when Linking Decoction *(yī guàn jiān)* is indicated, I would be concerned about potential injury to the qi and yin from Frigid Extremities Powder *(sì nì sǎn)*. If, on the other hand, the disorder is primarily owing to Liver constraint and qi stagnation, as when Frigid Extremities Powder *(sì nì sǎn)* should be used, I would be concerned about the enriching herbs in Linking Decoction *(yī guàn jiān)* blocking the normal movement of the body's qi.

DR. YU   I think that we should keep our focus on the clinic. In the clinic, do we not see this combination of Liver-Kidney yin deficiency and Liver constraint with qi stagnation? And do we not see cases, like the one above, in which the two pathodynamics seem to be equal in importance?

Please remember that I intentionally did not describe the patient's condition as Liver-Kidney yin deficiency accompanied by Liver constraint with qi stagnation, or the other way around. I specifically said that the two pathologies are both present and that it is impossible to differentiate primary and secondary.

In treating such a case, if I were to use only Linking Decoction *(yī guàn jiān)*, with or without additional Kidney-enriching herbs, the ability of the formula to enrich the Liver and Kidneys would be sufficient. However, we would only have the one associate herb, Toosendan Fructus *(chuān liàn zǐ)*, to dredge the Liver and move the qi. Given the simplicity of this approach and the mildness of the force of the herbs, how could we hope to use that formula by itself to eliminate the patient's fullness and stifling sensation or to dissipate her abdominal distention?

PHYSICIAN C   According to the description of Linking Decoction *(yī guàn jiān)* in *Medical Discourses of [Wei] Liu-Zhou (Liǔ-Zhōu yī huà)*, the formula enriches yin and dredges the Liver to treat Liver-Kidney yin deficiency and qi stagnation with symptoms such as pain in the chest, ribs, and epigastrium, acid regurgitation, along with bulging disorders, conglomerations, and gatherings. Given that the formula is specifically designed to enrich the Liver and Kidneys while simultaneously dredging the Liver and moving the qi, is it not superfluous to add Frigid Extremities Powder *(sì nì sǎn)* to it?

DR. YU Could that possibly be true? I think that if we examine the pathodynamic and the symptoms associated with yin deficiency and qi stagnation, we may find some answers to this thorny question. How should we view "Liver-Kidney yin deficiency with qi stagnation?" In Chapter 8 of the *Divine Pivot (Líng shū)*, it states that "when yin is deficient, there is no qi." The meaning of this is that when yin fluids are deficient, they cannot transform qi. When qi decreases, it loses its ability to move the blood. In turn, the blood is less able to moisten the channels and the organs. This cycle can lead to pain in the chest, ribs, and epigastrium. Pain of this type is characterized by its lack of severity, manifesting as dull or intermittent.

If we consider how the creator of Linking Decoction *(yī guàn jiān)*, Wei Liu-Zhou, viewed qi stagnation in the context of this formula, we can see that it is the product of reduced qi, and reduced qi is the product of Liver-Kidney yin deficiency. Thus, this type of "qi stagnation" can only be treated by using a foundation of herbs that enrich the Liver and Kidney yin and by including a small amount of qi-moving herbs that do not damage the yin. In this way, we can tonify without producing stagnation. Enriching the yin without including several substances to promote the proper movement of qi would be ill-advised tonification.

To return to our main discussion: are the qi stagnation symptoms in this case owing to reduced qi? Fullness and a stifling sensation in the epigastrium, frequent belching, and unbearable distention in the lower abdomen: these symptoms are all compatible with the pathodynamic of Liver constraint with qi stagnation. Liver constraint with qi stagnation, however, is absolutely not a matter of not enough qi, but of its overabundance.

Hopefully it is clear that the previous reference to reduced qi is in reference to physiology, whereas in the case we are discussing here, the qi is copious and overabundant, thus falling into the rubric of pathology. If my explanation is correct, one should be able to see that in this case, the addition of Frigid Extremities Powder *(sì nì sǎn)* was, in fact, not superfluous.

PHYSICIAN A I was paying particular attention to the fact that at the patient's second visit her dull costal pain, fullness and stifling sensation in the epigastrium, scorching heat, and bloating in the lower abdomen had all decreased in severity. The dull pain in the patient's chest was unchanged, however, and her stools were still dry.

I expected that you would add Hemp Seed Pill *(má zǐ rén wán)* and some herbs that invigorate the blood and unblock the collaterals to the original formula. I did not expect that by adding Lilii Bulbus *(bǎi hé)*, dry-fried Cassiae Semen *(chǎo jué míng zǐ)*, and wine-prepared Cistanches Herba *(jiǔ cōng róng)*, and substituting Aurantii Fructus immaturus *(zhǐ shí)* for Aurantii Fructus *(zhǐ ké)*, you would be able to resolve both the patient's chest pain and her dry stools. Can you explain this?

DR. YU When dull pain in the chest appears in Liver disease, it is because the Liver channel passes through the diaphragm and enters the Lung. When treating the Liver is ineffective, one must consider that the Lung has been directly affected by the disease process. In this case, deficiency fire produced by Liver-Kidney yin deficiency scorched the Lung. Lung dryness led to damage to the Lung collaterals and then to dull pain. Lung heat descended into the Large Intestine and the Intestines became dry, which gave rise to dry stools.

Lilii Bulbus *(bǎi hé)* clears and moistens the Lung collaterals. Dry-fried Cassiae Semen *(chǎo jué míng zǐ)*, wine-prepared Cistanches Herba *(jiǔ cōng róng)*, and Aurantii Fructus immaturus *(zhǐ shí)* moisten the Intestines and unblock the stool. From my experience, I can say that in cases of dull chest pain that are the result of deficiency fire scorching the Lung, leading to Lung dryness and damaging the collaterals, a large dosage of Lilii Bulbus *(bǎi hé)* quickly relieves the pain. Furthermore, constipation from Intestinal dryness responds quickly to large doses of dry-fried Cassiae Semen *(chǎo jué míng zǐ)* and wine-prepared Cistanches Herba *(jiǔ cōng róng)* with a small dose of Aurantii Fructus immaturus *(zhǐ shí)*. Very few cases do not respond to this treatment and there are very few relapses, which is why this combination is superior to Hemp Seed Pill *(má zǐ rén wán)*.

PHYSICIAN B   I have been thinking about something else. In this case, although there is the pathology of Liver constraint and qi stagnation, the signs of Liver-Kidney yin deficiency appear even more obvious. Thus, it seems to me that perhaps Frigid Extremities Powder *(sì nì sǎn)* is a little bit too drying. Is there not another formula that would dredge Liver qi, yet be a bit more balanced?

DR. YU   In Frigid Extremities Powder *(sì nì sǎn)* there are only four herbs: Bupleuri Radix *(chái hú)*, Paeoniae Radix alba *(bái sháo)*, Aurantii Fructus immaturus *(zhǐ shí)*, and Glycyrrhizae Radix *(gān cǎo)*. Exactly which of these is too drying? Even if there is concern about Bupleuri Radix *(chái hú)* "plundering Liver yin," we must remember that this formula also contains Peony and Licorice Decoction *(sháo yào gān cǎo tāng)*, which is sour, sweet, and transforms yin, so as to benefit yin. I think that the idea that the formula is "a bit too drying" is actually a misunderstanding.

If I might add another note, the nature of Toosendan Fructus *(chuān liàn zǐ)* is cold and it is extremely bitter and bad tasting. It should only be used in small quantities and for a limited amount of time. It is worth noting that although Wei Liu-Zhou included Toosendan Fructus *(chuān liàn zǐ)* in his original formula, when we read his case studies, we see that he substituted Tribuli Fructus *(cì jí lí)* for Toosendan Fructus *(chuān liàn zǐ)* in many of the formulas he prescribed. It may be that he reassessed the formula after recording it.

PHYSICIAN C   I have heard that in recent years you have used the combination of Linking Decoction *(yī guàn jiān)* and Frigid Extremities Powder *(sì nì sǎn)* quite often in the clinic. For what conditions have you employed this combination?

DR. YU   I have used this combination in the treatment of the recovery stage of acute hepatitis, chronic hepatitis, sequelae of hepatitis, menopausal syndrome (both female and male), chronic pelvic inflammatory disease, and neuroses. However, these are all Western medical names and you should not allow them to limit your use of this approach. Rather we need to pay attention to a patient's signs and symptoms. If a patient presents with signs and symptoms that indicate a combination of Liver-Kidney yin deficiency and Liver constraint with qi stagnation, this formula combination will yield reliable and rapid results.

4.6 **Bitter taste**

Bitter taste in the mouth for six months

A simple, inexpensive, and proven specialty treatment

簡便廉驗的專方專藥

■ CASE HISTORY

Case #1: *61-year-old man*

The patient complained of six months of bitter taste in the mouth, which didn't particularly worry him. However, about two weeks ago, after drinking an excessive amount of alcohol, the bitter taste intensified. The symptom was especially intense at night. He began tossing and turning and having difficulty sleeping.

A previous physician had prescribed three packets of Minor Bupleurum Decoction *(xiǎo chái hú tāng)* plus scorched Gardeniae Fructus *(jiāo zhī zǐ)*, Anemarrhenae Rhizoma *(zhī mǔ)*, and Prunellae Spica *(xià kū cǎo)*. The bitter taste in the mouth diminished slightly. The formula was then changed to Gentian Decoction to Drain the Liver *(lóng dǎn xiè gān tāng)* for three packets, but this was ineffective.

INTAKE EXAMINATION
DATE: October 5, 1985

The patient's tongue was red with a thin, yellow coating. His pulse was wiry, fine, and slightly rapid.

■ CASE HISTORY

Case #2: *30-year-old woman*

The patient reported that for the last year she had suffered from fullness and a stifling sensation in the epigastric region, abdominal distention, and bitter taste in the mouth. She would get hungry and want to eat, but following food intake, she would experience fullness and a stifling sensation in the epigastric region and unbearable abdominal distention. She also reported that she had copious belching and flatulence, felt flustered, and had nocturnal intestinal rumbling that was, at times, quite pronounced. Her symptoms were exaggerated when she ate oily or greasy foods, resulting in loose, unsatisfying bowel movements and a persistent bitter taste.

She had already taken more than 20 packets of Chinese herbs without effect. Examination by a Western medicine practitioner revealed that her stomach had prolapsed 6cm, but no other organic abnormalities were found in her stomach or intestines.

INTAKE EXAMINATION
DATE: June 13, 1985

The patient's tongue was pale and enlarged with a thin, white coating. Her pulse was wiry and sunken.

Differentiation of Patterns and Discussion of Treatment

PHYSICIAN A The pathodynamic of bitter taste is relatively simple: upward flaring of Gallbladder fire. Is that correct?

DR. YU That is correct, but we can go a step further. Everyone knows that bitter taste in the mouth is a cardinal symptom of Gallbladder disease. It can be seen in *shào yáng* diseases as a result of "Gallbladder fire flaring upward." Chapter 47 of the *Basic Questions (Sù Wèn),* entitled "On Strange Diseases," explains:

> In disease with a bitter taste in the mouth ... the disease name is Gallbladder singular [heat] (膽癉 *dǎn dān*). The Liver is the general in the center and receives its decisions from the Gallbladder and the throat serves as its envoy. When this person plans and considers so much that they cannot make a decision, the Gallbladder qi becomes deficient and qi overflows upward, causing a bitter taste in the mouth.

A passage in Chapter 44 of the same book also notes that "When the Liver qi is hot, the Gallbladder discharges and there is a bitter taste in the mouth." From this we can see that the secondary locus of the disease is in the Gallbladder and that the primary locus is in the Liver.

Because the Liver governs planning and consideration, when "[he or she] plans and considers so much that they cannot make a decision," then the Liver qi becomes constrained. Over time, constraint transforms into fire, which then floods the Gallbladder, leading to irregular function. Consequently, Gallbladder fire flares upward or Gallbladder qi swells upward giving rise to a bitter taste in the mouth.

PHYSICIAN B Line 263 of the *Discussion of Cold Damage (Shāng hán lùn)* states, "*Shào yáng* disease consists of a bitter taste in the mouth, dry throat, and vertigo." Bitter taste is the first of three primary symptoms recorded in the outline for *shào yáng* disease. Given that, can we still say that "the secondary locus of the disease is in the Gallbladder and that the primary locus is in the Liver?"

DR. YU We can understand this by remembering that Zhang Zhong-Jing states in the preface to his text that he "drew from the *Basic Questions (Sù Wèn)* and the *Nine Fascicles (Jiǔ juǎn)* [commonly thought to be another name for the *Divine Pivot (Líng shū)*]." The scholarship and the thought process in the *Discussion of Cold Damage (Shāng hán lùn)* have a direct relationship with the *Basic Questions (Sù Wèn)*.

But more importantly, we must consider clinical reality. Many of the patients we see who are considered to have *shào yáng* disease are people who normally experience Liver constraint, such that the Liver is not in a soothed state. Thus, when treating bitter taste in the mouth, while it is essential to clear Gallbladder fire and direct it downward, it is equally essential to dredge the Liver and spread out what has been constrained.

Treatment and Outcome

Case #1

This was a simple case of bitter taste in the mouth, which is referred to as "Gallbladder singular [heat] (膽癉 *dǎn dān*)."

The formula prescribed was a modification of the modern master Dr. Jian Yu-Guang's Bupleurum, Gentian, and Oyster Shell Decocotion *(chái dǎn mǔ lì tāng)*.

> Bupleuri Radix *(chái hú)* 10g
> Gentianae Radix *(lóng dǎn cǎo)* 10g
> Ostreae Concha *(mǔ lì)* 30g
> Puerariae Radix *(gé gēn)* 30g
> Glycyrrhizae Radix *(gān cǎo)* 6g

Instructions: two packets

About an hour after taking the first dose, the patient's bitter taste in the mouth was greatly reduced. After finishing the first packet, this symptom had resolved and he was sleeping peacefully.

A month later, after another round of drinking and eating spicy food, the patient's bitter taste returned. He cooked the unused packet from the initial visit, and by the end of that packet, his bitter taste had again resolved.

Over many years now, only infrequently has he experienced any recurrence of the bitter taste in the mouth. When he does, he takes a packet or two of the formula and it quickly disappears.

Case #2

This was a case of deficiency cold of the Spleen and Stomach with stagnation of turbid qi.

The formula prescribed was a modified combination of Regulate the Middle Decoction *(lǐ zhōng tāng)* plus Magnolia Bark, Fresh Ginger, Pinellia, Licorice, and Ginseng Decoction *(hòu pò shēng jiāng bàn xià gān cǎo rén shēn tāng)*.

> Codonopsis Radix *(dǎng shēn)* 15g
> Atractylodis macrocephalae Rhizoma *(bái zhú)* 12g
> Zingiberis Rhizoma *(gān jiāng)* 12g
> Glycyrrhizae Radix praeparata *(zhì gān cǎo)* 6g
> Poria *(fú líng)* 15g
> Ginger Magnoliae officinalis Cortex *(jiāng hòu pò)* 20g
> standard Pinelliae Rhizoma praeparatum *(fǎ bàn xià)* 10g
> Zingiberis Rhizoma recens *(shēng jiāng)* 10g

After three packets there was a significant reduction in the patient's epigastric fullness, stifling sensation, and abdominal distention. Her intestinal rumbling and flustered feeling had ceased, but the bitter taste in the mouth remained unchanged. She also reported frequent shortness of breath and aversion to cold.

To the above formula we added Astragali Radix *(huáng qí)* 30g and Aconiti Radix lateralis praeparata *(zhì fù zǐ)* 15g (precooked). After three packets, all of her symptoms had resolved, except for the bitter taste in the mouth, which had worsened.

At this point, I realized that there was constrained heat in the Liver and Gallbladder. The warming and heating herbs were beneficial to the Spleen and Kidneys, but not to the Liver and Gallbladder.

I went back to the original formula and added Bupleuri Radix *(chái hú)* 10g, Gentianae Radix *(lóng dǎn cǎo)* 3g, and Ostreae Concha *(mǔ lì)* 15g. After two packets, the bitter taste had significantly diminished. At that point, I removed the formula and just gave her the three medicinal substances that I had added to the original formula—the ingredients of Jian Yu-Guang's Bupleurum, Gentian, and Oyster Shell Decocotion *(chái dǎn mǔ lì tāng)*—as a stand-alone formula. After three packets, the bitter taste had resolved completely.

Disease	Primary Symptoms	Differentiation	Treatment Method	Formula
Gallbladder heat	Bitter taste in the mouth	Constrained fire in the Liver and Gallbladder	Clear and direct fire downward, dredge the Liver, and thrust out constraint	Bupleurum, Gentian, and Oyster Shell Decocotion *(chái dǎn mǔ lì tāng)*

Reflections and Clarifications

PHYSICIAN A   Certainly, bitter taste in the mouth is a common symptom, but it is fairly uncommon to have a patient come to the clinic with this as their chief complaint. As a result, many physicians do not pay it much attention. And yet you not only consider bitter taste in the mouth to be important, but you have specific formulas and medicinal substances to address it.

In the first case, bitter taste in the mouth was the primary symptom and you simply used Bupleurum, Gentian, and Oyster Shell Decoction *(chái dǎn mǔ lì tāng)*. In the second case, in which bitter taste in the mouth was an accompanying symptom, you used Bupleurum, Gentian, and Oyster Shell Decoction *(chái dǎn mǔ lì tāng)* in combination with other formulas. In both cases, the effect was excellent.

DR. YU   This formula was created by my teacher, Dr. Jian Yu-Guang. Bupleurum, Gentian, and Oyster Shell Decoction *(chái dǎn mǔ lì tāng)* contains only the three substances for which the formula is named. It fits the principle of "while it is essential to clear Gallbladder fire and direct it downward, it is equally essential to dredge the Liver and spread out that which has been constrained." The Liver likes to thrust out and prefers to ascend. Bupleuri Radix *(chái hú)* is bitter and neutral, it moves the Liver qi up and out so as to dredge the Liver and to spread out what has been constrained. The Gallbladder likes tranquility and prefers to descend. Gentianae Radix *(lóng dǎn cǎo)* is bitter and cold, it sinks into the yin and thrusts downward; it clears Gallbladder fire and directs it downward. Ostreae Concha *(mǔ lì)* is salty and cold, it enriches water and conserves wood and it restrains Gallbladder fire. Thus, as Zhang Xi-Chun wrote, "when water enriches wood, Liver and Gallbladder each achieve nourishment."

It is my experience that the treatment of bitter taste in the mouth proceeds most effectively with all three substances used together: Bupleuri Radix *(chái hú)* 10g, Gentianae Radix *(lóng dǎn cǎo)* 6-10g, and Ostreae Concha *(mǔ lì)* 15-30g. If you only use one or two, or you add a number of other medicinal substances, the effect will be diminished or will disappear altogether.

I have used this formula for many years and my experience has taught me that while, in general, this formula is quite effective, its effect in patients with deficiency cold, biliary reflux gastritis, or depression is far from ideal.

PHYSICIAN A   What is the approximate rate of efficacy of this formula?

DR. YU   In the appropriate cases, this formula will help about 80-90% of patients. Sadly, the opportunities to use this formula alone are few, since, as we discussed, simple cases of bitter taste in the mouth are rare. Also, my experience has taught me that while in general this formula is quite effective, it does not appear to be very useful in patients with underlying deficiency cold as well as those who suffer from biliary reflux gastritis or depression.

PHYSICIAN C   Although it is true that unadorned cases of bitter taste in the mouth are rare, the symptom of bitter taste shows up as a symptom in many different types of disorders. How should we think about that?

DR. YU   This is because the Gallbladder is yang wood, and the ministerial fire, which is contained within the Gallbladder, is distributed throughout the entire body. The other eleven organs receive this fire from the Gallbladder in order to live and thrive. As the *Yellow Emperor's Inner Classic (Huáng Dì nèi jīng)* states, "All eleven organs depend on the Gallbladder." Conversely, disease of any of the other eleven organs can impact the Gallbladder. Thus, bitter taste in the mouth, one of the principal symptoms of Gallbladder disease, can occur in many different disorders.

PHYSICIAN B   There are a lot of new ideas in this statement. Can you make it a bit more concrete for me?

DR. YU   Because the Liver and the Gallbladder are directly connected, Liver disease most readily affects the Gallbladder, and thus many patients with Liver disease complain of bitter taste in the mouth. In other cases, such as accumulation of damp-heat in the Spleen and Stomach, Heart fire flaring upward, Kidney fire flushing upward, or accumulation of Lung heat, once the heat impacts the Gallbladder, it will give rise to a bitter taste. These cases all belong to excess heat, which is easier to explain.

However, in the second case above, which pertains to Spleen-Stomach deficiency cold, the appearance of bitter taste in the mouth is due to the presence of constrained heat in both the Liver and Gallbladder. This situation is harder to explain and more readily leads to confusion.

Zhang Jing-Yue explained:

> When there is excessive thinking, overwork, or excessive sexual desire, there will often be a pattern of bitter taste in the mouth, dry mouth, and [the symptom of] food lacking taste. If the fault is not primarily with the Heart and Spleen, then it is with the Liver and Kidneys. When the Heart and Spleen are deficient, the qi of the Liver and Gallbladder overflows; this leads to a bitter taste in the mouth. When the Liver and Kidneys are deficient, the true yin is insufficient and this produces dry mouth.

This passage is actually describing the complex situation in which deficiency of either Heart and Spleen or Liver and Kidneys impacts the Gallbladder.

PHYSICIAN B   You like to use Bupleuri Radix *(chái hú)*, Gentianae Radix *(lóng dǎn cǎo)*, and Ostreae Concha *(mǔ lì)* to treat bitter taste in the mouth. Are there any other herbs that you like to use for this symptom?

DR. YU   From a theoretical perspective, any herb that clears and directs downward or restrains Gallbladder fire should be useful in the treatment of bitter taste in the mouth. Examples of these herbs include Artemisiae annuae Herba *(qīng hāo)*, Scutellariae Radix *(huáng qín)*, Bambusae Caulis in taeniam *(zhú rú)*, Indigo naturalis *(qīng dài)*, Artemisiae scopariae Herba *(yīn chén)*, Gardeniae Fructus *(zhī zǐ)*, Arisaema cum Bile *(dǎn nán xīng)*, and Pig Bile *(zhū dǎn zhī)*.

However, when encountering a bitter taste in the mouth, it is important to think carefully. Is the symptom a direct result of Gallbladder disease or is it the result of some other disease process impacting the Gallbladder? You should not solely clear heat in every case.

One example to consider is stomach pain that is accompanied by bitter taste. If Gallbladder fire is accosting the Stomach, use Left Metal Pill *(zuǒ jīn wán)*. If phlegm-dampness has transformed to heat, use Warm Gallbladder Decoction *(wēn dǎn tāng)* as the primary formula. Where the root is Liver-Kidney yin deficiency, use Enrich Water and Clear the Liver Drink *(zī shuǐ qīng gān yǐn)* as the primary formula. For Spleen-Stomach deficiency cold that is accompanied by Liver-Gallbladder constrained heat, use warming herbs to treat the deficiency cold and add a small amount of Coptidis Rhizoma *(huáng lián)*, as in Regulating Decoction with Coptis *(lián lǐ tāng)*. In summary, we should "pay attention to the pathodynamic and determine to which one each [case] belongs." Only then can we select the proper herbs and formulas.

I recall the case of a woman in her 40s who complained of a bitter taste in the mouth for six months. She had taken ten vials of Gentian Pill to Drain the Liver *(lóng dǎn xiè gān wán)*, which not only had no effect on the bitter taste, but also seemed to have caused dry mouth and constipation. Her tongue was pale red with a scanty, dry coating. Her pulse was wiry, sunken, and fine. I considered this to be a case of yin deficiency with Liver constraint. I gave her Linking Decoction *(yī guàn jiān)* combined with Frigid Extremities Powder *(sì nì sǎn)* to which I added dry-fried Cassiae Semen *(chǎo jué míng zǐ)* and wine-prepared Cistanches Herba *(jiǔ cōng róng)*. After two packets, the patient's bitter taste in the mouth was greatly reduced.

PHYSICIAN B   Given what you have said, in how many situations is Bupleurum, Gentian, and Oyster Shell Decocotion *(chái dǎn mǔ lì tāng)* actually useful?

DR. YU   Bupleurum, Gentian, and Oyster Shell Decoction *(chái dǎn mǔ lì tāng)* is an excellent formula for simple cases of bitter taste in the mouth in that it is an easy, inexpensive, and proven specialty treatment.

When bitter taste in the mouth is an accompanying symptom, using this simple formula within the larger pattern-based formula is a way of getting quick resolution of this symptom.

It should also be noted that my teacher, Dr. Jian of our Chinese medicine department, achieved excellent results using this formula for chronic cholecystitis when it fit the pattern of Liver-Gallbladder constrained heat.

In fact, by combining Bupleurum, Gentian, and Oyster Shell Decoction *(chái dǎn mǔ lì tāng)* with the appropriate base formula according to pattern identification, we can expand its use to treat chronic cholecystitis. For example, if it is phlegm-heat type, combine with Warm Gallbladder Decoction with Coptis *(huáng lián wēn dǎn tāng)*; for damp-heat type, pair it with Three-Seed Decoction *(sān rén tāng)*; for qi-constraint type, prescribe it with Bupleurum Powder to Dredge the Liver *(chái hú shū gān sǎn)*; and for Spleen-Stomach deficiency type, use it together with Six-Gentlemen Decoction plus Bupleurum and Peony *(chái sháo liù jūn zǐ tāng)*.

PHYSICIAN A   Have you used this formula to treat chronic cholecystitis?

DR. YU   Yes, I have used it frequently. For example, in February, 1983, I treated a 45-year-old woman named Zhao in Liaocheng, Shandong. She complained of right-sided upper abdominal distending pain that radiated to the shoulder and back. This symptom had persisted for 11 years and was accompanied by bitter taste in the mouth, belching, and indefinable epigastric discomfort. Her symptoms were exacerbated by the intake of oily, greasy foods, as well as by excessive thinking or anger. Her tongue was slightly red with a thin, yellow coating. Her pulse was wiry and rapid. She was diagnosed by x-ray with chronic cholecystitis. Although she had been treated with combined Chinese-Western medicine, the results had been unsatisfactory.

I considered that she had constrained heat in the Liver and Gallbladder and gave her an unmodified Bupleurum, Gentian, and Oyster Shell Decoction *(chái dǎn mǔ lì tāng)*. After six packets, she reported that the abdominal discomfort had signficiantly diminished and that the bitter taste in the mouth was gone. However, she also reported slightly loose stools, a bland taste in the mouth, poor appetite, and fatigue. I determined that the constrained heat in the Liver and Gallbladder was accompanied by deficiency of the Spleen and Stomach, so I gave her the same formula with Six-Gentlemen Decoction plus Bupleurum and Peony *(chái sháo liù jūn zǐ tāng)* plus Astragali Radix *(huáng qí)*. After 30 packets (one packet for two days), all of her symptoms had resolved. An ultrasound at that point showed no abnormalities in her gallbladder. I spoke to her again in 1986 and she had remained free of disease.

Over the years, as I have used Bupleurum, Gentian, and Oyster Shell Decoction *(chái dǎn mǔ lì tāng)* in conjunction with the appropriate pattern-based formula for chronic cholecystitis, the first symptom to resolve is often the bitter taste in the mouth. As I continue to use the formula to treat this symptom that is associated with other disease presentations, I have seen a very high efficacy rate. Thus, I have come to regard this formula as a proven specialty treatment for bitter taste in the mouth. As Xu Gan, the poet and philosopher who was a contemporary of Zhang Zhong Jing, wrote, "Nothing is more precious than experience; no words are more disposable than those not based on evidence." I hope that everyone can continue to advance the clinical applications of, and experiences with, this formula.

CHAPTER 5

Kidney System Disorders

5.1 Urinary tract stones

Urinary tract stones for a year

The origins of a "thousand-year flaw"

千載之缺憾,怎樣造成

■ CASE HISTORY

Patient: *45-year-old woman*

The patient presented with a one-year history of dull pain in her right lower back and abdominal regions, and sporadic dribbling urination. Numerous tests showed 1+ red blood cells and protein in her urine. An ultrasound revealed a single calculus in the upper end of her right ureter that was approximately 0.2 x 0.5cm.

In earlier attempts to treat her condition the patient had taken over 40 packets of various Chinese herbal formulas. Among these were formulas that unblock painful urinary dribbling and ones that invigorate the blood and transform stasis, soften hardness, and disperse knots. However, not only was the calculus not excreted, but her lower back pain increased and she began to gradually lose weight, eventually becoming emaciated. At that point she was afraid to continue taking Chinese herbs.

During the course of treatment, some of the doctors she had consulted appraised her situation differently and also included in her formulas herbs to tonify qi and nourish blood, such as Ginseng Radix *(rén shēn)*, or those that tonify the Kidneys and replenish essence. However, owing to the unpleasant side effects of each of the formulas, the patient stopped taking the herbs. This situation brought her to my clinic.

Intake Examination
DATE: September 5, 1986

The patient had a dull ache on the right side of her lower back and abdomen. Her urine was slightly yellow and her urination was mildly painful, rough, and dribbling. Her accompanying symptoms included reduced food intake, shortness of breath, weakness, dizziness, and tinnitus. Her tongue was pale and her pulse was sunken and frail.

Differentiation of Pattern and Discussion of Treatment

PHYSICIAN A   Urinary stones, called stony painful urinary dribbling (石淋 shí lín) in Chinese medicine, are generally treated with herbs that unblock painful urinary dribbling and expel stones. In severe cases these methods can be combined with agents to invigorate blood and transform stasis as well as those that soften hardness and dissipate knots. However, after taking 40 packets of herbs, not only were this patient's symptoms unresolved but she had become emaciated and weak, an indication that she was becoming more deficient. Although some of the formulas given to this woman contained tonifying herbs, even they caused side effects, leading the patient to stop treatment. It seems to me that, in this case, simultaneously attacking and tonifying was not the optimal approach.

DR. YU   Based on my experience, the primary symptom of patients with Kidney deficiency and urinary stones is a dull pain, or soreness, in the lower back and abdomen. Other symptoms include weakness in the legs and knees, and mental and physical fatigue. Some patients may also experience rough and painful urination, bloody or cloudy urine, and have a proximal pulse that lacks strength when strong pressure is applied.

These symptoms reflect deficiency of Kidney essence, or in this woman's case, exhaustion and damage of Kidney qi caused by long-term use of herbs that unblock painful urinary dribbling and expel stones. The appropriate treatment here is to secure the root by warming and tonifying Kidney qi, while enriching the Kidneys and fortifying essence. However, in cases where the formation of stones and chronic stagnation lead to the obstruction of collateral vessels, the inclusion of herbs to transform stasis and unblock the orifices will help to disperse and dispel stones.

Treatment and Outcome

With a preliminary diagnosis of Kidney deficiency urinary stones, I chose to modify a formula from the famous 12th-century physician Liu He-Jian called Roasted Kidney Pill (wēi shèn wǎn):

Eucommiae Cortex (dù zhòng)...12g
wine-prepared Cistanches Herba (jiǔ cōng róng)..........................15g
Morindae officinalis Radix (bā jǐ tiān) [with the center removed].........12g
Rehmanniae Radix preparata (shú dì huáng)..............................30g
Juglandis Semen (hé táo rén)...30g
Achyranthis bidentatae Radix (niú xi)....................................12g
Astragali Radix (huáng qí)..20g
Angelicae sinensis Radix (dāng guī).......................................6g

Manitis Squama slices *(chuān shān jiǎ)*[1] 6g
Vaccariae Semen *(wáng bù liú xíng)* 15g
Lysimachiae Herba *(jīn qián cǎo)* 15g
Lygodii Spora *(hǎi jīn shā)* [wrapped] 10g

Instructions: The patient was given six packets of the formula.

The patient returned the next day and reported that after only one dose of the decoction she had to stop because, about 30 minutes after taking it, she began experiencing roaring tinnitus. She also felt dizzy, as if she were about to fall, a sensation of qi flowing from her lower back and abdomen down toward the lower abdomen, and increased lower back pain. This was followed immediately by a feeling that things were blurry with disorientation that made it difficult to feel in control of herself. These symptoms lasted about 20 minutes. Thinking that perhaps there was some mistake with the formula, she was wary of taking any more and brought the remaining five packets back for me to check.

Even though this patient's reaction couldn't be predicted, the side effects she encountered can easily be understood using the theories of Chinese medicine. I decided to remove all the ingredients that transform stasis and unblock the orifices, so that only the following herbs were left (using the same dosage as in the formula above):

Eucommiae Cortex *(dù zhòng)* 12g
wine-prepared Cistanches Herba *(jiǔ cōng róng)* 15g
Morindae officinalis Radix *(bā jǐ tiān)* 15g
Rehmanniae Radix preparata *(shú dì huáng)* 30g
Juglandis Semen *(hé táo rén)* 30g
Astragali Radix *(huáng qí)* 20g
Angelicae sinensis Radix *(dāng guī)* 6g

After taking five packets of the modified formula the patient reported a decrease in lower back and abdominal pain and no side effects.

It has been said that "when the results are good, don't change the formula." The patient continued with 30 more packets of herbs, resulting in the resolution of her lower back and abdominal pain. Meanwhile, she also developed a healthy appetite and her energy returned to normal.

Although the patient didn't notice any passing of stones, a B-ultrasound failed to find any signs of calculi, and tests for red blood cells and protein in the urine were negative.

On follow-up six years later, she had continued to be in good health.

PHYSICIAN A   Dr. Yu, in my view, your diagnosis of urinary stones with Kidney deficiency was accurate and your combination of herbs to warm the Kidneys, boost qi, enrich the Kidneys and fortify essence with herbs to transform stasis and unblock the orifices was meticulously chosen. Thus, it came as a great surprise when the treatment caused side effects.

DR. YU   This is what's called "a mistake of the smallest kind can lead to a loss of great magnitude." However, in my years of treating urinary stones with Kidney deficiency,

....
1. *Translators' note:* Due to its designation as an endangered species, this substance is no longer available. Dr. Yu suggests increasing the amount of Vaccariae Semen *(wáng bù liú xíng)* to make up for the absence of this substance.

Disease	Primary Symptoms	Pattern	Treatment Method	Formula
Painful urinary dribbling syndrome (urinary stones)	Dull pain in the lower back and abdomen, dribbling urine	Kidney qi deficiency, depleted Kidney essence	Warm and tonify Kidney qi, enrich the Kidneys and fortify essence	Roasted Kidney Pill (wēi shèn wǎn) with modifications

this is the only case where I was unable to include herbs that transform stasis and unblock the orifices.

PHYSICIAN B   One case seems insufficient to be instructive. Can you give us a general protocol for treating Kidney-deficiency urinary stones?

DR. YU   For this disorder I often use the formula I used in this case, Roasted Kidney Pill *(wēi shèn wǎn)*. If the patient suffers from Kidney yin deficiency, with chest irritability, feeling hot at night, a tender, red tongue with no coating, and a pulse that is fine, rapid, and forceless, I remove Astragali Radix *(huáng qí)* and Angelicae sinensis Radix *(dāng guī)* and add Rehmanniae Radix *(shēng dì huáng)* and Two-Solstice Pill *(èr zhì wán)*. If the patient tends toward yang deficiency, with symptoms of chills, urinary frequency, an enlarged and pale tongue with teeth marks, and a pulse that is sunken, slow, and forceless, I add Cervi Cornu degelatinatum *(lù jiǎo shuāng)* and Psoraleae Fructus *(bǔ gǔ zhī)*. If the patient's chills are severe, I include Cinnamomi Cortex *(ròu guì)* and Aconiti Radix lateralis preparata *(zhì fù zǐ)*, removing them once this symptom has been alleviated.

If the patient has blood in the urine, I include Succinum *(hǔ pò)* powder and Notoginseng Radix *(sān qī)* powder, mixed into the hot decoction. In cases where the patient's urine is cloudy, I add Dioscoreae hypoglaucae Rhizoma *(bì xiè)* and Acori tatarinowii Rhizoma *(shí chāng pú)*. When there is pain on the lower abdomen, I often combine Roasted Kidney Pill *(wēi shèn wǎn)* with Peony and Licorice Decoction *(sháo yào gān cǎo tāng)*. If, during the period when the patient is taking herbs, the abdominal and lower back pain increases and they have pain radiating from these areas down to the lower abdomen, this indicates that the stone is moving downward and a large dose of Peony and Licorice Decoction *(sháo yào gān cǎo tāng)* can be used to relax tension and alleviate pain. At the same time one can help the body to guide the urinary stone downward and expel it by combining Peony and Licorice Decoction *(sháo yào gān cǎo tāng)* with Rhei Radix et Rhizoma *(dà huáng)* to guide downward and expel the urinary stones. Fortifying essence and boosting qi should be the primary treatment method, while transforming stasis and unblocking the orifices can be thought of as adjunctive. This approach is invariably effective for the treatment of Kidney-deficiency urinary stones.

Note that when treating urinary stones in people with Kidney deficiency it can be extremely difficult to clearly distinguish whether the patient leans toward yang deficiency or yin deficiency. Therefore, when writing a formula, one should not create a prescription that is skewed too strongly toward one or the other. Avoid making a formula that is overly warm and drying, which may damage the yin, or a formula that is overly enriching of yin, which may damage the yang. A formula based on fortifying essence and boosting qi along with a balanced tonification of yin and yang provides a solid foundation. A balanced formula is one to which, after a careful examination of the patient's signs and symptoms, herbs for warming yang or enriching yin can be added, as noted above. The goal of treatment is to gradually balance and stabilize yin and yang, allowing the body to recover its innate ability for self-regulation. In this way the formula can be beneficial for eliminating and preventing stones.

PHYSICIAN C Over the past ten or more years there has been an occasional article about using Kidney tonification to effectively treat urinary stones, but the protocol for treatment of this pattern is still in the exploratory phase. How did you gain such insight into this issue?

DR. YU I wouldn't go so far as to say that I have had any special insights. Instead, it has been more a matter of studying modern masters and putting their approaches into practice. Looking back at the 1950s, most doctors were consistently following the treatment principle of clearing heat, eliminating dampness, unblocking painful urinary dribbling, and expelling stones. It was difficult to find anyone whose treatments went beyond the bounds of convention, and patient recovery rates were very low. Not until the 1960s, when people began to use herbs to invigorate blood, transform stasis, soften hardness, and dissipate nodules, did results begin to markedly improve. Nevertheless, people with constitutional deficiencies (particularly those with diminished renal function due to hydronephrosis and hydroureter) often cannot tolerate the use of attacking agents, and for them, calculi within the urinary system are often not expelled. As treatment progresses the kidneys grow weaker and their condition worsens. These methods were popular for years and the results were mixed. It wasn't until the 1970s that people realized it was time to change tactics. Finally, like a beacon of light, an experiment conducted at the Shanghai No. 1 Medical College's Huashan Hospital shed light on the matter. Researchers used two different methods to treat hydronephrosis due to obstructing urinary stones.

The two methods they employed were that of Kidney tonification and that of separation and draining. Each group consisted of 12 subjects of similar age with stones of similar location and size. The group given Kidney tonification was prescribed the following herbs:

Dipsaci Radix *(xù duàn)*
Taxilli Herba *(sāng jì shēng)*
Ligustri lucidi Fructus *(nǚ zhēn zǐ)*
Ecliptae Herba *(mò hàn lián)*
Rehmanniae Radix *(shēng dì huáng)*
Psoraleae Fructus *(bǔ gǔ zhi)*
Epimedii Herba *(yín yáng huò)*
Morindae officinalis Radix *(bā jǐ tiān)*
wine-prepared Cistanches Herba *(jiǔ cōng róng)*
Juglandis Semen *(hé táo rén)*

The result showed that in the patients receiving the Kidney-tonifying formula, the overall excretory functions of the subject's kidneys as well as their ability to expel stones was superior to those treated with herbs that separate and drain.

I have found other examples of this approach in recent medical journals. The approach of a Dr. Lu is another example of the tonifying principle. He was deeply impressed by the case of a patient who began to experience kidney failure after more than one month of treatment with a formula called Stone Expulsion Decoction *(pái shí tāng)*. It was an example of how using just the attacking method can severely exhaust the normal qi. As a result, when treating urinary stones in patients with Spleen and Kidney yang deficiency (especially those with Kidney deficiency), he included a large dosage of Cervi Cornu degelatinatum *(lù jiǎo shuāng)* to warm the Kidneys and strengthen yang along with herbs that expel stones, invigorate blood, transform stasis, and unblock the collaterals. The usefulness of this formula was later confirmed by another study conducted with 12 subjects, all of whom fully recovered.

Another example is that of a Dr. Wang and his colleagues who used a formula called Cervi Gold Drink *(lù jīn yǐn),* which contains the following ingredients:

Cervi Cornu degelatinatum *(lù jiǎo shuāng)*............................ 30-60g
Lysimachiae Herba *(jin qián cǎo)*.. 30g
Malvae Fructus *(dōng kuí guô)* 30g
Lygodii Spora *(hǎi jin shā)*... 30g
Talcum *(huá shí)*.. 20g
Succinum *(hǔ pò)* 6g
Plantaginis Semen *(chē qián zǐ)*.. 10g
Pyrrosiae Folium *(shí wéi)*.. 10g
Polygoni avicularis Herba *(biǎn xù)*...................................... 10g

The test included 46 subjects with urinary stones, and had an efficacy rate of 82.6%. Because there is no record, past or present, mentioning the calculi expelling or dissolving properties of Cervi Cornu degelatinatum *(lù jiǎo shuāng),* the doctors in this study decided to observe what happened if they eliminated it from the formula. Surprisingly, none of the test subjects expelled their stones. There are many other similar examples of this which I won't discuss now, but summarizing more than ten years of clinical reports I can say that Kidney tonification is a very effective method for eliminating urinary stones in patients with Kidney deficiency. In addition, for those with minimal signs of Kidney deficiency, or those with urinary stones not due to Kidney deficiency, the addition of one or two herbs to tonify the Kidneys will increase the efficacy of the formula. You may wonder why this is beneficial. According to preliminary research, herbs that tonify the Kidneys, whether it be those that warm the Kidneys and boost qi or those that enrich the Kidneys and fortify essence, are able to stimulate Kidney qi, promote improved renal function, and strengthen peristalsis in the renal pelvis and ureter. Improvement in these functions then helps to reduce hydronephrosis and push the stones downward and out of the urinary tract. Additionally, specific Kidney-tonifying herbs such as Juglandis Semen *(hé táo rén)* have some ability to dissolve stones.

PHYSICIAN D   Dr. Yu, you have referenced modern "sages" but why haven't you referenced the ancient sages?

It seems to me that when treating urinary stones with Chinese medicine, of first and foremost importance is the process of studying the legacy of our tradition and drawing on the experience of our predecessors. The ancient physicians certainly had abundant experience in treating stony painful urinary dribbling. Prior to the Tang dynasty, physicians had already made the observation that there were various patterns associated with painful urinary dribbling, each with its own unique characteristics. In addition to the general symptoms of dribbling and painful urination, increased urinary frequency, and pain that reaches from the lower abdomen to the navel, stony painful urinary dribbling is characterized by the expulsion of pebble-like stones in the urine. Another example is that of Zhang Zhong-Jing's description in Chapter 13 of the *Essentials from the Golden Cabinet (Jīn guì yào lüè)* of "millet-like urine." Further, the *Treasury Classic (Zhōng cáng jīng)*, attributed to Hua Tuo, not only describes "sand and pebble like [substances] expelled with urine," but also surmises that "the formation of small stones comes from damage to the normal qi and the gradual deepening and accumulation of pathogenic heat." The author also provides a vivid analogy: "as with boiling water becoming salty if the flame is too high and there is not enough water, the salt will gradually form stones." As early as the Sui dynasty (6th century), Chao Yuan-Fang maintained that the deficiency and heat that leads to stones is specifically the result of "Kidney deficiency and Bladder heat."

For thousands of years these ideas have been the final word in later generations' understanding of the location and basic pathodynamic of stony painful urinary dribbling. For more than a thousand years since then no one has put forth any different ideas. It seems then that the fundamental treatment method would be to tonify Kidney deficiency and clear Bladder heat. How is it, then, that you give all the credit for insight into this illness to modern physicians?

DR YU It sounds as if I am under suspicion of forgetting my roots. It is worth repeating that Chinese medicine seeks consistency and synthesis within the structure of principles, strategies, formulas, and medicinal substances. If it is, as you say, that the pathodynamic is Kidney deficiency and Bladder heat (principle), then it must be that the fundamental treatment strategy should be to tonify Kidney deficiency and clear Bladder heat. If this is the case, then what formula and substances would best represent this method?

Looking at the medical literature we see that the first recorded formulas for treatment of stony painful urinary dribbling are found in the Tang-dynasty works *Important Formulas Worth a Thousand Gold Pieces (Qiān jīn yào fāng)* and *Arcane Essentials from the Imperial Library (Wài tái mì yào)*. The formulas therein consist of substances that clear heat, resolve dampness, unblock painful, dribbling urination, and expel stones. It is here that we find that the specific formulas and herbs employed reflect the beginnings of a divide between what had previously been assumed (in the Sui dynasty and before) to be the pathodynamic, and the treatment method applied. Later generations didn't concern themselves much with Kidney deficiency and instead chose the principles of clearing heat, resolving dampness, unblocking painful urinary dribbling, and expelling stones as the foundation of their treatments. Of course, each generation produces its own outstanding talent, and physicians who were able to shake off conventions were not uncommon. Examples include the Song-dynasty physician Chen Wu-Ze and his combination of Astragali Radix *(huáng qí)*, Ginseng Radix *(rén shēn)*, and fresh daikon to treat the five types of painful urinary dribbling with stones and unbearable pain; the Qing-dynasty physician You Zai-Jing who advocated the use of herbs that release constraint, move qi, break up blood stasis, and enrich yin; and the modern master Zhang Xi-Chun who combined agents that soften hardness and disperse knots with those that tonify qi and enrich yin.

Even though such ideas rectified errors and inspired new ways of approaching treatment, there was still a discontinuity between the general principle for addressing the pathodynamics of stony painful urinary dribbling and the formulas and herbs used to treat it. This has continued through a thousand years of medical history. So you can see that despite attributing the idea of treating urethral stones by tonifying the Kidneys to modern sages, I am in no way guilty of forgetting my roots.

PHYSICIAN A   Thank you. Your explanation has helped to resolve my confusion and given me a whole new perspective. Nevertheless, I am still not clear about one thing. This historical division you speak of as a "thousand-year flaw" between the overall treatment principle for stony painful urinary dribbling and the formulas and herbs that have been used historically to treat it—how did it come about?

DR. YU   We cannot blame the ancients for this inconsistency. Based on the primary symptoms described in the literature, we can presume that what was in prior times referred to as stony painful urinary dribbling is probably close to what is now termed bladder or urethral calculi. These disorders most commonly involve accumulation of damp-heat. Even though Kidney deficiency may be at the root of urinary stones, this underlying pattern is often not pronounced. Chinese medicine emphasizes treatment based on pattern differentiation, indicated by the principle "observe the pulse and symptoms and treat with the appropriate method." So in a case of damp-heat accumulation in the Bladder, treatment should be directed primarily at damp-heat, while treatment of the underlying Kidney deficiency can be ancillary or addressed later.

In the modern clinic, the common treatment for stones in the bladder or urethra is also to clear heat, dispel dampness, unblock painful urinary dribbling, and expel stones. This is frequently effective. As Chinese medicine is handed down from generation to generation we should build on this basis and continue to improve upon and develop the knowledge passed down to us.

PHYSICIAN A   Based on what you say, it is not possible to equate the problem of urinary stones to what the ancients called stony painful urinary dribbling.

DR. YU   That's correct! The modern term urinary stones refers not only to calculi in the bladder and urethra, but also those within the kidney and ureter. The primary symptoms of acute stage kidney or ureter stones (when the movement of the stones is most apparent) include renal colic and hematuria. During the chronic stage (when there is much less movement of stones) the primary symptoms include lower back pain or intense pain upon fist percussion to the area around the kidneys. Patients may report excreting stones in their urine, but this is not considered a necessary symptom for diagnosis of urinary stones. These symptoms are very different than those indicated for stony painful urinary dribbling. How can we call them the same disease? Consequently, how can we justify using the same treatment principles as those used for stony painful urinary dribbling?

The lower back pain associated with chronic stones in the kidneys or ureter is usually a dull pain, or soreness, which is a clear sign of Kidney qi depletion. If there is concern that tonifying the Kidneys won't be effective, then there should be even more concern in using herbs to clear heat, resolve dampness, resolve painful urinary dribbling, and expel stones.

From a different perspective, there is a long history of discourse on the topic of lower back pain due to Kidney deficiency as well as an incredible abundance of clinical experience in its treatment. Nevertheless, the ancients were unable to thoroughly understand the basic pathology of calculi in the urinary tract. This lack of understanding led to further misconceptions along the road of history, even to this day. Such misconceptions can be attributed to the limited level of scientific understanding of the times, and differences between the theoretical systems of Chinese and modern medicine.

As the famous rustic poet Tao Qian wrote about seventeen-hundred years ago, "You can't argue with what's been done, but I know the future's there to be sought." Why is it that modern practitioners, when treating urinary stones, feel the need to match a modern disease name with one from Chinese medicine or to force a match when none exists? At the same time, why do they refuse to include the method of Kidney tonification in their therapeutic armamentarium?

PHYSICIAN B   Despite the fact that Kidney tonification may be useful for treating urinary stones, it seems there is less and less need for Chinese medicine therapy because of modern methods for treating stones, such as surgery or extracorporeal shock wave lithotripsy.

DR. YU   This is the law of natural selection. Those who adapt survive and those who do not are eliminated.

Nevertheless, these methods cannot replace the unique benefits and advantages of Chinese medicine's approach. We must be careful to neither stand still complacently and refuse to make progress nor to underestimate our abilities. By weeding through the chaff to bring forth the new we will be completely up to this challenge.

5.2 **Impotence**

Erectile dysfunction

The essence of the saying, "Commoners go with the flow, immortals go against it."

"順則凡，逆則仙"的真諦

■ CASE HISTORY

Patient: *35-year-old man*

One year prior to coming to the hospital the patient returned from a business trip and found that although he strived to make love with his wife, he was only able to achieve a weak erection. He attributed the problem to fatigue, but when the situation repeated itself the following day he privately blamed himself. His wife also chided him.

He tried some over-the-counter patent medicines, one called Male Treasure and the other, Masculine Lion Pill. He took these for one month, but after finding them ineffective, sought the help of a doctor.

The physician diagnosed the patient with Kidney deficiency and prescribed a modification of Restore the Right [Kidney] Pill *(yòu guī wán)*. The patient took ten packages of the formula and then sought another doctor because he failed to see any improvement. The second doctor diagnosed qi deficiency with Liver constraint and prescribed a modification of Tonify the Middle to Augment the Qi Decoction *(bǔ zhōng yì qì tāng)* combined with Rambling Powder *(xiāo yáo sǎn)*. Ten packets of the formula only slightly improved his condition.

Seeking better results, he found an experienced doctor at a private clinic through the recommendation of a friend. Despite spending a great deal of money and taking herbs (the herbs were not disclosed) for almost six months, the patient still had difficulty achieving a firm erection and at times was completely unable to do so. He remembered the promotional poster that hung over this doctor's clinic door that read, "Secret family recipe for treating male impotence, 100% effective!" and a large calligraphic sign inside that stated, "With miraculous and rejuvenating cures, Hua Tuo is again in this world." This increased his concern that his case was hopeless. His wife was also extremely worried, and when the patient decided to consult me, she made a point of accompanying him.

Intake Examination
DATE: March 16, 1986

The patient's affect was depressed. His symptoms included lumbosacral aches and pain as well as periodic discomfort in the chest and lateral costal regions. His tongue was normal and his pulse was wiry and fine.

Differentiation of Patterns and Discussion of Treatment

PHYSICIAN A   In the many discussions of impotence (literally, 'yang wilting' 陽痿 *yáng wěi)* throughout history, most physicians have emphasized the cause as deficiency impairment of essence-qi. The Ming-dynasty physician Zhang Jing-Yue was even more explicit when he established the theory of Kidney yang deficiency:

> When men have impotence and failure to achieve erection, this is most commonly due to debilitated fire at the gate of vitality. ... Those with debilitated fire account for seven to eight [cases out] of ten, while those [cases] with abundant fire are seldom seen.

In this instance the patient had been taking Kidney-warming, yang-invigorating formulas for quite some time with no positive results. This shows that the patient's problem was not one of debilitated fire. When he took formulas that tonified qi and dredged the Liver, however, he began to see some improvement. This indicates the involvement of Liver constraint.

My question is, how do we diagnose erectile dysfunction due to Liver constraint?

DR. YU   When a patient with impotence doesn't have any obvious signs of Kidney deficiency, damp-heat, blood stasis or phlegm stasis, it is important to get a detailed patient history. This history should include lifestyle, overall health, relationship status, and, in particular, their sexual activity. This, taken into account with their accompanying symptoms and tongue and pulse, should provide enough information to determine whether or not Liver constraint is a major or attendant cause of the disorder.

In this case the patient had just come home from a business trip and, despite being exhausted, mustered what energy he could to be intimate with his wife, only to be unable to maintain a firm erection. He would have been wise to have rested for a few days and allow his primal qi to recover, but the patient was not one to take care of himself and he also lacked basic knowledge about sexual health. This, coupled with his wife's chiding, led to the emotional stress which was the origin of his Liver constraint. What followed was an extended period of ineffective treatments that caused him to become increasingly worried and anxious. When the patient came in to see me he was depressed, had discomfort in his chest and lateral costal regions, a normal tongue, and a pulse that was fine and wiry. How could this be other than Liver constraint?

The patient's lumbosacral aches and pain were a manifestation of Liver constraint that had then affected the Kidneys, leading to the Kidney qi becoming both deficient and stopped up.

Because the patient's condition was due to a combination of pathodynamics, the best course of action was to use a combination of treatment methods: soothe Liver constraint, unjam the Kidneys, and tonify Kidney deficiency.

Treatment and Outcome

We considered this to be constrained Liver qi, failed dredging function, and deficient and jammed Kidney qi and so decided to use a modification of Settle the Menses Decoction (*dìng jīng tāng*) from *Fu Qing-Zhu's Women's Disorders* (*Fù Qīng-Zhǔ nǚ kē*) as follows:

> wine-fried Cuscutae Semen *(jiǔ chǎo tù sī zǐ)* 30g
> wine-fried Paeoniae Radix alba *(jiǔ chǎo bái sháo)* 30g
> wine-washed Angelicae sinensis Radix *(jiǔ xī dāng guī)* 30g
> Rehmanniae Radix preparata *(shú dì huáng)* 15g
> Morindae officinalis Radix *(bā jǐ tiān)* 15g
> Poria *(fú líng)* 10g
> Bupleuri Radix *(chái hú)* 10g
> Tribuli Fructus *(cì jí lí)* 10g
> bran-fried Aurantii Fructus *(fū chǎo zhǐ ké)* 10g
> Glycyrrhizae Radix *(gān cǎo)* 5g
> Scolopendra *(wú gōng)* [roasted until crisp, ground into
>   a powder with one-half of the powder taken with each
>   dose of the strained decoction] .... 1 piece
>   (approximately 8cm long, head and legs left on)

In order to gain the confidence of the patient and ensure him that his condition was treatable, I explained the cause and pathology of his condition, as well as how the formula was composed. I also urged his wife to be supportive of her husband and to have patience because results may not come as quickly as she would like.

After taking three packets of the formula the patient was able to achieve mildly firm erections.

Since the formula seemed effective we didn't alter it, except to prescribe it in powder form. The patient was prescribed six packets of the formula to be roasted over a low flame until crisp and then ground into a fine powder. Ten grams of the powder were to be taken three times each day, washed down with warm water.

After one month of taking this formula the patient was healthy and enjoying a satisfying sex life.

Six months later he came in to our clinic be treated for an unrelated condition and said that his erectile dysfunction problems had not returned.

Disease	Primary Symptoms	Differential Diagnosis	Treatment Method	Formula
Impotence	Erectile dysfunction, depression, lumbo-sacral aches and pains	Liver qi constraint leading to an inability to dredge properly, jammed and deficient Kidneys	Soothe Liver constraint, unjam the Kidneys, tonify Kidney deficiency	Settle the Menses Decoction (dìng jīng tāng)

Reflections and Clarifications

PHYSICIAN B   Dr. Yu, your consideration of Liver constraint as a primary pathology involved in impotence is something the ancients have overlooked. Modern textbooks on Chinese medicine have also omitted Liver constraint when discussing the possible etiology and pathodynamics of impotence. The spectrum of potential pathologies included in textbooks is limited to debilitated fire at the gate of fire, Heart and Spleen impairment, fear injuring the Kidneys, and downward pouring of damp-heat.

DR. YU   Treatment of the Liver for impotence has a theoretical foundation in the *Inner Classic (Néi jīng)*. Chapter 10 of the *Divine Pivot (Líng shū)* states that "The vessel of Liver leg *jué yīn* … follows the thigh, enters the [pubic] hair and passes by the genitals." Zhang Jing-Yue said that the Liver "links to all sinews and unites them, allowing them to be utilized for robust movement." The male genitals are classified as belonging to the sinews and thus are governed by the Liver.

It does appear, however, that physicians prior to the Ming dynasty did overlook Liver constraint when discussing the patterns, causes, diagnosis, and treatment of impotence. The Qing-dynasty physician Shen Jin-Ao, who was particularly skilled at the inquiry aspect of examination, revealed this secret:

> also if ejaculation is done improperly, or if restraint is engaged in, this can damage the sinew convergence … or those who are despondent or depressed, these damage the Liver and Liver/wood becomes unable to thrust outward properly, this also leads to yin wilting [which is another name for impotence] and an inability to achieve erection.

In recent years there has been an increase in the number of articles discussing the treatment of impotence from the perspective of patterns such as Liver constraint, blood stasis, and phlegm with blood stasis. These articles raise interesting ideas that merit reflection. I say this because men in China who suffer from impotence are fond of using

Kidney-warming, yang-fortifying medicinal substances. Furthermore, many patients are anxious about resolving their condition and it is quite common for them to seek out strange and exotic medicines or unusual treatments. This has been the case since antiquity. Among these are 'spring medicines' (春藥 *chūn yào*). This name is a euphemism for aphrodisiac and implies a return to youth. These help men achieve erections or promote arousal. Although such products may provide quick relief, long-term use will damage essence and blood and have deleterious effects.

Many doctors rely on expensive and rare medicinal substances for the treatment of impotence. Cervi Cornu pantotrichum *(lù róng)*, Cervi Testes et Penis *(lù biān)*, and Callorhini Testes et Penis *(hǎi gǒu shèn)* are examples. But the etiology and pathodynamics behind impotence are not limited to Kidney yang deficiency and debilitation. Furthermore, the ancient sages such as Zhang Jing-Yue have already given clear instructions on the treatment method for Kidney yang deficiency impairment: "those who are good at tonifying yang, seek yang within yin. When yang receives assistance from yin there are endless transformations."

PHYSICIAN A   Is impotence due to Liver constraint common?

DR. YU   Based on my experience over the years, I would say that a sizable percentage of impotence is owing to Liver constraint. Regrettably, the medical community in China was rather slow to engage in research on sexual health and consequently there is not a lot of available material on the subject. According to the contemporary book *Sexual Medicine* by Wu Jie-Ping, "Impotence is the most common sexual dysfunction in men." The etiology of impotence can be divided into that caused by organic changes in the body and that caused by psychological issues. Psychological impotence makes up 85-90% of all cases. In my opinion, a large portion of what Western medicine calls psychological impotence falls within the scope of what Chinese medicine identifies as impotence from Liver constraint.

PHYSICIAN A   Dr. Yu, your diagnosis was Liver qi constraint leading to an inability to dredge properly, and jammed and deficient Kidneys. You defined the problem as a compound illness and treated it very effectively in a relatively short amount of time with Settle the Menses Decoction *(dìng jīng tāng)*. This illustrates that in the clinic it is important not to have any predetermined notions and instead do your best to think outside the box and avoid hackneyed ideas. Still, the treatment method you referred to as "unjamming the Kidneys" sounds suspiciously like something you formulated just for the sake of being different.

DR. YU   Fu Qing-Zhu used this method when treating irregular menstruation and he presented a wonderful discussion of his reasoning:

> The Liver is the child of the Kidneys, so when the Liver is constrained the Kidneys are also constrained; when the Kidneys are constrained then its qi will not diffuse. [Menstruation arriving] early or late or stopping and continuing is [dependent on] free flow or obstruction of the Kidneys. Some say that when the Liver is constrained the Kidney qi does not respond. But this is not necessarily true. Those who say this do not realize the intimate relationship between a child and mother. When a child is ill, the mother will invariably respond with feelings

of care and support. When the Liver is constrained the Kidneys, like a friend, cannot but have a strong connection. This is the principle of the Kidneys being unable to have a strong connection to Liver constraint. Whether Liver qi is open or closed up, and then whether the Kidney qi leaves or stays, are intertwined and vice versa. How can there be any doubt about this? The treatment method should be one of soothing Liver constraint, which is equivalent to opening up Kidney constraint.

You see, I am in no way trying to be different for the sake of being different. I am choosing what is good and following it; transposing the treatment principles from one condition to another. One thing worth noting is that in his discussion of the relationship between Liver constraint and Kidney constraint, Fu Qing-Zhu leaves out any reference to Kidney deficiency. However, let us look at the ingredients he relied on when he created Settle the Menses Decoction *(dìng jīng tāng)*:

Cuscutae Semen *(tù sī zǐ)*	30g
Paeoniae Radix alba *(bái sháo)*	30g
Angelicae sinensis Radix *(dāng guī)*	30g
Rehmanniae Radix preparata *(shú dì huáng)*	15g
Dioscoreae Rhizoma *(shān yào)*	15g
Poria *(fú líng)*	9g
Schizonepetae Spica *(jīng jiè suì)*	6g
Bupleuri Radix *(chái hú)*	1.5g

One can see that this is actually Rambling Powder *(xiāo yáo sǎn)* with the removal of Atractylodis macrocephalae Rhizoma *(bái zhú)*, Menthae haplocalycis Herba *(bò hé)*, Zingiberis Rhizoma recens *(shēng jiāng)*, and Glycyrrhizae Radix *(gān cǎo)*, and the addition of Cuscutae Semen *(tù sī zǐ)*, Rehmanniae Radix preparata *(shú dì huáng)*, Dioscoreae Rhizoma *(shān yào)*, and Schizonepetae Spica *(jīng jiè suì)*. Fù included large dosages of herbs to tonify the Kidney and increase essence.

It would probably be beneficial to flesh out areas of the theory that Fu Qing-Zhu left unclear; that is, menstrual blood comes from the Kidneys and the root of a regular menstrual cycle is Kidneys that have abundant essence. Consequently, when soothing Liver constraint and unjamming the Kidneys, it is necessary to tonify the Kidneys and replenish the essence. When making use of Settle the Menses Decoction *(dìng jīng tāng)* to treat impotence due to Liver constraint, it is more important to emphasize this aspect of the formulation than when applying it to irregular menstruation.

PHYSICIAN C   Are you saying that those with Liver constraint impotence invariably have Kidney deficiency?

DR. YU   To say "invariably" would be an overstatement; "mostly" would be more accurate. Everyone is familiar with the statement in Chapter 8 of the *Basic Questions (Sù wèn)* that the Kidneys "hold the office of strong accomplishment and that skills and expertise issue from them." When a person's Kidney essence is abundant, the Kidney qi will flourish and the ability of "strong accomplishment" will come naturally. If simple Liver constraint leads to a one-time incidence of erectile dysfunction, once the circumstances change the person will usually recover without medical help.

Impotence becomes a serious problem in those who suffer from Liver constraint only when they have Kidney essence deficiency to begin with, or if they have an underlying "deficient root." This is the reason why, in most situations, a treatment that soothes the Liver and resolves constraint must be combined with substances to tonify the Kidneys and replenish essence.

PHYSICIAN B   If the patient has impotence with a simple pattern of Liver constraint, what formula would you use?

DR. YU   Prominent modern physicians use Bupleurum Powder to Dredge the Liver *(chái hú shū gān sǎn)* with the addition of Tribuli Fructus *(cì jí lí)*. This is an effective treatment, and if Scolopendra *(wú gōng)* is added, the results will be even more rapid.

PHYSICIAN C   What is your reason for adding Scolopendra *(wú gōng)* to the formula you gave this patient?

DR. YU   A contemporary physician, Chen Yu-Mei, developed a formula called Elixir to Overcome Wilting (抗痿靈 *kāng wěi líng*) to treat impotence. It consists of the following substances:

>   Scolopendra *(wú gōng)*
>   Angelicae sinensis Radix *(dāng guī)*
>   Paeoniae Radix alba *(bái sháo)*
>   Glycyrrhizae Radix *(gān cǎo)*

The primary medicinal substance in the formula is Scolopendra *(wú gōng)*. Based on my experience, including this item in the formula increases its efficacy.

In fact, the modification of the formula I gave the patient in this case contains the ingredients of Elixir to Overcome Wilting *(kāng wěi líng)* within it. Dr. Chen's heavy dosage of Scolopendra *(wú gōng)* to treat impotence is borrowed from the Republican-era physician Zhang Xi-Chun. Master Zhang once praised Scolopendra *(wú gōng)* by saying that "its motility and penetrating strength is most swift. Whether internally in the yin and yang organs or externally in the channels and collaterals, Scolopendra *(wú gōng)* is able to unblock any place where the qi and blood have congealed."

Dr. Chen's use of Scolopendra *(wú gōng)* to open the congestion of qi and blood in the Liver channel and quickly firm up erections is a good example of learning from one's predecessors.

PHYSICIAN B   There is one thing about which I still have a question. There must be no small number of formulas from recent and ancient history to reference when thinking about treating Liver constraint and impotence. You chose to utilize a formula from Fu Qing-Zhu that he used to treat irregular menses. I have trouble understanding why you chose a formula for women's health to treat a male disorder.

DR. YU   An essential teaching of Daoism asserts that "Commoners go with the flow, immortals go against it, only those in the middle get mixed up." There is deep meaning in these words. How can the truth be made clear in only a few words? Nevertheless, I do believe that through experience and further investigation the time will come when you have a great moment of insight.

5.3 Umbilical pain

Umbilical pain

Off by a small margin

差別就那麼一點點

■ CASE HISTORY

Patient: *58-year-old man, farmer*

The patient came to the clinic because of dull umbilical pain that had persisted for more than one month. The pain was continuous but had not increased in intensity since it began, and felt better with warmth and pressure.

The patient had, at one point, tried steaming and washing his umbilicus with a decoction of aged mugwort, Artemisiae argyi Folium *(ài yè),* and also placing fresh scallion bulbs, Allii fistulosi Bulbus *(cōng bái)* that had been pulverized with salt and warmed by dry-frying, into his navel. These techniques brought temporary relief, but the dull pain soon returned.

He had seen a doctor who gave him two packets of Mume Decoction *(wū méi tāng),* but the formula didn't bring him any relief. The doctor changed formulas, giving him two packets of Regulate the Middle Decoction plus Aconite *(fù zǐ lǐ zhōng tāng).* The patient felt some improvement at first, but after a few days the pain returned.

The patient's condition was clearly owing to a cold pattern, but why were the internal and external warming treatments inadequate? If we look closer at his case we can better understand how his problem developed. The patient described himself as a person who has long been averse to cold, and the previous autumn, while he had been caring for a citrus orchard for ten days or so, he was living in a drafty thatched cottage. While there, he frequently went outside to check on the orchard in shoes that had thin soles. He said that he had often felt chilled.

Further compounding his misery, the patient became deeply frightened one day when, owing to his inattention, a fire broke out in the cottage and burned it to the ground. Following that trauma he was bed-ridden for several days and it was then that the dull pain in his abdomen began.

INTAKE EXAMINATION
DATE: December 15, 1985

The patient had a dull complexion, frigidly cold hands and feet, borborygmus, loose stools, and a pale tongue with a white, slippery coating. His pulse was sunken and slow.

Differentiation of Pattern and Discussion of Treatment

PHYSICIAN A   Dull pain in the umbilicus is not a serious disorder and is not commonly seen. Nor is it mentioned in Chinese medicine textbooks. What makes this case difficult for me to understand is that if we look at the etiology, the nature of the illness, the patient's constitution and his tongue and pulse, it seems to be a clear case of yang deficiency of the Spleen and Kidneys. Would not Regulate the Middle Decoction plus Aconite *(fù zǐ lǐ zhōng tāng)* be an effective choice of formula?

DR. YU   The umbilicus is the location of CV-8 *(shén què)*. Pain at CV-8 *(shén què)*, referred to as umbilical pain in Chinese medical books, is within the scope of *shào yīn* abdominal pain.

The man in this case study is almost 60 years old and constitutionally fears cold. It seems obvious that he suffers from Kidney yang insufficiency. Furthermore, his working conditions, exposure to the elements, and the shock and fear he felt after the fire contributed to his development of cold hands and feet, borborygmus, loose stools, pale tongue with a white, slippery coating and a sunken, slow pulse. Added together these are clear signs of Kidney yang deficiency debilitation with cold congealing at the site of CV-8 *(shén què)*.

By looking at the symptoms of deficiency cold and examining the pulse and tongue it is easy to broadly identify a pattern of Spleen and Kidney yang deficiency. The precise location of the patient's pain, however, doesn't support that diagnosis. The abdomen is divided into sections, the area from the epigastrium to just above the umbilicus is termed the greater abdomen and is associated with *tài yīn*. In this case, the patient's pain was centered in his umbilicus, which is not part of the greater abdomen, and thus is not included, or primarily included, in the realm of the *tài yīn/* Spleen organ. Although Regulate the Middle Decoction plus Aconite *(fù zǐ lǐ zhōng tāng)* does warm and tonify both the Spleen and Kidneys, its focus is on warming and tonifying Spleen yang with a secondary goal of warming Kidney yang. The formula doesn't precisely fit with the pathodynamic in this case, and for that reason the results were subpar.

By analyzing the patient's signs and symptoms we can see that his condition is one of depleted Kidney yang and cold congealing in the umbilicus.

Treatment and Outcome

We prescribed a formula based on the experiences of my teacher, Jiang Er-Xun, and his teacher, Chen Ding-San, called True Warrior Decoction *(zhēn wǔ tāng)* plus Trigonelle Semen *(hú lú bā)*.

> Aconiti Radix lateralis preparata *(zhì fù zǐ)* [pre-cooked for one hour] 30g
> Atractylodis macrocephalae Rhizoma *(bái zhú)* 15g
> Poria *(fú líng)* 15g
> Paeoniae Radix alba *(bái sháo)* 12g
> Zingiberis Rhizoma recens *(shēng jiāng)* 15g
> Trigonelle Semen *(hú lú bā)* 30g

After finishing three packets of the formula the patient no longer experienced dull umbilical pain, his hands had become warm, and the intestinal rumbling and loose stools that he had been experiencing were resolved. One year later the patient reported no recurrence of umbilical pain.

Disease	Primary Symptoms	Differential Diagnosis	Treatment Method	Formula
Umbilical pain	Dull pain in the umbilicus	Kidney yang depletion with cold congealing at CV-8 (shén què)	Warm the Kidneys, eliminate cold, bind up yin, and harmonize yang	True Warrior Decoction (zhēn wǔ tāng) plus Trigonelle Semen (hú lú bā)

Differentiation of Pattern and Discussion of Treatment

PHYSICIAN A   When treating abdominal pain, it seems that determining the exact location of the pain is essential. There is not a lot of emphasis given to this aspect of treatment in the textbooks. Could you shed more light on the subject for us?

DR. YU   What is called the abdomen in Chinese medicine refers to the area from the epigastrium down to the border of the pubic bone. However, the abdomen can be divided into more distinct zones. From the epigastrium to the upper border of the umbilicus is called the greater abdomen, and pertains to *tài yīn*. From the umbilicus down to the pubic bone is called the lesser abdomen and pertains to *shào yīn*-Kidneys. The area to the left and right of the umbilicus pertains to the Penetrating vessel, while the area lateral to each side of the small abdomen is called the lower abdomen and pertains to the *jué yīn*-Liver.

If the location of the patient's abdominal pain isn't pinpointed, thereby determining which organs and channels are involved, it is almost impossible to determine a clear plan of treatment. The practitioner then loses confidence in his or her diagnosis and treatment.

PHYSICIAN B   Dr. Yu, I was surprised by the efficacy of the formula you chose to use, True Warrior Decoction *(zhēn wǔ tāng)*. This is a formula that warms yang and promotes urination and is used to treat yang deficiency edema. In this case, the patient didn't have any symptoms of yang deficiency edema. Why, then, did you choose this formula?

DR. YU   You are correct to point out that True Warrior Decoction *(zhēn wǔ tāng)* can be used to treat yang deficiency edema. To say that it can only be used for this condition, however, would be too limiting.

Strictly speaking, True Warrior Decoction *(zhēn wǔ tāng)* is a formula that treats Kidney yang depletion pathogenic water disorders. Pathogenic water, also known as water-qi, can flood outward resulting in edema, gush upward producing dizziness or wheezing and coughing, or pool internally and cause intestinal rumbling and loose stools (as in this case). The patient's umbilical pain, however, was not due to pathogenic water, but rather stemmed from Kidney yang deficiency-depletion with cold congealing at CV- 8 *(shén què)*.

I chose True Warrior Decoction *(zhēn wǔ tāng)* because the combination of Aconiti Radix lateralis preparata *(zhì fù zǐ)* and Paeoniae Radix *(sháo yào)* not only warms Kidney yang and eliminates cold congealment, but moreover enters yin and breaks up knots, binds up yin, and harmonizes yang. Such actions are in complete accordance with the underlying pathodynamic of *shào yīn* abdominal pain.

Wu Yi-Luo, a Qing-dynasty physician and author of *Practical Established Formulas (Chéng fāng qiè yòng)*, was very insightful when he said that True Warrior Decoction *(zhēn wǔ tāng)* "treats *shào yīn* cold damage abdominal pain." It has long been established clinically that this formula can be used not only to treat Kidney yang deficiency-depletion pathogenic water disorders, but also can be applied to Kidney yang deficiency depletion with internal pain owing to cold congealment.

PHYSICIAN B   Why did you add a large dosage (30g) of Trigonelle Semen *(hú lú bā)*?

DR. YU   This is based on the experience of my teacher's teacher, Chen Ding-San. There are also historical writings about its use. The *Comprehensive Outline of the Materia Medica (Běn cǎo gāng mù)*, for example, says that the nature and flavor of Trigonelle Semen *(hú lú bā)* is "bitter, extremely warm, and non-toxic" and that it treats "deficiency and cold qi in the primal viscera." The term "primal viscera" here refers to the Kidneys. Both Dr. Chen and Dr. Jiang obtained consistent results when using True Warrior Decoction *(zhēn wǔ tāng)* with the addition of a large amount of Trigonelle Semen *(hú lú bā)* to treat umbilical pain due to yang deficiency and cold congealment.

PHYSICIAN A   I have two questions. The first is in regards to your assertion that the application of True Warrior Decoction *(zhēn wǔ tāng)* can be expanded to treat internal pain with a pattern of yang deficiency with cold congealment. My question is: in the case at hand, how effective would True Warrior Decoction *(zhēn wǔ tāng)* have been without the addition of Trigonelle Semen *(hú lú bā)*?

My second question is: if the use of an unmodified True Warrior Decoction *(zhēn wǔ tāng)* would not have been particularly effective, what results would be achieved by substituting other herbs able to treat deficiency and cold qi in the primal viscera—such as Cinnamomi Cortex *(ròu guì)*, Curculiginis Rhizoma *(xiān máo)*, Foeniculi Fructus *(xiǎo huí xiāng)*, and Caryophylli Flos *(dīng xiāng)*—for Trigonelle Semen *(hú lú bā)*?

DR. YU   Based on Dr. Jiang's experience, True Warrior Decoction *(zhēn wǔ tāng)* with Trigonelle Semen *(hú lú bā)* brings quick relief, minimal recurrence of symptoms, and results that are superior to the use of an unmodified True Warrior Decoction *(zhēn wǔ tāng)*.

As for the quality of results to be obtained by adding agents other than Trigonelle Semen *(hú lú bā)* to warm the Kidneys and dispel cold, I suggest that everyone begin experimenting with other substances when the chance occurs. Allow me to say one more thing. In patients who have yang deficiency and cold congealment which gives rise to pain in the lesser abdomen, when that pain is below the umbilicus rather than centered on it, an unmodified True Warrior Decoction *(zhēn wǔ tāng)* is quite effective.

CHAPTER 6

Disorders of the Body Structure and Channels

6.1 **Atrophy**

Paralysis of the lower extremities lasting 14 days

Using an incomparable classic formula to treat the acute symptom of wind disablement

治風痹急症，用曠世經方

■ CASE HISTORY

Patient: *36-year-old man, farmer*

The patient had been generally healthy, but one day contracted an external pathogen that manifested with fever, headache, fatigue, and cough. He took both Chinese and Western medicines off and on, and once his symptoms resolved he gave the matter no further thought. On October 14, however, while he was pumping water at a pump, he experienced soreness, weakness, and lack of feeling in his legs, all of which progressively worsened. About four hours later this developed into a complete loss of feeling in both of his legs along with obstructed urination. The patient's mental state remained unaffected.

He was immediately taken to the local hospital where they took a sample of his cerebrospinal fluid for analysis. He was diagnosed with acute myelitis after the tests revealed elevated protein and white blood cell counts in his cerebrospinal fluid. The patient was given steroids, vitamins, and various neural nutrients to address his symptoms. At the same time he took Chinese herbs, including three packets each of Major Large Gentian Decoction (dà qín jiāo tāng) and Three Painful Obstruction Decoction (sān bì tāng), and four packets of Tonify the Yang to Restore Five-tenths Decoction (bǔ yáng huán wǔ tāng). These treatments were ineffective.

INTAKE EXAMINATION
DATE: October 24, 1986

At present the patient's legs showed signs of flaccid paralysis, such as lack of muscle tone and negative deep tendon reflexes. He was also unable to urinate on his own, and his bowel movements were very difficult.

Because the patient had difficulty transferring to the hospital where I work, his family members came, bringing only his medical records and asking if I could write a formula for him.

Treatment and Outcome

DR. YU   Based on his signs and symptoms, the patient's condition was given the Chinese medicine diagnosis of wind disability (風痱 fēng féi).

He was given Extend Life Decoction (xù mìng tāng) in its original form from the *Essentials of the Golden Cabinet (Jīn guì yào lüè)*. Note that this formula later became known as Major Extend Life Decoction (dà xù mìng tāng), which is how we will refer to it from here on.

Ephedrae Herba (má huáng)	9g
Cinnamomi Ramulus (guì zhī)	9g
Angelicae sinensis Radix (dāng guī)	9g
Codonopsis Radix (dǎng shēn)	9g
Gypsum fibrosum (shí gāo)	9g
Zingiberis Rhizoma (gān jiāng)	9g
Glycyrrhizae Radix (gān cǎo)	9g
Chuanxiong Rhizoma (chuān xiōng)	4.5g
Armeniacae Semen (xìng rén)	12g

After finishing only two packets of the formula the patient reported that he had recovered sensation in his legs. He was able to get out of bed and walk and both his bowel movements and urination were relatively smooth.

We changed the formula to a modified combination of Eight-Treasure Decoction (bā zhēn tāng) and Tonify the Yang to Restore Five-tenths Decoction (bǔ yáng huán wǔ tāng). He took ten packets of that formula and recovered fully.

PHYSICIAN A   This is an unusual case. Had it not been one of your personal cases I would have found it difficult to believe. The fact that the patient fully recovered leads me into a maze of doubts.

First is the question of diagnosis. Given that the patient was unable to come to your clinic in person, I am wondering how you arrived at the Chinese medicine diagnosis of wind disablement based solely on his medical history and the Western medical diagnosis of acute myelitis.

DR. YU   There are reasons for diagnosing this patient's disorder as wind disablement. First, let us define the disorder. Historically, there are numerous references to this illness in the medical literature. Chapter 21 of the *Divine Pivot (Líng shū)*, "On Feverish Diseases," states that "Disablement is an illness [characterized by] a body without pain, [but with] flaccid limbs, and mild mental confusion." The 17th-century text *Required Readings from the Medical Tradition (Yī zōng bì dú)* elaborates:

> Disablement means the same as incapacitated. Disablement means a deep-seated pathogen [leading to] unilateral withering ... the arms and legs become crippled and cannot move, hence the name, disablement. The term disablement (痱 *féi*) can be used whether one side of the body is incapacitated or both.

In the 12th-century text *Comprehensive Records of Sagely Benevolence (Shèng jì zǒng lù)* it is written that "The disorder 'disablement' (痱 *féi*) is also known by the character 廢 *(fèi)*, 'useless' or 'abandoned.' The flesh is not like flesh [neither looks normal nor functions normally], there is no pain in the body, and the limbs are weak, flaccid, and of no use."

These passages reveal that physicians throughout history had similar understandings of this illness. Wind disablement is characterized by sudden paralysis (hemiplegia or paraplegia), lack of generalized pain, and no signs or only mild signs of cognitive dysfunction.

In this case the patient's legs gradually began to feel sore, weak, and numb as he was doing physical labor. After about four hours he had completely lost sensation in his legs, but his mind was functioning normally. The symptoms and onset of the patient's illness align completely with the characteristics of wind disablement.

This type of sudden paraplegia is entirely different from the paralysis that results from disorders such as stroke or hysteria.

PHYSICIAN A   I feel clear on how to diagnose wind disablement, but I'm not clear as to the reasons behind your choice of this unusual formula.

DR. YU   The formula I used, Major Extend Life Decoction *(dà xù mìng tāng)*, was recorded in Chapter 5 of the *Essentials of the Golden Cabinet (Jīn guì yào lüè)*. There it is said that the formula "Treats disablement from wind attack, when the body structure cannot support itself, the mouth is unable to speak and [the patient] is confused about the location of any pain. There may be restrictions from increased tension that makes it impossible to twist to the sides."

This formula was selected on the basis of formula-pattern correspondence, following the principle set forth by Zhang Zhong-Jing: "When *this* presentation occurs, use *this* formula." If the presenting signs and symptoms correspond with those listed for the formula, then that formula can be used with confidence, unencumbered by the various pattern-differentiation and treatment systems developed by later generations of physicians.

Disease	Primary Symptoms	Differential Diagnosis	Treatment Method	Formula
Wind disablement	Sudden paralysis of the legs	Sudden loss of the Spleen and Stomach's ability to regulate ascent and descent	Regulate the Spleen and Stomach yin and yang, and restore the body's ability to regulate proper ascent and descent	Major Extend Life Decoction (dà xù mìng tāng)

Differentiation of Pattern and Discussion of Treatment

PHYSICIAN A   I have analyzed the nature, flavor, and function of each of the nine herbs in this formula and honestly cannot understand the mechanism by which it works. How could a formula like this quickly cure paraplegia? If I may be candid, do you think the remarkable results could possibly be a coincidence or just plain luck?

DR. YU   Your question is certainly a pointed one. I will give you some background on the use of Major Extend Life Decoction (dà xù mìng tāng) in the treatment of wind disablement so that you can decide for yourself if the results in this case were due to luck.

In the 1930s, when my teacher Jiang Er-Xun had just begun studying medicine, he came across a 50-year-old man who was surnamed Tang. He was a well-built man who loved drinking alcohol. One day, while he was sitting in a teahouse, his arms and legs suddenly became flaccid and paralyzed; he immediately fell to the ground. The man had no cognitive dysfunction or speech impediment. He could not find a doctor who could determine what was wrong with him.

Dr. Jiang's teacher, Chen Ding-San, examined the patient and said, "This illness is called wind disablement and the appropriate formula is one from *Records of Proven Formulas from Past and Present (Gǔ jīn lù yàn fāng)* called Extend Life Decoction (xù mìng tāng)." The man took one package of the formula and the next day was immediately cured. Now, during that era, the salt sold in the markets was a type of crude table salt called "snowflake salt" that contained relatively high levels of barium chloride. After consuming this salt for long periods, some people would suddenly suffer paralysis of their arms and legs. At the time, however, the cause was unknown. Dr. Chen used this formula to treat many people and the results were often quite rapid.

In 1950, Dr. Jiang had a patient, surnamed Qiao, who was in the prime of his life. One day he was suddenly unable to move his legs. The legs had no itching or pain. He could not get out of bed. He asked for Dr. Jiang's immediate help. Dr. Jiang gave him this formula and after two packages he was able to get out of bed and walk.

In August of 1965, Dr. Jiang used this formula in combination with acupuncture to successfully treat a person with a severe case of wind disablement. The patient was an 18-year-old boy who came down with what had been diagnosed as acute myelitis and Guillain–Barré syndrome. The patient experienced numbness in his arms and legs and partial paralysis, but the most pressing concern was that he was losing his ability to breathe and swallow.

At the hospital the patient was given antibiotics, an IV drip, vitamins, continuous injections of lobeline with camphor water, and oxygen therapy. After six days of emergency treatment the patient began to develop paroxysmal dyspnea with gasping, and appeared that he might stop breathing at any moment. At times he had no pupillary reflex, or would become non-responsive as if he was asleep, and would occasionally lack any response to stimuli. Realizing the improbability of being able to rescue the boy, the doctors, on multiple occasions, told the patient's family that their son did not have long to live. At this point his family called home and told their relatives to make preparations for the boy's funeral. However, the family felt they hadn't yet done all they could do and so requested that Dr. Jiang see their son.

Dr. Jiang treated the patient with this formula as well as with acupuncture. After only one packet of the formula the patient's more severe symptoms were quickly resolved. After five packets, all his symptoms had disappeared. In order to consolidate the treatment, Dr. Jiang followed with herbs aimed at regulating and tonifying qi and blood.

So you can see that the swift efficacy of the treatment in our case was not the result of coincidence or luck, but rather the fruition of knowledge and experience passed down from Chen Ding-San and Jiang Er-Xun.

PHYSICIAN C   Based on what you have said, can we surmise that the ability of this formula to treat wind disablement is not limited to the Western disease category of acute myelitis?

DR. YU   That is correct. In addition to acute myelitis and barium chloride poisoning mentioned previously, Major Extend Life Decoction *(dà xù mìng tāng)* can also be used to treat polyneuritis. There was once a Western medical doctor studying with Dr. Jiang who used this formula to treat more than a dozen cases of polyneuritis and obtained excellent results.

PHYSICIAN A   The composition of herbs that make up this formula is quite unique, and the mechanism behind them is difficult to understand. I'm curious as to how Dr. Chen understood them.

DR. YU   Dr. Jiang was also very surprised after witnessing the amazing results of Dr. Chen's treatment and asked Dr. Chen to clarify how the formula worked. Dr. Chen replied that "The Spleen governs the four limbs. So when the limbs become paralyzed, this indicates the illness is in the Spleen and Stomach. The combination of Gypsum fibrosum *(shí gāo)* and Zingiberis Rhizoma *(gān jiāng)* is directed at regulating the yin and yang of the Spleen and Stomach."

Dr. Jiang replied that "Previous physicians have all agreed that Ephedrae Herba *(má huáng)* and Cinnamomi Ramulus *(guì zhī)* are used to disperse external wind-cold, and Gypsum fibrosum *(shí gāo)* is used to clear heat that has developed from wind, while Zingiberis Rhizoma *(gān jiāng)* is used as a paradoxical assistant to counteract the cold, cooling Gypsum fibrosum *(shí gāo)*. Dr. Chen, I am having trouble understanding your unique perspective." Dr. Chen replied that "This formula has inconceivable subtlety and cannot be understood by those without deep experience." Dr. Jiang then continued to seek an answer.

PHYSICIAN A   Did Dr. Jiang gain any insight into the "inconceivable subtlety" of this formula?

DR. YU   He did. Dr. Jiang's explanation of the dynamic behind wind disablement is based on the following passage from Chapter 29 of the *Basic Questions (Sū wèn)*:

> Why is [it said that] when the Spleen is diseased the four limbs become useless? Qi Bo replied: "The four limbs all are supplied qi from the Stomach, but when [its qi] does not arrive in the channels [directly]. It is due to the Spleen, as it allows [them] to be supplied. Now when the Spleen is diseased and it is unable to properly move the fluids on behalf of the Stomach. When the four limbs don't receive the qi of food and liquids, their qi will diminish daily, and the vessels will be impeded. The sinews, bones, muscles, and flesh will lack qi to enliven them, and thus become useless."

PHYSICIAN B   Common knowledge tells us that impairment and atrophy of the limbs is owing to the limbs not being supplied the qi of food and liquids due to chronic deficiency of the Spleen and Stomach, and that the manifestation of such problems would be gradual. In a case such as this, where the illness manifests so quickly, isn't it a bit implausible to suggest that the illness resides in the Spleen and Stomach?

DR. YU   It seems as if I will have to clarify Dr. Jiang's tricks of the trade. According to Dr. Jiang, it is significant that the classics say, "[W]hen the Spleen is diseased the four limbs become useless" and not "When the Spleen is deficient the four limbs become useless." There is a difference between diseased and deficient and one must not confuse the two. Unfortunately, doctors today, compelled by Li Dong-Yuan's theory of internal damage to the Spleen and Stomach, overemphasize deficiency.

Dr. Jiang explained that there are at least two situations where Spleen disease leads to the inability to use the arms and legs. One is the gradual decrease of the qi of food and liquids received by the arms and legs due to long-term deficiency of the Spleen and Stomach. The other situation is one where the Spleen and Stomach are not deficient, but instead are suddenly unable to regulate the ascending and descending functions. Wind disablement is attributed to the latter.

PHYSICIAN C   If this is the case, then the obvious treatment would be to restore the functions of the Spleen and Stomach to direct upward and downward properly. But Major Extend Life Decoction *(dà xù mìng tāng)* doesn't contain any herbs to assist with the Spleen's raising up of the qi or the Stomach's function of directing the qi downward. In other words, there is a disconnect between the treatment method and the herbs applied. How do you explain this?

DR. YU   When you say that there are no herbs in the formula to help with the Spleen and Stomach's respective functions of raising up and directing downward, I assume you are referring to herbs that Li Dong-Yuan commonly used to achieve these goals?

PHYSICIAN C   Yes.

DR. YU   That selection of herbs involves a completely different line of reasoning. Let me continue with Dr Jiang's thoughts. According to Dr. Jiang, it is important to respect the inherent natures of the Spleen and Stomach when treating wind disablement. The Spleen prefers what is dry and unyielding and should be treated with yang medicinal substances that aid ascension. The Stomach, on the other hand, prefers what is moist and yielding and therefore should be treated with yin medicinal substances that promote directing downward. Zingiberis Rhizoma *(gān jiāng)* is acrid, warm, unyielding, and drying. It is said to be both conserving and dispersing. It has a strong ability to warm, raise, disseminate, and unblock. Gypsum fibrosum *(shí gāo)* on the other hand is acrid, cold, yielding, and moistening, and it has a heavy quality as well as a sinking and descending nature.

These two herbs comprise the core of the formula. They serve to regulate yin and yang and the Spleen and Stomach; they help the Spleen to direct upward and the Stomach to direct downward, to restore normal qi transformation. Thus, the four limbs gain nourishment from the qi of food and liquids. This process is the root of the treatment of wind disablement. If one is able to clearly discern the physiological characteristics of the Spleen and Stomach and the nature of their pathologies, as well as the mechanisms behind the combined use of cold and hot Gypsum fibrosum *(shí gāo)* and Zingiberis Rhizoma *(gān jiāng)*, then the wondrous cures attained by this formula do not seem so unimaginable.

The remainder of the formula consists of Ginseng Radix *(rén shēn)*, Glycyrrhizae Radix *(gān cǎo)*, Chuanxiong Rhizoma *(chuān xiōng)*, Angelicae sinensis Radix *(dāng guī)*, which constitute half of Eight-Treasure Decoction *(bā zhēn tāng)*. Note that Angelicae sinensis Radix *(dāng guī)* and Chuanxiong Rhizoma *(chuān xiōng)* comprise a formula called Buddha's Hand Powder *(fó shǒu sǎn)*, a formula whose blood-invigorating function is superior to its ability to tonify blood. Although wind disablement is not due to long-term deficiency, the fact that the arms and legs are disabled means that they aren't receiving the qi of food and liquids. When qi is insufficient, the transportation of blood is hindered. Consequently, once you tonify qi and invigorate blood the momentum will shift to facilitate proper movement.

Ephedrae Herba *(má huáng)*, Cinnamomi Ramulus *(guì zhī)*, Armeniacae Semen *(xìng rén)*, and Glycyrrhizae Radix *(gān cǎo)* make up Ephedra Decoction *(má huáng tāng)*. This formula is designed to expel wind-cold from the exterior, and if wind disablement is due to wind-cold, it is ideal. However, even in wind disablement cases where wind-cold is not part of the pattern, Ephedra Decoction *(má huáng tāng)* is still effective, as it also disseminates Lung qi. Because the Lung governs the qi of the entire body, when Lung qi moves freely and smoothly, it not only facilitates the smooth flow of qi in the channels (the Lung governs the hundred vessels), but also assists the Spleen and Stomach as they direct upward and downward respectively. Furthermore, there is a classic formula called Return the Ethereal Soul Decoction *(huán hún tāng)*, now more commonly known as Three-Unbinding Decoction *(sān ǎo tāng)*, that consists of Ephedrae Herba *(má huáng)*, Glycyrrhizae Radix *(gān cǎo)*, and Armeniacae Semen *(xìng rén)*; it is used to treat a condition called sudden death. There are clear explanations of this formula in the traditional literature. If one gets stuck on just the functions of individual herbs, it is very difficult to understand the essence of Major Extend Life Decoction *(xù mìng tāng)*.

6.2 **Painful obstruction**

Intense calf pain for 25 days

Standing on the shoulders of our predecessors

站在前醫的肩膀上

■ CASE HISTORY

Patient: *46-year-old man*

The patient had the habit for more than ten years of bathing in cold water in all seasons. During this time he seldom had been ill. Two months prior to coming to the hospital, he had traveled around northern China on business and in the process twisted the lateral aspect of his left ankle several times (though never a true sprain). After returning home, he sat for long periods and was exposed to cold, as he often stayed up through the night. This resulted in a pain in the muscle of his left calf, which he didn't give much thought to at the time. About a month later, at dusk, the pain in his leg suddenly intensified and his calf muscle began to periodically spasm. The patient was afraid to straighten his leg and was unable to stand.

The next day he applied a hot compress and a liniment to his calf followed by the commercial medical plaster Musk and Tiger Bone Plaster *(shè xiāng hǔ gǔ gāo)*. He also took a combination of aspirin and acetaminophen as well as ibuprofen. The patient's spasms and pain gradually diminished, but in the middle of the night worsened to the extent that he lay awake moaning until dawn.

The following morning the patient asked a doctor of Chinese medicine to come see him. The doctor administered moxibustion and acupuncture and also gave him Peony, Licorice, and Aconite Accessory Root Decoction *(sháo yào gān cǎo fù zǐ tāng)* using large dosages of the herbs. Two packets of the formula brought mild relief.

He also went to see a surgeon who listed the possible causes of his condition as calcium deficiency, gout, sprain of the calf muscle, a meniscus injury, and cruciate ligament damage. But laboratory tests showed that his blood calcium and uric acid levels were within normal range, and X-rays revealed no abnormalities in his joints. Unable to arrive at a clear diagnosis, the doctor decided to address the symptoms with anti-inflammatory drugs, pain killers, and vitamin supplements.

At this point the patient felt he had no choice but to seek the help of an old Chinese medicine doctor. After a thorough examination and careful consideration the doctor said, "This is an injury to the sinews of the calf due to an invasion of wind-cold." The doctor's treatment consisted of the following protocol:

1. A decoction of a modified Soothe the Sinews and Invigorate the Blood Decoction *(shū jīn huó xùe tāng)* containing:

   Notopterygii Rhizoma seu Radix *(qiāng huó)*
   Angelicae pubescentis Radix *(dú huó)*

Chuanxiong Rhizoma *(chuān xiōng)*
Saposhnikoviae Radix *(fáng fēng)*
Gentianae macrophyllae Radix *(qín jiāo)*
Achyranthis bidentatae Radix *(niú xī)*
Olibanum *(rǔ xiāng)*, Myrrha *(mò yào)*
Daemonoropis Resina *(xuè jié)*

The patient took one packet per day with Notoginseng Radix *(sān qī)* powder, Yunnan Bai Yao, and an herb-infused tincture for the treatment of trauma.

2. Application of a decoction of herbs that dispel wind, disperse cold, eliminate dampness, and invigorate blood, as a steam and wash. This was applied to the affected area three times a day.

3. Moxibustion and acupuncture twice a day to related points on the left calf and foot.

After 23 days of treatment, there was minimal improvement in the patient's condition.

INTAKE EXAMINATION
DATE: January 5, 1987

The patient's left lower leg and foot were sensitive to cold and his calf muscles had atrophied. The patient did not dare to straighten his leg as the calf would spasm when he did so. If the patient slept on his right side the pain was slightly better, but if he slept on the painful leg or on his back, the pain was unbearable. The pain was worse during the afternoon and at night and the patient would experience spasms from time to time. His condition was better in the morning. He could, in a stooped position, take a few steps with a cane. Nevertheless, he was unable to stand up straight, because if he did so the pain would intensify. His appetite was fine and there was nothing particularly abnormal about his pulse or tongue.

Treatment and Results

PHYSICIAN A   This patient's condition came about during the winter, which makes me think of the teaching from Chapter 74 of the *Basic Questions (Sù wèn)*: "All cold, gathering in, and contraction belong to the Kidneys." It seems clear that this patient's pattern is one of cold congealment due to yang deficiency causing pain due to blockage.

The first doctor the patient saw prescribed Peony, Licorice, and Aconite Accessory Root Decoction *(sháo yào gān cǎo fù zǐ tāng)* to warm the yang and nourish yin, relax tension, and relieve pain. After two packets of the formula his pain had improved slightly, which indicates that the original diagnosis was not that far off the mark. If, at that time, the treatment principle had been modified to one focused on warming yang and dispersing cold, I am sure the patient would have recovered quickly.

Regrettably, however, the patient changed doctors, thus changing course completely to a treatment based on damaged sinews. Despite the combination of methods applied, the patient's symptoms persisted because the herbs didn't fit the pattern. I think there is a lesson to be learned here.

DR. YU   Given the patient's medical history and his previous treatments, I believe the older Chinese medicine doctor's diagnosis of damaged sinews in the calf due to invasion by wind-cold was very insightful. The intensity of the spasms and pain in the patient's leg made it clear that his condition had already transformed into a pattern of painful obstruction (痹 *bì*). This is painful obstruction owing to yang deficiency, overabundant yin, and cold congealing in the collaterals of the leg.

PHYSICIAN B   When you say that the doctor's diagnosis of damaged sinews in the calf due to invasion by wind-cold was insightful, I assume you are taking into consideration that:

1. The patient had previously twisted his ankle numerous times.

2. The intense spastic pain in the calf was the result of the site of these chronic sinew injuries being suddenly affected by wind-cold.

3. The yang-warming, yin-nourishing, tension-relaxing, analgesic effects of Peony, Licorice, and Aconite Accessory Root Decoction *(sháo yào gān cǎo fù zǐ tāng)* were not in the end particularly effective.

Is this correct?

DR. YU   Yes, that's correct. In addition, I felt that the patient's long-term habit of bathing in cold water was significant (as was his habit of drenching himself in cold water during the heat of summer whenever he had sweated profusely). We should note that showering with cold water in itself is not bad — it is not really a problem if the person finishes up by showering with very hot water. In this way the cold water can be invigorating for the body, but the last drenching with hot water will prevent any lingering effects of cold on the body. I don't believe that this patient followed that procedure. This, combined with the fact that the patient was seldom ill, raises the possibility that there was the underlying unseen danger of cold congealing and stagnating in the collaterals of his body. It is not uncommon for people who rarely get colds or other minor diseases to be more vulnerable to severe problems. This is because the cold is never really discharged from the exterior of the body by the process of recovering from colds or flus, and it ends up lodging deeper inside the body. There, it can be triggered to cause intense problems by any pathogen that is strong enough to penetrate the body's defenses.

These elements, along with the patient's recurrent left-leg trauma, constituted the underlying factors, while the invasion by wind-cold was the precipitating factor. These factors came together to form a pattern of yang deficiency, overabundant yin, and cold congealing in the collaterals of the leg which eventually led to painful obstruction. In Chapter 33 of the *Basic Questions* it states that, "Where a pathogen collects, the qi must [first] have been deficient." Unfortunately, later writers such as the Qing-dynasty's Zhang Lu, in his *Comprehensive Medicine According to Master Zhang (Zhāng shì yī tōng)*, added the misguided notion, "When [a pathogen] lingers and does not go away, its qi is therefore in excess." Is this not like adding a dog's tail to a mink coat?

The appropriate treatment for painful obstruction from yang deficiency, yin overabundance, and cold congealing in the collaterals is to warm yang, disperse yin, dispel cold, and unblock the collaterals.

The treatment we prescribed was:

1. A formula using the rationale underlying Balmy Yang Decoction *(yáng hé tāng)* as

a model, combined with Ephedra, Asarum, and Aconite Accessory Root Decoction *(má huáng xì xīn fù zǐ tāng)*:

Ephedrae Herba *(má huáng)*.. 50g
Rehmanniae Radix preparata *(shú dì huáng)*............................. 100g
Asari Radix et Rhizoma *(xì xīn)*.. 30g
Aconiti Radix lateralis preparata *(zhì fù zǐ)* [precooked].................. 100g

Instructions: Three packets in all. Directions for preparation and consumption of the formula and dietary restrictions were as follows:

1. Aconiti Radix lateralis preparata *(zhì fù zǐ)* should be boiled and cooked over moderate heat for one hour[1] before adding the rest of the herbs, then simmer at the boiling point for another 40 minutes, being sure to use enough water to cover all the herbs. The formula should then be cooked a second time, and the liquid from each decoction combined to make about 500ml of decoction. The decoction made from one packet of herbs was to be taken in five equal parts throughout the day. The patient also was told not to eat foods containing vinegar, fruit, or any other raw or cold-natured foods.

2. Soak 500g of Corni Fructus *(shān zhū yú)* in two liters of distilled spirits for at least seven days and save for later use.

SECOND VISIT: After one packet of the formula the pain in the patient's left calf significantly diminished. After finishing the third packet the patient was able to extend his leg while sitting or lying down and to walk for short distances using a cane. He was still unable to stand for long periods of time. Since the formula was effective, three more packets were prescribed.

THIRD VISIT: The pain in the patient's leg was now gone and he was able to stand for longer periods of time as well as walk a few hundred steps without his cane. His only complaint was that his left leg felt heavy and inflexible. He was advised to drink the Corni Fructus *(shān zhū yú)* tincture he had previously prepared. He was instructed to take 50ml of the tincture twice a day, after lunch and dinner respectively, and to continue this for 15 days. Follow-up one month later revealed that the patient had fully recovered.

Note that the normal dose for this type of tincture is 20-50ml once a day, after dinner. The larger dose was used here because the problem was relatively severe, the patient had a strong constitution, and he also happened to enjoy drinking alcohol.

Differentiation of Pattern and Discussion of Treatment

PHYSICIAN A   Given that the diagnosis is painful obstruction due to yang deficiency with yin overabundance and cold congealing in the collaterals of the leg, Peony, Licorice, and Aconite Accessory Root Decoction *(sháo yào gān cǎo fù zǐ tāng)* didn't match the pathodynamic. Nevertheless it did bring the patient some mild relief. Why was that?

1. *Translators' note:* At present, Dr. Yu recommends adding 30g of both Glycyrrhizae Radix *(gān cǎo)* and Zingiberis Rhizoma recens *(shēng jiāng)* when precooking the Aconiti Radix lateralis praeparata *(zhì fù zǐ)* for an hour.

Disease	Primary Symptoms	Pattern	Treatment Method	Formula
Painful Obstruction	Severe pain in the left calf	Yang deficiency with yin over-abundance, cold congealing in the collaterals of the leg	Warm yang, reduce yin, dispel cold, and unblock the channels	A formula based on Balmy Yang Decoction (yáng hé tāng) combined with Ephedra, Asarum, and Aconite Accessory Root Decoction (má huáng xì xīn fù zǐ tāng)

DR. YU The patient's mild, temporary relief was due to the ability of Aconiti Radix lateralis preparata (zhì fù zǐ) to warm the yang and disperse cold. Peony, Licorice, and Aconite Accessory Root Decoction (sháo yào gān cǎo fù zǐ tāng) is discussed at line 68 of the *Discussion of Cold Damage (Shāng hán lùn),* and states, "If after inducing sweating, the disease is not released and instead there are chills, deficiency is the reason. Peony and Licorice Decoction (sháo yào gān cǎo tāng) governs." This is a pattern of post-sweating dual deficiency of yin and yang that is treated with herbs that support yang and augment yin.

This formula is not suited, however, for a pattern of yang deficiency with yin over-abundance because the acrid and warm nature of Aconiti Radix lateralis preparata (zhì fù zǐ) is impeded by the sour and cold nature of Paeoniae Radix (bái sháo). Continuing with the formula would make further warming of yang and dispersing of cold very difficult.

PHYSICIAN B Dr. Yu, you're obviously astute at learning from the errors of others. Your choice of Balmy Yang Decoction (yáng hé tāng) and Ephedra, Asarum, and Aconite Accessory Root Decoction (má huáng xì xīn fù zǐ tāng) to warm yang, disperse yin, dispel cold, and unblock the collaterals matched the patient's pattern well. I am confused, however, by your statement declaring that you used Balmy Yang Decoction (yáng hé tāng) as an inspiration when in fact you only used two herbs from the formula: Ephedrae Herba (má huáng) and Rehmanniae Radix preparata (shú dì huáng). Also, you used a very large dosage of Ephedrae Herba (má huáng): 50g. Weren't you concerned that such a large dosage would cause the patient to sweat profusely and thus devastate his yang?

DR. YU Balmy Yang Decoction (yáng hé tāng) is drawn from the 18th-century work *Complete Compendium of Patterns and Treatments in External Medicine (Wài kē zhèng zhì quán shēng jí).* It contains Rehmanniae Radix preparata (shú dì huáng), Sinapis Semen (bái jiè zǐ), Cervi Cornus Colla (lù jiǎo jiāo), Cinnamomi Cortex (ròu guì), Zingiberis Rhizoma carbonatum (jiāng tàn), Ephedrae Herba (má huáng), and Glycyrrhizae Radix (gān cǎo). It is very effective at warming yang, tonifying the Kidneys, dispersing cold, and unblocking stagnation, and is a specific remedy for yin-cold patterns that present as yin-type flat abscesses, bone-adhering abscesses, spreading sores, and crane's knee wind. The famous late-Qing physician Ma Pei-Zhi praised this formula saying, "This formula is without peer in treating yin-type patterns."

Early in my career I liked to use this formula to treat yin-cold patterns such as yin-type flat abscess, painful obstruction, cold-type asthma, and leg and lower back pain due to yang deficiency. I was suspicious, however, that the original dosages of some of the herbs in the formula were responsible for the relatively slow results I was observing. I consequently began to gradually increase the dosage of Ephedrae Herba *(má huáng)* until I was using about 30g (the original formula called for 1.5g). The formula then became noticeably more effective. Over time I began to increase the dosage even further. Later, I began to follow the example of the famous Republican-era doctor Zhu Wei-Ju,[2] who added Aconiti Radix lateralis *(fù zǐ)* and Asari Radix et Rhizoma *(xì xīn)* to the formula, which means that it then contained the ingredients of Ephedra, Asarum, and Aconite Accessory Root Decoction *(má huáng xì xīn fù zǐ tāng)*, thus strengthening the formula's ability to warm yang and disperse cold. In this format I found the formula to bring speedy results.

In recent years I have been carefully trying to experiment with the formula in order to find the most effective combination of herbs and dosages, putting particular emphasis on trying to simplify the formula while maintaining its effectiveness. As a result, of all the herbs in Balmy Yang Decoction *(yáng hé tāng)* I came to only use Ephedrae Herba *(má huáng)* and Rehmanniae Radix preparata *(shú dì huáng)*, which are in fact the primary herbs of the formula.

I discovered that generally speaking, in severe cases of yang deficiency with cold congealment and painful obstruction in the collaterals, Ephedrae Herba *(má huáng)* must be used in a dosage approaching 50g while Rehmanniae Radix preparata *(shú dì huáng)* must be used in a dosage of 100g or more before the formula will begin to be highly effective in breaking and dispelling yin-cold as well as unblocking the collaterals and invigorating blood. I have also become convinced of the veracity of the statement written in the *Complete Compendium of Patterns and Treatments in External Medicine (Wài kē zhèng zhì quán shēng jí)*: "When Ephedrae Herba *(má huáng)* is combined with Rehmanniae Radix preparata *(shú dì huáng)* it unblocks the collaterals and does not discharge exterior pathogens."

Furthermore, experience has shown me that if Ephedrae Herba *(má huáng)* is cooked for 40 minutes or more, even 100g of it won't induce sweating. There need not be any concern about causing profuse sweating and devastating the yang. Keep in mind that after an extended period of cooking, the ability of even large doses of Ephedrae Herba *(má huáng)* to induce sweating and resolve the exterior is almost completely nonexistent. However, its ability to unblock the collaterals and invigorate the blood is undamaged.

Nowadays, people most often use Ephedrae Herba *(má huáng)* for its ability to induce sweating and resolve the exterior, while they overlook its ability to unblock the collaterals and invigorate blood. Its ability to do so is in fact recorded in the *Divine Husbandman's Classic on Materia Medica (Shén nóng běn cǎo jīng)* where it says that Ephedrae Herba *(má huáng)* "breaks up fixed abdominal masses, hardness, accumulations, and clusters."

PHYSICIAN C The sentence is so confusing that the reference to these functions, and noth-

....

2. *Translators' note:* Zhu Wei-Ju belonged to what has recently been called the *Huǒ Shén pài* 火神 派—Fire God current—and was nicknamed Zhu fu-zi for his copious use of Aconiti Radix lateralis *(fù zǐ)*.

ing else, was removed from the quotation in this classic in the fifth edition of the official *Materia Medica* textbook entry about Ephedrae Herba *(má huáng)*.

DR. YU   It's not just modern day people who have been confused by this. Even three famous physicians from the Qing dynasty—Chen Xiu-Yuan, Zhang Yin-An, and Ye Tian-Shi—who wrote annotations to the *Divine Husbandman's Classic on Materia Medica (Shén nóng běn cǎo jīng)* had varying opinions about the meaning of this line.

Chen Xiu-Yuan wrote:

> Fixed abdominal masses, hardness, accumulations, and clusters are internal diseases and are due to yin-cold qi that has congealed within the yin aspect, accumulating over days and months. The sweating induced by Ephedrae Herba *(má huáng)* causes [the pathogen] to be expelled from the yin aspect by way of the yang. Thus, the fixed abdominal masses, hardness, accumulations, and clusters disperse. This is due to the ability of Ephedrae Herba *(má huáng)* to induce sweating.

If it is the case that the ability of Ephedrae Herba *(má huáng)* to affect concretions comes from its acrid, warm, diaphoretic nature, then why don't other warm and acrid diaphoretics have some similar functions?

Zhang Yin-An noted that, "Because Ephedrae Herba *(má huáng)* expels heat and cold from the body's exterior, it enables the qi of the *tài yáng* to enter and exit from within earth, [thus] fixed abdominal masses, hardness, accumulations, and clusters disappear." This is a poor explanation that is overly abstruse and lacks instructional value.

Ye Tian-Shi wrote:

> Fixed abdominal masses, hardness, accumulations, and clusters are the result of cold qi congealing and knotting. Cold is yin and the nature of cold is hardness. Ephedrae Herba *(má huáng)* is bitter and so enters the Heart, which governs the blood, while its warm nature dispels cold. With the cold dispelled and the blood invigorated the accumulations and clusters will dissipate.

The deduction that Ephedrae Herba *(má huáng)* invigorates blood and disperses cold based on its bitter and warm properties seems reasonable, but there are many bitter and warm herbs that also enter the Heart and disperse cold. Do they all have the ability to break up fixed abdominal masses, hardness, accumulations, and clusters?[3]

You can understand then that, from a theoretical perspective, it becomes very difficult to determine whether or not Ephedrae Herba *(má huáng)* can break up fixed abdominal masses, hardness, accumulations, and clusters. As a consequence, we practicing physicians need to avoid the tangles and confusion of theory and instead focus on our clinical practice by continuously testing to determine what is truly effective and what is not.

PHYSICIAN C   Regarding the dosage you gave of Asari Radix et Rhizoma *(xì xīn)*, the ancients said that no more than a *qián* (~3g) should be used. The fifth edition of the

---

3. *Translators' note:* All of these quotations are drawn from the *Divine Husbandmen's Classic on Materia Medica: Combined Annotations of Three Physicians (Shén nóng běn cǎo jīng)*, compiled in the early 20th century by Guo Ru-Cong.

standard *Materia Medica* textbook used in China sets the standard for usage of Asari Radix et Rhizoma *(xì xīn)* between one and three grams. In this case study you surprisingly used 30g. If a serious problem had occurred, what would you have done?

DR. YU The *Divine Husbandman's Classic on Materia Medica (Shén nóng běn cǎo jīng)* states that Asari Radix et Rhizoma *(xì xīn)* treats "contractions and spasms of the hundred joints, wind-damp painful obstruction, and dead flesh." The *Rectification of the Meaning of Materia Medica (Běn cǎo zhèng yì)* says of Asari Radix et Rhizoma *(xì xīn)* that, "Internally it disseminates [qi through] the collateral vessels and dredges the hundred joints, externally it moves through the pores to directly get to the muscles and skin." It is indeed a very powerful herb!

Asari Radix et Rhizoma *(xì xīn)* is an herbaceous plant that is historically said to be nontoxic. If we only use three grams or less, and disregard the severity of the patient's condition, how would we obtain such significant results? The amount of Asari Radix et Rhizoma *(xì xīn)* I have used in decoctions ranges from 3g to 60g, and I have never seen any toxic side effects.

Who knows how many people have been deceived from ancient times to the present by the adage, "Asari Radix et Rhizoma *(xì xīn)* should not surpass one *qián*." Even some very famous physicians have not been able to unravel this ball of confusion. An example is the important early 20th-century physician Zhang Xi-Chun who said, "There is a saying that no more than one *qián* of Asari Radix et Rhizoma *(xì xīn)* should be used. As many physicians of later generations disagreed with this idea, I myself am unsure whether to disregard it or not." I believe the adage regarding the proper dosage of Asari Radix et Rhizoma *(xì xīn)* might come from the 11th-century text *Alternative Statements in Materia Medica (Běn cǎo bié shuō)* where it says, "If using powdered Asari Radix et Rhizoma *(xì xīn)* alone, do not use more than half of one *qián*, otherwise the breath will become obstructed and if not unblocked, death will ensue." This is absolutely true and should not be ignored because it refers to ground Asari Radix et Rhizoma *(xì xīn)* that is taken orally, but not to Asari Radix et Rhizoma *(xì xīn)* that has been decocted.

According to modern research, Asari Radix et Rhizoma *(xì xīn)* contains both volatile and nonvolatile oils. Animal testing has confirmed that some of the components of the volatile oils, methyl butyrate and saffrole, can cause initial excitation of the respiratory center of the central nervous system followed by respiratory paralysis. Once Asari Radix et Rhizoma *(xì xīn)* is decocted for an extended period of time, however, the toxic volatile oils are almost completely dissipated while the beneficial oils remain intact. Hence, if Asari Radix et Rhizoma *(xì xīn)* is cooked properly, there should be no concerns about negative consequences.[4]

PHYSICIAN A A basic tenet of Chinese medicine states, "Where there is free flow there is no pain. Where there is pain there is absence of free flow." The principle when treating painful conditions should be to free the flow of qi and blood and it is generally thought that this implies that astringent medicinal substances should be absolutely avoided. However, Dr. Yu, once the patient's symptoms were almost completely resolved you

---

4. See the *Translators' notes* at the end of this chapter.

gave him a strong tincture made from the sour and astringent herb Corni Fructus *(shān zhū yú)* for the final stage of his treatment. This is something I have not seen before.

DR. YU   The *Divine Husbandmen's Classic of Materia Medica (Shén nóng běn cǎo jīng)* says that Corni Fructus *(shān zhū yú)* "drives out cold and damp painful obstructions." In the notes on Corni Fructus *(shān zhū yú)* in the *Materia Medica* textbook used in China nowadays, this line is omitted. Examples of this usage can be seen in the writings of Zhang Xi-Chun, who frequently used Corni Fructus *(shān zhū yú)*, usually in a large dosage, to treat pain in the Heart, abdomen, body (trunk), and limbs.

....

Translators' notes:

Asari Radix et Rhizoma *(xì xīn)*   There is concern recently about the aristolochic acid (AA) content of Asari Radix et Rhizoma *(xì xīn)*. Asarum belongs to the Aristolochia family and has been found to contain varying amounts of AA. In general, the aerial portions of the plant contain much higher amounts of AA than the roots and rhizomes. In addition, the amount of AA found in the below-ground portion of the plant is quite small and varies according to the age of the plant, the conditions under which it is grown, and the exact variety used. Further, a large portion of the AA found in the roots will not survive the cooking process. Thus, if the correct source material is used and correctly processed, an AA-free Asari Radix et Rhizoma *(xì xīn)* can be produced. In this way the concern about AA in concentrated granules can be eliminated. For legal import into the United States, this item must be tested for AA and proven to have no detectable amount. Practitioners would be wise to request a copy of the AA test on any given lot of Asari Radix et Rhizoma *(xì xīn)* they prescribe for their patients to avoid liability regarding this issue. And to avoid the AA issue altogether, an herb such as Clematidis Radix *(wēi líng xiān)* can be used as a substitute for Asari Radix et Rhizoma *(xì xīn)* in cases like the one presented here.

Ephedrae Herba *(má huáng)*   Ephedrae Herba *(má huáng)* is currently forbidden for import into the United States and several other Western countries. Its inclusion in dietary supplements is also forbidden. Its use by practitioners of Chinese medicine resides in a grey area. When we asked Dr. Yu about a replacement for this herb owing to its unavailability to Western practitioners, he shook his head, smiled, and had no answer. This led to an interesting discussion of the difficulty of practicing Chinese medicine in the absence of this herb.

EXTERNAL MEDICINE

CHAPTER 7

Skin Disorders

7.1 Itching

Itching lasting six months

Success and failure hinge on a single action

成敗在此一舉

■ CASE HISTORY

Patient: *57-year-old woman*

The patient presented with itching over her entire body which was worse at night and detrimental to her sleep. She had taken sedatives and allergy-alleviating Western medicines and found temporary relief. The itching returned when the patient stopped taking the drugs.

She therefore sought help from a doctor of Chinese medicine and was given modified Eliminate Wind Powder from the *Orthodox Lineage (xiāo fēng sǎn)*. She took four packets of the formula accompanied by a steam-wash consisting of Sophorae flavescentis Radix *(kǔ shēn)*, Cnidii Fructus *(shé chuáng zǐ)*, Kochiae Fructus *(dì fū zǐ),* and Dictamni Cortex *(bái xiān pí)*. The itching ceased. Two weeks later, the itching returned. She used the same formula (and steam-wash) as before, with no positive result. Then, items such as Scolopendra *(wú gōng)*, Scorpio *(quán xiē)*, and Bombyx batryticatus *(bái jiāng cán)* were added to the formula and four packets were consumed. The patient's whole-body itching worsened.

The patient was introduced to a doctor at a distant village who gave her a formula consisting of a large dosage of Ephedrae Herba *(má huáng)*, Asari Radix et Rhizoma *(xì xīn)*, Aconiti Radix lateralis praeparata *(zhì fù zǐ)*, Zingiberis Rhizoma *(gān jiāng)*, Cinnamomi

Cortex *(ròu guì)*, Cinnamomi Ramulus *(guì zhī)*, Caryophylli Flos *(dīng xiāng)*, Evodiae Fructus *(wú zhū yú)*, etc. The dosages were about three times normal. The patient, who had a cursory knowledge of Chinese medicine, was astonished, but was assured by the doctor who explained that "when the constrained fire is discharged, don't worry and continue to take the herbs. After the flare we can prescribe herbs to clear and resolve toxicity to bring about an immediate cure." Consoled by this explanation, the patient took one packet of herbs. She experienced dry mouth and tongue, and severe itching. The doctor said that "the herbs have already gotten to the disease, don't quit halfway." The patient forced herself to take two more packets of the herbs. Her body felt as if it was singed with fire and her itching became extreme both day and night. The doctor followed with large dosages of Coptis Decoction to Resolve Toxicity *(huáng lián jiě dú tāng)* and Five-Ingredient Drink to Eliminate Toxin *(wǔ wèi xiāo dú yǐn)* to clear heat and resolve toxicity. The patient took six packets but saw no improvement.

The patient had no alternative but to once again take Western tranquilizing and anti-allergy medications. She felt dazed all the time and still had frequent itching. This condition dragged on for six months.

INTAKE EXAMINATION
DATE: May 25, 1999

The patient's complexion was dark and lusterless. She had scratch marks all over her body with scabs everywhere. Her skin was rough and thick. The patient's mouth was dry and she was constipated. Her tongue was dark red with a thin, yellow coating and scanty fluids. Her pulse was wiry, sunken, and rough.

Differentiation of Patterns and Discussion of Treatment

PHYSICIAN A   In this case, the second application of Eliminate Wind Powder from the *Orthodox Lineage (xiāo fēng sǎn)* to dispel wind and nourish blood failed to bring about results. This demonstrated that the pattern had changed from the original. Thus, the second doctor struck out on a new path and decided to use the method of 'discharging constrained fire.' One could make the argument that the doctor's error was excessive dosages of the hot, acrid herbs. This was a case of "going too far is as bad as not going far enough," which brought about injurious results. Do you agree?

DR. YU   This is poor judgment! It is well known that the reference in Chapter 73 of the *Basic Questions (Sù wèn)* to the treatment method 'discharging constrained fire' refers to the idea that a fire pathogen constrained in the interior should not be treated with bitter and cold herbs, but rather treatment should capitalize on 'fire's own tendency to blaze upward' by applying light, clearing, dispersing herbs to discharge, disperse, vent, and diffuse suppressed fire.

For example, *Secrets from the Orchid Chamber (Lán shì mì cáng)* treats fire constrained in the interior with symptoms of heat in the five centers and irritability-heat by using Decoction for Fire from Constraint *(huǒ yù tāng)*. This formula builds on the ability of Peony and Licorice Decoction *(sháo yào gān cǎo tāng)* to nourish and enrich the Spleen. To this it adds Cimicifugae Rhizoma *(shēng má)*, Bupleuri Radix *(chái hú)*, Saposhnikoviae Radix *(fáng fēng)*, and Puerariae Radix *(gé gēn)* to raise yang and disperse fire. Furthermore, the *Supplemented Collections on Patterns and Treatments* *(Zhèng zhì huì bǔ)* treats fire constrained in the interior that gives rise to heat in the extremities, irritability and heat in the five centers, and reddened skin. It does this by using Coptidis Rhizoma *(huáng lián)*, Forsythiae Fructus *(lián qiào)*, and Gardeniae Fructus *(zhī zǐ)* to drain fire. It couples these herbs with Cimicifugae Rhizoma *(shēng má)*, Bupleuri Radix *(chái hú)*, Puerariae Radix *(gé gēn)*, and Menthae haplocalycis Herba *(bò hé)* to raise yang and disperse fire. Note that the herbs that raise yang and disperse fire are used in very small dosages in these texts.

The method of herb use in these sources is clearly different from the use of large dosages of only hot, acrid, harsh herbs that is exhibited in this case. How could one be confused with the other? Even if we understand the correct meaning of 'discharging constrained fire' as outlined above, that approach is completely unsuitable for this case. The reason for this is that the patient is an older woman whose condition is a chronic one that continually flares up and worsens at night. The diagnosis for this type of condition is blood deficiency and Liver exuberance for which the treatment principle is to nourish blood, calm the Liver, dispel wind, and moisten dryness. One could consider a modification of the combination of Linking Decoction *(yī guàn jiān)* and Two-Solstice Pill *(èr zhì wán)*.

I believe that in this example the efficacy of Eliminate Wind Powder from the *Orthodox Lineage (xiāo fēng sǎn)* on the first encounter was entirely owing to the formula's inclusion of Sesami Semen nigrum *(hēi zhī má)*, Angelicae sinensis Radix *(dāng guī)*, and Rehmanniae Radix *(shēng dì huáng)* to nourish and invigorate blood. This is in step with the saying, "When treating wind, first treat the blood; once the blood moves, the wind will be extinguished by itself." Two weeks later when the itching reappeared the formula was ineffective, even with the inclusion of the bug medicinal substances such as Scolopendra *(wú gōng)*, Scorpio *(quán xiē)*, and Bombyx batryticatus *(bái jiāng cán)*. This was because the long-term nature of the disorder had damaged the patient's yin and blood, and long-term use of the wind and damp-dispelling and heat-clearing herbs in Eliminate Wind Powder from the *Orthodox Lineage (xiāo fēng sǎn)* further consumed yin and blood. Thus, the formula's disadvantages began to outweigh its advantages. At this point in the disease progression, the proper treatment would have been to employ herbs to strongly nourish yin and cool blood, using a prescription in the category of combined Linking Decoction *(yī guàn jiān)* and Great Tonify the Yin Pill *(dà bǔ yīn wán)*.

If one takes into account the static heat now lurking deeply in the blood aspect, the treatment should be to clear heat, cool the blood, and disperse stasis.

Use augmented Rhinoceros Horn and Rehmannia Decoction *(xī jiǎo dì huáng tāng)*:

fresh Bubali Cornu *(shuǐ niú jiǎo)*[1] [cook separately
   and then add to strained decoction] .... 200g[2]
Rehmanniae Radix *(shēng dì huáng)* 30g
Paeoniae Radix rubra *(chì sháo)* 30g

---

1. *Translators note:* Due to fear of spreading mad cow disease, water buffalo horn and other bovine products cannot be imported to the United States, so this product is difficult to obtain there.

2. Reduce the dosage by half when using the dried product.

Moutan Cortex *(mǔ dān pí)*.. 15g
Arnebiae/Lithospermi Radix *(zǐ cǎo)* 30g
Salviae miltiorrhizae Radix *(dān shēn)* 30g
Polygoni cuspidati Rhizoma *(hǔ zhàng)*.................................... 30g
Notoginseng Radix *(sān qī)* [powdered and mixed
   into hot decoction just before drinking]............................... 30g

The patient was instructed to take three packets, and if she saw improvement, to continue taking another three to six packets, and to stop taking the Western medications.

SECOND VISIT: After taking one packet of herbs the patient felt the itching over her body decline. She continued taking four more packets. Itching during the day all but disappeared, as did her mouth dryness. Her stools became normal. At night she still had difficulty sleeping because of intermittent itching and scratching. One could clearly see that her body still had scratch marks and scabbing. Her skin was still as rough and thick as it was in the initial exam. Her tongue, however, was no longer dark red; it was closer to a tender red with no coating. Her pulse was sunken, wiry, fine, and rapid.

This fits the picture of a pattern of insufficiency of the Heart and Kidneys with yin deficiency and exuberant fire. The appropriate treatment is to nourish the Heart, enrich the Kidneys, and restrain and hold back the deficiency fire. We prescribed modified Emperor of Heaven's Special Pill to Tonify the Heart *(tiān wáng bǔ xīn dān)* as follows:

Rehmanniae Radix *(shēng dì huáng)*.. 30g
Scrophulariae Radix *(xuán shēn)*... 15g
Salviae miltiorrhizae Radix *(dān shēn)* 30g
Glehniae Radix *(běi shā shēn)* 15g
Ophiopogonis Radix *(mài mén dōng)* 15g
Poria *(fú líng)*.. 15g
prepared Polygalae Radix *(zhì yuǎn zhì)* 6g
Ziziphi spinosae Semen *(suān zǎo rén)* 30g
Prunellae Spica *(xià kū cǎo)*.. 30g
Schisandrae Fructus *(wǔ wèi zǐ)* 10g
Margaritiferae Concha usta *(zhēn zhū mǔ)*................................. 30g

After taking three packets, the patient's nighttime itching declined and her sleep improved, but even after eight packets she still had some nighttime itching. The above formula was combined with Cinnamon Twig Decoction *(guì zhī tāng)* by adding Cinnamomi Ramulus *(guì zhī)* 10g, Paeoniae Radix alba *(bái sháo)* 12g, and Glycyrrhizae Radix praeparata *(zhì gān cǎo)* 6g. After taking four packets of this modified formula, the nighttime itching was almost completely gone and the scratch marks and scabs started to disappear. After six more packets the pattern resolved. In a follow-up visit four months later the patient reported no recurrence of this disorder.

Reflections and Clarifications

PHYSICIAN A   You said that the herbs in Eliminate Wind Powder from the *Orthodox Lineage (xiāo fēng sǎn)* that dispel wind, eliminate dampness, and clear heat can consume yin and blood, but we have frequently seen you use modified versions of that formula when you treat skin disorders.

Disease	Main Symptoms	Differential Diagnosis	Treatment Method	Formula
Itching	The skin over the entire body feels as if it is singed. Itching is unbearable at night.	Static heat lurking deeply in the blood aspect	Clear heat, cool the blood, and disperse stasis	Rhinoceros Horn and Rehmannia Decoction (xī jiǎo dì huáng tāng)

DR. YU Actually, I said that *long-term use* of the drying herbs in the formula can consume yin and blood. Eliminate Wind Powder from the *Orthodox Lineage (xiāo fēng sǎn)* is recorded in Chen Shi-Gong's Ming-dynasty text *Orthodox Lineage of External Medicine (Wài kē zhèng zōng)*. It contains Schizonepetae Herba *(jīng jiè)*, Saposhnikoviae Radix *(fáng fēng)*, and Cicadae Periostracum *(chán tuì)* to strongly dispel wind; Atractylodis Rhizoma *(cāng zhú)* and Akebiae Caulis *(mù tōng)* to eliminate dampness; Gypsum fibrosum *(shí gāo)*, Anemarrhenae Rhizoma *(zhī mǔ)*, Sophorae flavescentis Radix *(kǔ shēn)*, and Glycyrrhizae Radix *(gān cǎo)* to clear heat and resolve toxicity, and Sesami Semen nigrum *(hēi zhī má)*, Angelicae sinensis Radix *(dāng guī)*, and Rehmanniae Radix *(shēng dì huáng)* to nourish and invigorate the blood.

The subtle magic of this formula lies in its use of Sesami Semen nigrum *(hēi zhī má)*, Angelicae sinensis Radix *(dāng guī)*, and Rehmanniae Radix *(shēng dì huáng)* to nourish and treat the blood. Why is that so? It's not just because it adheres to the principle of "when treating wind, first treat the blood; once the blood moves the wind will be extinguished by itself." These herbs also fulfill the mandate to "first calm the places that have not been affected by a pathogen." Moreover, to a certain extent, they also moderate the potential drying and yin-damaging side effects of the herbs in the formula that dispel wind, eliminate dampness, and clear heat.

The scope of treatment of this formula is quite broad. It can address all wind, heat, and dampness that seeps into the blood vessels to give rise to wind papules (風疹 *fēng zhěn)*, eczema (濕疹 *shī zhěn)*, scabies-like disorders (疥瘡 *jiè chuāng)*, and simple pruritus. If the patient is strong, one can use a relatively large dosage of Sophorae flavescentis Radix *(kǔ shēn)* 15-20g and add Arnebiae/Lithospermi Radix *(zǐ cǎo)* 15-20g.

One shortcoming of Eliminate Wind Powder from the *Orthodox Lineage (xiāo fēng sǎn)* is that it is extremely bitter and difficult to drink. This difficulty can be offset by taking the formula in small, frequent doses throughout the day. Also, the dregs can be re-used as an effective steam-wash. In fact, my hospital has a special wash formula for skin disorders (designed by my teacher, Dr. Jiang) called Master Jiang's Speedy Recovery from Itching Formula (江氏癢述泰 *Jiāng shì yáng shù tài)*. It is essentially a modification of Eliminate Wind Powder from the *Orthodox Lineage (xiāo fēng sǎn)*.

Schizonepetae Herba *(jīng jiè)*...10g
Saposhnikoviae Radix *(fáng fēng)* 10g
Cicadae Periostracum *(chán tuì)*..10g
Arctii Fructus *(niú bàng zǐ)* 10g
Sophorae flavescentis Radix *(kǔ shēn)* 10g
Tetrapanacis Medulla *(tōng cǎo)* 6g
Atractylodis Rhizoma *(cāng zhú)*...10g

Rehmanniae Radix *(shēng dì huáng)*.. 20g

Gypsum fibrosum *(shí gāo)* 30g

Glycyrrhizae Radix *(gān cǎo)*... 6g

Anemarrhenae Rhizoma *(zhī mǔ)* 10g

Tribuli Fructus *(cì jí lí)*.. 20g

Dictamni Cortex *(bái xiān pí)*... 20g

Mume Fructus *(wū méi)*... 30g

Arnebiae/Lithospermi Radix *(zǐ cǎo)* 10g

Carthami Flos *(hóng huā)* 6g

There was a rural doctor in our city about 20 years ago who treated neurodermatitis with a secret formula that was ground to a powder to prevent anyone from discerning its contents. Fortunately, this doctor liked to drink alcohol, and one night after several rounds of liquor and some prodding, he unexpectedly revealed that the formula was Eliminate Wind Powder from the *Orthodox Lineage (xiāo fēng sǎn)* with Two-Marvel Powder *(èr miào sǎn)* plus Arnebiae/Lithospermi Radix *(zǐ cǎo)*, Gastrodiae Rhizoma *(tiān má)*, Bubali Cornu *(shuǐ niú jiǎo)*, Sesami Semen nigrum *(hēi zhī má)*, and Mori Folium *(sāng yè)*.

It should be pointed out that dermatology patients suffering from wind, dampness, and heat pathogens can exhibit a wide range of pulses. The tongue picture, however, is generally clear: a distinctly red or reddish tongue body with a yellow-greasy or yellow-pasty coating. If the tongue material is tender red and the coating is thin, yellow, and either lacking or without moisture altogether, it is appropriate to remove Atractylodis Rhizoma *(cāng zhú)*, Akebiae Caulis *(mù tōng)*, and Sophorae flavescentis Radix *(kǔ shēn)* from the formula and add a large dosage of gentle, moistening herbs that extinguish wind such as Paeoniae Radix alba *(bái sháo)*, Polygoni multiflori Radix *(hé shǒu wū)*, Polygonati odorati Rhizoma *(yù zhú)*, and Mori Fructus *(sāng shèn)*. If, after giving several packets of this formula, one sees no improvement, it may be wise to change course and consider if the pattern is possibly blood deficiency with Liver exuberance.

In summary, the causes of itching can be complex, but wind-heat-dampness and blood deficiency Liver exuberance are the two most commonly seen patterns. Once you understand the differentiation of these two patterns, you are in a good position.

PHYSICIAN B   After this patient was prescribed a large dosage of acrid and hot herbs her pattern had developed into lurking, static heat in the blood aspect and her condition became serious. When we received the patient at the clinic we prescribed Rhinoceros Horn and Rehmannia Decoction *(xī jiǎo dì huáng tāng)* with Bubali Cornu *(shuǐ niú jiǎo)* substituted for Rhinocerotis Cornu *(xī jiǎo)*. We used 200g of fresh Bubali Cornu *(shuǐ niú jiǎo)* to subdue the power of the disorder. Why did we use such a large dosage?

DR. YU   This is something that I stumbled upon last year when I was treating a patient suffering from a serious allergic reaction to allopurinol.[3] The patient presented with severe peeling dermatitis covering the entire body. This was a pattern of heat toxicity entering into the blood and nutritive levels, which fit within the scope of treatment of Rhinoceros Horn and Rehmannia Decoction *(xī jiǎo dì huáng tāng)*. The normal 50g

....

3. *Translators' note:* Allopurinol is a drug primarily given for treatment of gout. Serious dermatologic disorders are a known side effect.

dosage of Bubali Cornu *(shuǐ niú jiǎo)* was ineffective, so we increased it to 200g and got exceptional results.

It is worth pointing out that there are times when one should use hot herbs in the treatment of itching skin disorders. However, the large collection of extremely acrid and hot herbs used in this case was clinically irresponsible. It created an injurious situation by depleting the patient's blood and damaging her yin.

PHYSICIAN B   After the patient took several packets of modified Rhinoceros Horn and Rehmannia Decoction *(xī jiǎo dì huáng tāng)* her daytime itching was almost completely eliminated. Her tongue body turned from dark red to something akin to tender red. But because her sleep was still disturbed by itching, you changed the formula to a modified version of Emperor of Heaven's Special Pill to Tonify the Heart *(tiān wáng bǔ xīn dān)* to improve her sleep and thereby relieve her nighttime itching. That is easy to understand. What is difficult to understand, however, is why, when the continued use of Emperor of Heaven's Special Pill to Tonify the Heart *(tiān wáng bǔ xīn dān)* was unable to eradicate the itching, there was no alternative other than to combine the formula with Cinnamon Twig Decoction *(guì zhī tāng)* to completely get rid of it.

DR. YU   You say that the reason for using Emperor of Heaven's Special Pill to Tonify the Heart *(tiān wáng bǔ xīn dān)* in the patient's second visit is easy to understand. What is your understanding of this?

PHYSICIAN B   Chapter 74 of the *Basic Questions* notes that "pain, itching, and sores all pertain to the Heart." The Heart governs the blood, so in the initial visit we used modified Rhinoceros Horn and Rehmannia Decoction *(xī jiǎo dì huáng tāng)* to clear heat, cool the blood, and disperse stasis with the aim of improving the Heart's function of governing the blood. On the follow-up visit we used Emperor of Heaven's Special Pill to Tonify the Heart *(tiān wáng bǔ xīn dān)* to enrich yin, clear heat, nourish the Heart, and quiet the spirit in order to further improve the Heart's ability to govern the blood.

DR. YU   The use of Emperor of Heaven's Special Pill to Tonify the Heart *(tiān wáng bǔ xīn dān)* to enrich yin, clear heat, nourish the Heart, and quiet the spirit was mainly intended to restore the Heart's function of storing the spirit. If a heat pathogen harasses the Heart, the Heart becomes irritated and the spirit restless, and a restless spirit gives rise to itching. When guided back to its lair, the spirit is quieted and also stored. Once the spirit is stored, the itching ceases.

Because, in this case, continued use of Emperor of Heaven's Special Pill to Tonify the Heart *(tiān wáng bǔ xīn dān)* was unable to completely resolve the patient's itching, it was necessary to address the deeper etiology by coupling the formula with Cinnamon Twig Decoction *(guì zhī tāng)*. Cinnamon Twig Decoction *(guì zhī tāng)* is the first formula mentioned in the *Discussion of Cold Damage (Shāng hán lùn)* and is the ancestor of all formulas. Within the formula are two others, Cinnamon Twig and Licorice Decoction *(guì zhī gān cǎo tāng)* and Peony and Licorice Decoction *(sháo yào gān cǎo tāng)*. The former is acrid and sweet; it transforms yang to adjust yin. The latter is sour and sweet; it transforms yin to adjust yang. The combination of the two gives Cinnamon Twig Decoction *(guì zhī tāng)* the capacity to adjust and harmonize the yin and yang of the entire body. In regard to the body, yin and yang relate to the blood and qi, and blood and qi relate to the nutritive and protective aspects. The ancients glowingly praised the ability of Cinnamon Twig Decoction *(guì zhī tāng)* to address external disorders by releasing the muscle layer and harmonizing the nutritive and protective aspects, and to address internal disorders by transforming qi and adjusting yin and yang. From a clinical viewpoint, a large number of chronic, stubborn, and complex patterns are lingering and difficult to cure. Although they have a complex disease origin and disease dynamic (equally so based on a Western medical etiology), in the final analysis these disorders fall into the category of disharmony between the nutritive and protective aspects. This disharmony may be between the blood and qi, between the yin and yang, or a combination of the two. If this is true, in general, about long-term complex disorders, it should also be true of stubborn pruritus.

Ten years ago there was a 41-year-old nurse in our hospital who had had hives for over a year. She had used both Western and Chinese medicine (including steroids), but only got temporary relief. When she stopped treatment the symptoms returned. This person had an allergic-type constitution; also, when she was young she had her gallbladder removed. Dr. Jiang knew that the common treatment of Eliminate Wind Powder from the *Orthodox Lineage (xiāo fēng sǎn)* had already been tried without success. He gave the patient a series of formulas such as Warming and Clearing Drink *(wēn qīng yǐn)*, Augmented Rambling Powder *(jiā wèi xiāo yáo sǎn)*, Emperor of Heaven's Special Pill to Tonify the Heart *(tiān wáng bǔ xīn dān),* and Allergy Decoction *(guò mǐn jiān)*,[4] also without any effect. He then thought about the situation and said, "Let's try Cinnamon Twig Decoction *(guì zhī tāng)* with Notoginseng Radix *(sān qī)*." The formula included the following:

Cinnamomi Ramulus *(guì zhī)*..10g
Paeoniae Radix alba *(bái sháo)*...12g
Glycyrrhizae Radix praeparata *(zhì gān cǎo)* 5g
Jujubae Fructus *(dà zǎo)* 10g
Zingiberis Rhizoma recens *(shēng jiāng)*..5g
Notoginseng Radix *(sān qī)* [powdered and mixed
      with strained hot decoction] 5g

Instructions: one packet per day

After taking six packets there was no change in the patient's condition. After six more packets she began to see results. The patient continued to take this formula for another month and her outbreaks of hives ceased completely. It is difficult to determine if these results are reproducible. Nonetheless, I was inspired by this case and subsequently, when treating stubborn itching skin disorders, for a period of time I often included Cinnamon Twig Decoction *(guì zhī tāng)* to harmonize the nutritive-protective, qi-blood, and yin-yang. While I no longer do this as a matter of course, in certain patients this treatment strategy can observably increase efficacy.

....

4. *Translators' note:* Allergy Decoction (過敏煎 *guò mǐn jiān)* is a formula by the modern physician Zhu Chen-Yu. It contains 10g each of Saposhnikoviae Radix *(fáng fēng)*, Stellariae Radix *(yín chái hú)*, Mume Fructus *(wū méi)*, Schisandrae Fructus *(wǔ wèi zǐ)*, and Glycyrrhizae Radix *(gān cǎo)*.

PHYSICIAN C This is a case where pruritus, which was mistakenly treated with hot herbs, became a serious disorder. I believe that the mistreatment was the result of the doctor's misunderstanding of the five-phase treatment principle of discharging constrained fire. For those with only basic knowledge of Chinese medicine, these types of misconceptions are difficult to avoid. Even among those with a deeper understanding, opinions of these ambiguous principles vary. Thus, in my opinion, one is better off not taking a chance with questionable treatment principles and possibly ending up with unexpected results. What is your opinion?

DR. YU The scientific aspects of five-phase doctrine are not always apparent. In Chinese medicine it is considered just a reasoning tool. Since it is a tool, one must determine if it is applicable in each specific situation.

Let's first examine an instance where employing five-phase theory is inappropriate. In the *Discussion of Warm-Heat Pathogen [Disorders] (Wēn rè lun),* Ye Tian-Shi of the Qing dynasty famously said, "The warm pathogen is received in the upper [body], [it] first invades the Lung, adverse transmission [is to the] Pericardium." In his commentary to the text, Zhang Xu-Gu makes an effort to explain why transmission to the Pericardium is called adverse. His explanation is based on the five-phase theory of mutual control: "The Heart pertains to fire and the Lung to metal, fire overcomes metal, [so] a Lung disease contrarily transmitting to the Heart is called adverse transmission." While this explanation is seemingly logical according to five-phase theory, it has no place here because, in the context of Ye Tian-Shi's writings, normal transmission is from the upper burner downward: the pathogen proceeds from the protective aspect to the qi aspect to the nutritive aspect and then to the blood aspect. The Qing-dynasty physician Wang Meng-Ying pointed this out by stating that the theory of warm disease posits that

> the pathogen moving downward from the qi aspect is normal, pathogens entering the nutritive aspect and sinking inward is adverse. ... If [one does] not [begin with] this [concept of] normal [transmission], how [can one] conceive adverse [transmission]? Master Zhang is not capable of deeply investigating, and uses the engendering and restraining cycle to explain [this passage,] following neither [Ye Tian-Shi's] original intention nor that of the classic text. Has he not read the book of the gentleman from Yue?

Wang issued this strong refutation although he must have known that Zhang Xu-Gu was a famous physician and had written the well-known text *A Stick to Awaken Physicians (Yī mén bàng hè).* He harshly criticized Zhang and even derided him for apparently not having read the gentleman from Yue's (another name for Bian Que) *Classic of Difficulties (Nàn jīng).* In trying to clarify this profound concept of Chinese medicine, Zhang's strained use of the five-phase theory left him open to ridicule and proved that sometimes, even a wise man makes mistakes.

Now let us discuss an appropriate usage of five-phase theory. In the *Essentials from the Golden Cabinet (Jīn guì yào lüè),* Zhang Zhong-Jing writes, "Seeing Liver disease, one knows that the Liver transmits to the Spleen [so one] should first firm up the Spleen." This profoundly reveals the link between the phases of earth and wood and the origin, nature, and course of disease. To the current day this principle guides clinical practice. Comment on Zhang Zhong-Jing's text by later practitioners explains that

"When wood is exuberant it overwhelms earth. One should preemptively tonify earth to prevent this." The early-modern practitioner Zhang Xi-Chun stated, "When wood is exuberant it overwhelms earth, and when wood is deficient it cannot dredge earth. Both of these meanings are reflected in the statement that one ought to first firm up the Spleen." This is truly exceptional insight.

One could also ask if, in five-phase theory, exuberance in wood results in deficiency in earth, does deficiency in earth necessarily give rise to exuberance in wood? Not inevitably. In the clinic, there is no lack of cases of incessant dizziness associated with the pattern of earth deficiency/wood shaking. One needs to prescribe formulas in the Six-Gentlemen Decoction *(liù jūn zǐ tāng)* family to strengthen the Spleen and harmonize the Stomach to relieve the dizziness. This is deficiency of both wood and earth.

If we abide too strictly by the statement in Chapter 74 of the *Basic Questions* that "all wind, falling down, and dizziness pertain to the Liver", our perspective is overly constrained. Likewise, contradictory five-phase treatment principles like "earth does not engender metal/nurture earth to engender metal"; "wood and fire torment metal/clear metal to restrain wood"; and also "water cannot moisten wood/nourish water to moisten wood" cannot be interpreted too strictly. While the meaning of each statement is quite clear, none of them should be interpreted either too strictly or too loosely; each has a degree of clinical value in specific situations.

In summary, there are a few ways in which five-phase theory can be helpful in clinical practice. Not only can they be used to simplify complex situations, but understanding them can make some situations so familiar that we can recognize them right away and easily deal with them. Following the winding paths of these theories can sometimes take us to places of deep insight. Furthermore, many important practitioners over the millennia have utilized these theories, and, as Confucius said, "When you see a worthy [person], you should think to emulate them." Finally, in this context we must not fall into the trap of "not eating because we are afraid we might choke" and thereby avoid all dealings with five-phase theories just because some of them are hard to swallow.

7.1.1 Itching

Exfoliative dermatitis

A fast car on a familiar drive can suddenly go off the road
(A routine task runs into difficulty)

輕車熟路居然走不通

■ CASE HISTORY

Patient: *65-year-old male*

The patient, under treatment for gout, had taken allopurinol and suffered generalized itching. The itching started after seven days, and by day ten had become so severe that he went to the emergency room at his local hospital and was admitted. At this time he had superficial edema and his skin was dry and red. The rash was most severe above the waist.

The patient was evaluated by a specialist at the West China University of Medical Sciences and was diagnosed with generalized exfoliative dermatitis owing to allopurinol sensitivity. He was treated for two weeks with injections of the imported steroid methylprednisolone sodium succinate, along with intravenous drips of antibiotics and vitamins, together with symptomatic treatments.

The patient's condition did not change and he was then prescribed modified Eliminate Wind Powder from the *Orthodox Lineage (xiāo fēng săn)*. Passage of stool and urine declined. He was then prescribed a modification of Eight-Herb Powder for Rectification *(bā zhèng săn)* and took two packets. His stool and urine stopped completely and the patient's consciousness became cloudy. When informed of the seriousness of the patient's condition, his family rushed him to my clinic.

INTAKE EXAMINATION
DATE: November 28, 1998

The patient's face and body was red and swollen. The rash was extremely itchy and included large patches of exfoliated skin. His abdomen was distended and tympanic. He had not urinated or defecated for three days. He drifted in and out of consciousness. The patient's tongue was enlarged and red with an underlying purple tinge and was covered with a thick, grayish-yellow coating with little moisture. His pulse was large and forceless.

Differentiation of Patterns and Discussion of Treatment

PHYSICIAN A   Can you please describe the critical manifestation of generalized exfoliative dermatitis?

DR. YU   The disorder presents with large patches of exfoliated skin throughout the body. The upper limbs look as if one had removed a pair of opera gloves and the skin had come off with them. The lower limbs are similar, substituting knee socks for opera gloves in the metaphor. The peeling process can be repeated several times.

The most difficult aspect of this disorder, however, is that over the body where the skin exfoliates there appear areas of foul-smelling, damp erosions and fissures that are extremely difficult to treat.

When infectious skin lesions combine with cardiac, hepatic, or renal damage the prognosis is not favorable. I am familiar with two such cases treated with Western medicine by well-known doctors. Both cases of exfoliative dermatitis resulted from use of allopurinol on young patients suffering from renal or cardiac problems (aside from its use to treat gout, allopurinol has also been used to treat chronic kidney disease and chronic heart disease). In both cases, the patients died owing to cardiac or renal failure.

Allopurinol is a common and effective medication for gout. However, up to now its serious side effects have not received enough attention. According to the Western medical literature, occurrence of serious allopurinol sensitivity is exceptionally rare. However, because the prognosis for those unfortunate few who do develop exfoliative dermatitis from allopurinol is so poor, it is best not to let one's guard down when encountering a patient taking this drug. One should alert the patient of this possible side effect and caution him or her, in order to preclude a serious outcome, to immediately cease taking the drug and to promptly seek treatment if any skin rash appears.

PHYSICIAN B Drug sensitivity reactions are generally considered to be equivalent to wind, heat, and dampness in Chinese medicine and are treated with formulas to disperse wind, clear heat, and resolve dampness. The use of Eliminate Wind Powder from the *Orthodox Lineage (xiāo fēng sǎn)* in the current case is an example of this.

DR. YU In the initial stages, if the patient has a weak constitution or if the pattern includes dampness and damp-heat accumulation symptoms that are especially pronounced, it is easy for those symptoms to conceal the presence of heat toxin deep in the body at the nutritive and blood levels.

This disorder has a very rapid progression, and to effectively treat it, one must have a careful plan and promptly dispatch herbs to clear the nutritive level, resolve toxicity, and cool and disperse the blood.

PHYSICIAN A We understand that the fundamental approach to this disorder in the clinic is to clear the nutritive level, resolve toxicity, and cool and disperse the blood. In this case, however, because the patient had a blockage of both urine and stool, it was a critical situation that called for immediate action in unblocking the urination and bowels.

DR. YU Not long after the patient was admitted through the emergency room he was seen by a Chinese medicine doctor who observed that he was overweight and had a thick, greasy tongue coating. He accordingly diagnosed the case as one of damp-heat and prescribed a modification of Eliminate Wind Powder from the *Orthodox Lineage (xiāo fēng sǎn)* to dispel wind, clear heat, and resolve dampness. This gradually depleted the patient's blood, damaged his yin, and subsequently slowed the passage of urine and stool.

Chapter 65 of the *Basic Questions (Sù wèn)* instructs that for "inhibited urine and stool [one must] treat the branch." By instructing us on the treatment of those in urgent need, the text presents us with a fundamental principle. The word 'treat' (治 *zhì*) in this sentence has been the subject of intense study, and in no way does it condone blindly purging or unblocking. In the current case, for example, where internal collection of damp-heat and major damage to the yin and thick fluids combine, the use of common treatments to unblock urination and the bowels, for example, Eight-Herb Powder for Rectification *(bā zhèng sǎn),* led to a precarious situation.

Treatment and Outcome

After careful consideration I decided the best approach was Polyporus Decoction *(zhū líng tāng)*, with its ability to both nourish yin and promote urination, combined with herbs like Armeniacae Semen *(xìng rén)*, Eriobotryae Folium *(pí pá yè),* and Platycodi Radix *(jié gěng)* that diffuse and unblock Lung qi while avoiding damage to the yin. Here, using herbs to unblock Lung qi is an example of applying the principle of "removing the cover of the vessel in order to pour from the spout", that is, to free the urine and stool. This principle is a reference to facilitating urination by diffusing the Lung qi. The Lung is the "cover" of the yin organs, and by unblocking Lung qi, the Lung is then able to clarify the fluids and send them downward through the water pathways. Treatment of edema with urinary difficulty is the most common application of this treatment principle. Furthermore, because of the interior-exterior relationship between the Lung and Large Intestine, diffusing Lung qi and causing it to descend can also help unblock the bowels.

While the proper treatment would generally be to cool and disperse blood, nourish yin, and enrich the Kidneys, in this case it is best to address the blockage of stool and urine, which, being a critical condition, requires immediate attention. Thus, it is appropriate to engender yin and promote urination, diffuse the qi of the Lung, and unblock the bowels.

We prescribed a modification of Polyporus Decoction (*zhū líng tāng*) as follows:

Asini Corii Colla *(ē jiāo)* [dissolve into hot decoction]....................20g
Polyporus *(zhū líng)*...15g
Poria *(fú líng)*..15g
Alismatis Rhizoma *(zé xiè)*..30g
Talcum *(huá shí)*..30g
Armeniacae Semen *(xìng rén)* 15g
Platycodi Radix *(jié gěng)* 6g
Eriobotryae Folium *(pí pá yè)*.......................................30g
Plantaginis Semen *(chē qián zǐ)* [wrap separately before decocting] 30g
Polygoni cuspidati Rhizoma *(hǔ zhàng)*...............................30g
dry-fried Raphani Semen *(chǎo lái fú zǐ)*............................30g

Two packets were prescribed to be cooked into a thick decoction and spoon-fed to the patient frequently throughout the day. A thick decoction is one that is initially boiled twice in the normal way. After the strained decoctions of the two cookings are combined, the liquid is further cooked over a low flame until the desired volume is reached. In this case, the volume was reduced down to about three cups for one day's consumption. The patient's Western medication was not altered.

SECOND VISIT: The patient was spoon-fed the decoction beginning at 6 p.m. the evening after the first visit. At 2 a.m. the next morning he urinated once. Then at 6 a.m. he defecated and his consciousness cleared. The tide had been turned on a dangerous condition.

The formula was changed to a modified Rhinoceros Horn and Rehmannia Decoction (*xī jiǎo dì huáng tāng*) in order to strongly clear the toxic heat that had penetrated deeply into the nutritive and blood levels.

fresh Bubali Cornu *(shuǐ niú jiǎo)* [cook separately for
    two hours then add to drained decoction] ....50g[5]
Rehmanniae Radix *(shēng dì huáng)*..................................30g
Moutan Cortex *(mǔ dān pí)*..15g
Paeoniae Radix rubra *(chì sháo)*.....................................30g
Arnebiae/Lithospermi Radix *(zǐ cǎo)* 30g
Ecliptae Herba *(mò hàn lián)*..30g
Leonuri Herba *(yì mǔ cǎo)* 30g
Agrimoniae Herba *(xiān hè cǎo)*......................................30g

....

5. Reduce the dosage by half when using the dried product.

Instructions: If the formula is ineffective, the dosage of Bubali Cornu *(shuǐ niú jiǎo)* can be increased up to 200g.

THIRD VISIT: The patient took five packets of the above prescription without a noticeable change in his condition. The patient's steroids were then reduced; his condition rapidly declined and large patches of skin began to exfoliate, the itching became unbearable, and he became extremely agitated.

Following the previously given instructions, the amount of Bubali Cornu *(shuǐ niú jiǎo)* was increased to 200g. It was double-boiled for two hours and then strained; the remaining liquid, about 100ml, was then divided into three doses and added to the liquid decocted from the other herbs in the formula. Also, the patient's steroid medication was gradually restored to its previous dosage.

After five packets of herbs, exfoliation throughout the body was stabilized and the skin's redness and itching also markedly decreased. After 20 packets the patient's skin had returned to normal.

The remaining symptoms included a deficiency type of superficial edema of the face, shortness of breath, lack of strength, confused dreams, reduced food intake, loose stools, dry mouth with no desire to drink, a pale, purple tongue with a thin, white coating, and a wiry, weak pulse.

These symptoms indicated Spleen deficiency with sinking qi and inadequate intake and transport of nourishment. To address this situation, the prescription was changed to a modified combination of Raise the Sunken Decoction *(shēng xiàn tāng)* and Ginseng, Poria, and White Atractylodes Powder *(shēn líng bái zhú sǎn)*. After eight packets of this combination, the patient's food intake and sleep improved greatly.

TWO-YEAR FOLLOW-UP REPORT

The patient, following the doctor's advice, had continued to take prednisone for three months and was then gradually weaned from it. He had numerous follow-up examinations and the functions of his internal organs (heart, liver, kidneys) were all normal. Further, his bone density was normal and he was declared healthy and free of disease.

Disease	Main Symptom	Pattern Differentiation	Treatment Method	Formula
Exfoliative dermatitis	Large patches of exfoliated skin throughout the body	Heat toxin deeply entering the nutritive and blood aspects	Clear the nutritive, resolve toxicity, and cool and disperse blood	Rhinoceros Horn and Rehmannia Decoction *(xī jiǎo dì huáng tāng)*

Reflections and Clarifications

PHYSICIAN A   In this case the patient was advanced in years and the Western medical staff was quite concerned. Prior to coming to our clinic he was twice classified as critical. Fortunately, his heart, liver, kidneys, and other internal organs were all functioning normally. After we administered Chinese herbs, although we were unable to prevent large patches of skin exfoliation over the patient's body, he did not experience any of the dangerous outcomes we have spoken of. Nonetheless, people have attributed his recovery to the administration of imported methylprednisolone.

DR. YU   Correct. Chinese herbs cannot replace methylprednisolone. But the use of methylprednisolone cannot prevent the occurrence of severe outcomes. There is no denying that once Chinese herbs were applied, the serious symptoms abated and the tide was turned.

Regarding this case we also need to give credit to the clinically correct line of thinking that was followed. Why is it that the Chinese medical attention the patient received previously yielded less than ideal results? This was because the standard thinking about allergic rashes owing to drugs is that they are associated with wind, heat, and dampness and the usual treatment employs herbs to disperse wind, clear heat, and resolve dampness. I would say that this fast car on that familiar drive just went off the road! When taking a fast car along a familiar road, a not-so-small miscalculation can lead to an even larger deviation from the correct path. This case reminds us that severe reaction to allopurinol resulting in large patches of exfoliative dermatitis is due to blood that is consumed and agitated by heat toxin entering deeply into the blood and nutritive aspects.

We resolutely stand by the method of using a large amount of Rhinoceros Horn and Rehmannia Decoction *(xī jiǎo dì huáng tāng),* adding large dosages of substances that cool the blood, stop bleeding, and resolve toxicity such as Arnebiae/Lithospermi Radix *(zǐ cǎo)*, Ecliptae Herba *(mò hàn lián),* and Agrimoniae Herba *(xiān hè cǎo).* The large dosage (up to 200g) of fresh Bubali Cornu *(xiān shuǐ niú jiǎo)* in the formula is essential for addressing the serious heat toxin in the nutritive and blood aspects.

PHYSICIAN B   Regarding this formula, you have said that in this case the pattern of heat toxin lurking deep within the nutritive and blood aspects arises from an allergic reaction to a drug. The heavy dosage of Bubali Cornu *(shuǐ niú jiǎo)* is an example of striking two birds with one stone. It cools blood and resolves toxicity and also counteracts allergies. Does Bubali Cornu *(shuǐ niú jiǎo)* truly have this latter function?

DR. YU   Bubali Cornu *(shuǐ niú jiǎo)* has gained renown recently as a miraculous medicinal substance. It is credited with the functions of aiding the recovery of the sovereign Heart, sheltering the essence-spirit, and quieting and settling the ethereal and corporal souls. Its ability to change the nature of the spirit-essence and aid in the recovery from serious disorders by altering the nature of the qi affected by pathogens has led to its designation as a substance that Chapter 13 of the *Basic Questions (Sù wèn)* calls "altering the essence and changing the qi."

Long-term clinical study has revealed that the causes of allergic disorders are complex, but it is hard to ignore the observation that allergic disorders readily occur in those whose spirit-essence loses shelter, and in those patients whose ethereal and corporal souls are unsettled. This being the case, we do have the sense that Bubali Cornu *(shuǐ niú jiǎo)* has an ability to counteract allergies.

Later we had a chance to once again test the formula in a similar circumstance.

The patient was a 36-six-year-old male who had a robust constitution. Due to a long-standing case of gout, he had been taking allopurinol off and on for several years and the results had been acceptable. When he occasionally experienced itching, he would stop taking the allopurinol and take imported anti-allergic drugs. In 1999 just prior to Chinese New Year, the patient had taken allopurinol for an uninterrupted two weeks when he experienced redness of the face, head, and entire body along with intense itching and peeling skin. He went to the emergency room where he was diagnosed with generalized exfoliative dermatitis. His treatment by Western medicine mimicked that of the original case. At that time, the patient in the first case was still in the hospital and was happy to introduce this new patient to my department.

Because of the experience we had had with the first case, we quickly gave the patient a modified Rhinoceros Horn and Rehmannia Decoction *(xī jiǎo dì huáng tāng)* including 200g of Bubali Cornu *(shuǐ niú jiǎo)*. He took 12 packets and his itching gradually abated until it ceased completely. The skin redness lessened and the peeling was under control. For financial reasons, the patient's family requested he leave the hospital. After leaving the hospital the patient, following the doctors' advice, took methylprednisolone. He also took 30 more packets of herbs. All of his symptoms disappeared and, at the time of this writing, have not returned.

PHYSICIAN B In the original case, when the patient suffered from blockage of the stool and urine, you prescribed Polyporus Decoction *(zhū líng tāng)* from the *Discussion of Cold Damage (Shāng hán lùn)* modified by adding such herbs as Armeniacae Semen *(xìng rén)*, Platycodi Radix *(jié gěng)*, and Eriobotryae Folium *(pí pá yè)* to diffuse and unblock the Lung qi while not damaging yin. You said that the aim of this formula was to unblock bowel movements and promote urination by applying the principle of "removing the cover of the vessel in order to pour from the spout." In Chinese medical textbooks this principle is mentioned only for promoting urination. How is it that it also unblocks the bowels?

DR. YU The Lung governs qi and has an interior-exterior relationship with the Large Intestines. When Lung qi diffuses, Intestinal qi is unblocked. Thus, removing the cover of the vessel not only unblocks urination but also unblocks the bowels.

When I treat habitual constipation and find that formulas to enrich the Spleen and direct Stomach qi downward are less than effective, I like to add herbs such as Armeniacae Semen *(xìng rén)*, Platycodi Radix *(jié gěng)*, and Eriobotryae Folium *(pí pá yè)* to diffuse and unblock Lung qi. This frequently brings good results.

Once I treated a woman who had a dry cough at night. Her stools were dry and she only had one bowel movement a week. Because she had no way to cook herbs, I suggested she simply use 60g of prepared Asteris Radix *(zhì zǐ wǎn)* and 6g of Cicadae Periostracum *(chán tuì)* steeped in a teapot of water and consumed as one would drink tea throughout the day. After two days of this regimen, her stools moved normally and her cough was greatly diminished. This is another example of employing the principle of "removing the cover of the vessel in order to pour from the spout" to unblock the bowels.

7.2 Herpes zoster

A case of herpes zoster

Avoid detours by taking a careful history

詳詢治療史,避免走彎路

■ CASE HISTORY

Patient: *60-year-old woman*

Two weeks prior to her visit the patient experienced stabbing pain on the left side of her ribcage. This progressed to blisters that exuded fluid. She took several medications including polyinosinic-polycytidylic acid injection, acyclovir, and vitamin B12 for seven days. This treatment was accompanied by physical therapy, all to no effect. The patient then took six packets of modified Gentian Decoction to Drain the Liver *(lóng dǎn xiè gān tāng)* but again saw no noticeable improvement.

INTAKE EXAMINATION

The skin on the patient's left ribcage was flushed red. A burning-hot rash wrapped around a ribbon of mung-bean sized vesicles. She was irritable and had dry mouth with a bitter taste. Her stools were dry. She had a dry tongue with a coating that was dry, thin, and yellow. The tip and sides of the tongue displayed small red dots and her pulse was wiry, fine, and rapid.

Differentiation of Patterns and Discussion of Treatment

PHYSICIAN A   In classical Chinese medicine what in Western medicine is called herpes zoster is called descriptive names such as linking snake sores (蛇串瘡 *shé chuàn chuāng*) or waist-wrapping cinnabar fire (纏腰火丹 *chán yāo huǒ dān*). It is a commonly occurring disorder that most often strikes in the spring or autumn months. The groupings of blistering, hot, and painful sores most often manifest along the course of the intercostal nerves, or on the ribs themselves, following the Liver or Gallbladder channels. This disorder is often seen in the company of a slippery and rapid pulse and a red tongue with a yellow coating. Chinese medicine views it as damp-heat in the Liver and Gallbladder and typically treats it with Gentian Decoction to Drain the Liver *(lóng dǎn xiè gān tāng)*.

DR. YU   Since the patient had already tried six packets of Gentian Decoction to Drain the Liver *(lóng dǎn xiè gān tāng)* with no improvement, it was time to take a different tack. After that formula was ineffective, how could we continue to throw good herbs after bad? A new path was needed.

One must not simply diagnose according to the pulse alone, but must also carefully examine the patient's treatment history. When seeing a patient who has taken herbs for a time with no results, one must review the treatment history and clearly view the detour taken and thus avoid continuing on the same mistaken path.

PHYSICIAN B   Well said! In the clinic this type of case is a frequent occurrence. The patient complains of pain in the chest and ribs and the doctor reflects briefly and declares "constrained and knotted Liver qi" and with an unthinking pen prescribes a formula of Bupleurum Powder to Dredge the Liver *(chái hú shū gān sǎn)*. When this is ineffective, he announces that the pattern is "qi stagnation and blood stasis" and prescribes Drive out Stasis from the Mansion of Blood Decoction *(xuè fǔ zhú yū tāng)*. When this also fails to improve the patient's condition, and the pain increases and blistering sores appear, the doctor suddenly realizes that this, after all, is herpes zoster and follows convention to prescribe Gentian Decoction to Drain the Liver *(lóng dǎn xiè gān tāng)*. When this too has no effect, the doctor recommends Western medicine. This process causes the condition to drag on and become entrenched. Although the blistering sores gradually disperse, the nerve pain continues and the patient is left with postherpetic neuralgia.

DR. YU   This is not an exaggeration. I will cite an example to dispel any doubts about the truth of this. There is a doctor in my town who is more than seven decades old. His body is strong and vigorous. When his herpes episode began it resembled a flu or cold but then he quickly developed rib pain, and soon after, groups of small blistering sores appeared. He was prescribed three packets of Gentian Decoction to Drain the Liver *(lóng dǎn xiè gān tāng)*, to no avail, and then that was combined with Western medications for one week. At that time the patient began to suffer extremely painful vesicles along the course of his trigeminal nerve. He continued treatment with Western medicine and Chinese herbs for more than ten days and the vesicles gradually receded. However, the pain in the intercostal and trigeminal nerves continued and became almost unbearable. During the day he would groan unceasingly and at night would cry out in pain. Later, he came to my clinic for treatment and I used Chinese herbs to treat him. Herbal treatment continued for more than three months, during which time the pain gradually diminished and eventually ceased.

PHYSICIAN A   Since what Dr. Yu says is correct, in order to avoid misdiagnosis and mistaken treatment we must recognize that the treatment plan should depend on differentiation of the patient's constitution. From our observations in the clinic we can say that herpes zoster patients generally have a yang-flourishing body (陽旺軀 *yáng wàng qū)*, that is, a vigorous constitution or what is colloquially called a fire constitution. Only after employing the four diagnostic techniques of observation, inquiry, listening, and palpation, and especially inquiring about the disease history, the treatment history, lifestyle, family history, etc., can we then accurately differentiate the patient's constitutional type.

When a patient presents with a vigorous constitution and pain in the chest and ribs, they usually exhibit a yang, hot, excess pattern. Thus, employing formulas that use acrid and aromatic herbs that deplete qi, and acrid warm herbs that exacerbate fire, is like adding oil to a fire. In addition, formulas that move qi, invigorate the blood, and relieve pain will also be unsuitable for this pathodynamic and will clearly be ineffective.

DR. YU   That is correct! When treating herpes zoster one must integrate differentiation of the pattern of the disease as well as differentiation of the constitution and the disease pattern. In this way we can quickly and accurately diagnose and treat the patient. As herbal treatment should be the focus, once one matches the herbs and the pattern, quick and decisive treatment will totally avoid or at least mitigate any accompanying or postherpetic neuralgia.

As a young doctor I initially treated herpes zoster following the common custom of prescribing Gentian Decoction to Drain the Liver *(lóng dǎn xiè gān tāng)*. I treated many cases of herpes zoster, sometimes effectively and sometimes not. Of the cases with only slightly beneficial or completely fruitless results, most had a history of mistaken treatment or missed opportunities for treatment.

Later, while thumbing through Cheng Guo-Peng's Qing-dynasty text *Awakening of the Mind in Medical Studies (Yī xué xīn wù)*, I came across a passage where Cheng elaborated on the dynamics of the function of Trichosanthes Fruit Powder *(guā lóu sǎn)*:

> [This formula is] for chronic fire from constraint, [where] Liver qi [is] parched, tight, and unable to diffuse; thus blisters arise on the skin and give rise to distention and pain. The classics *[Classic of Difficulties (Nàn jīng), 14]* say: "For those with injury to the Liver, relax the middle." Trichosanthis Fructus *(guā lóu)* is sweet, moderating, and moistening yet does not adversely affect constraint; also, it is like [using] oil to clean things, [because it is] slippery and non-stagnating. It is effective.

When Cheng Guo-Peng says "chronic fire from constraint, [where] Liver qi [is] dry and tense and unable to diffuse," is this not describing the fundamental disease dynamic that underlies herpes zoster? The special characteristics of Trichosanthis Fructus *(guā lóu)*, the main ingredient in Trichosanthes Fruit Powder *(guā lóu sǎn)*, make it a perfect fit for this pattern.

I use Trichosanthes Fruit Powder *(guā lóu sǎn)* regardless of whether the pattern is Liver channel excess fire or damp-heat in the Liver or Gallbladder. On countless occasions it has achieved quick and reliable results without the occurrence of postherpetic neuralgia. After many years of clinical experience, I am entirely convinced that this formula matches the fundamental disease dynamic of herpes zoster and is the perfect specialized formula to use for this disorder. If one differentiates both the disease and the pattern and then integrates Trichosanthes Fruit Powder *(guā lóu sǎn)* with a formula that addresses the differentiated pattern, one will consistently get excellent results.

The original formula prescribes one large fruit of Trichosanthis Fructus *(guā lóu)*. Because nowadays it is difficult to find a large Trichosanthis Fructus *(guā lóu)*, I generally use Trichosanthis Semen *(guā lóu rén)* 30-50g and Trichosanthis Pericarpium *(guā lóu pí)* 15-20g in addition to Glycyrrhizae Radix *(gān cǎo)* and Carthami Flos *(hóng huā)* 10g each. After seeing some improvement in the patient's condition, one can consider reducing the dosages of the main herbs.

PHYSICIAN B The Qing-dynasty doctor Wang Xue-Quan also sings the praise of the special functions of Trichosanthis Fructus *(guā lóu)*. In his text *Jottings from Repeated Celebration Hall (Chóng qìng táng suí bǐ)* he states, "Trichosanthis Fructus *(guā lóu)* moistens dryness and opens up knots, flushes away heat and scours out phlegm; everyone knows this. What they do not know is that it is also especially good at soothing Liver constraint, moistening Liver dryness, calming Liver counterflow, and moderating Liver tension."

DR. YU   Though Wang Xue-Quan does not clearly indicate his source, the *Jottings from Repeated Celebration Hall (Chóng qìng táng suí bǐ)* was published after the *Awakening of the Mind in Medical Studies (Yī xué xīn wù)*. Thus, Wang's mention of the special ability of Trichosanthis Fructus *(guā lóu)* to soothe Liver constraint, moisten Liver dryness, calm Liver counterflow, moderate Liver tension, etc. is simply reprinted from Cheng Guo-Peng's commentary on Trichosanthes Fruit Powder *(guā lóu sǎn)*.

PHYSICIAN A   I have witnessed that some Chinese medicine doctors, when faced with a severe case of herpes zoster, even in the initial stages, won't dare to use Chinese herbs alone, but ask the patient to combine Chinese herbs with Western medical treatment.

DR. YU   When I treat this disorder, unless there is a serious, undesired reaction to treatment, I use only Chinese herbs.

Treatment and Outcome

After comprehensive analysis of the patient's treatment history and her list of attending symptoms such as chest irritability, dry mouth, a bitter taste, dry stool, etc., we diagnosed this case as injury to the Liver yin by fire toxin. The proper treatment was to drain fire, resolve toxicity, enrich the Liver, and moisten dryness.

The chosen formula was Trichosanthes Fruit Powder *(guā lóu sǎn)* with Rhinoceros Horn and Rehmannia Decoction *(xī jiǎo dì huáng tāng)*, with Bubali Cornu *(shuǐ niú jiǎo)* substituted for Rhinocerotis Cornu *(xī jiǎo)*, plus Linking Decoction *(yī guàn jiān)*:

Trichosanthis Semen *(guā lóu rén)* [stir-fried]..............................50g
Trichosanthis Pericarpium *(guā lóu pí)*..20g
Carthami Flos *(hóng huā)* 10g
Glycyrrhizae Radix *(gān cǎo)*..10g
Bubali Cornu *(shuǐ niú jiǎo)* [pre-cook 30 minutes].......................30g
Moutan Cortex *(mǔ dān pí)*...10g
Paeoniae Radix rubra *(chì sháo)* 15g
Rehmanniae Radix *(shēng dì huáng)*..30g
Glehniae Radix *(běi shā shēn)* 30g
Tribuli Fructus *(cì jí lí)*...15g

Instructions: Four packets were prescribed and Western medicine treatment was halted.

SECOND VISIT: The patient's skin was slightly red and the blisters more than half-way dried, the burning heat in the rib area had decreased greatly, as had the stabbing pain. Bowel movements were smooth and the patient's tongue was red with red dots on the tip and sides and a thin, yellow coating. The pulse was fine and wiry.

Because the formula was effective, it was left unchanged with the exception of reducing the Trichosanthis Semen *(guā lóu rén)* to 30g and Trichosanthis Pericarpium *(guā lóu pí)* to 10g. Four more packets were prescribed.

THIRD VISIT: The patient's skin was approaching normal and the blisters were almost all gone. Only the stabbing pain in the ribs remained unchanged.

This is depletion of Liver yin and entrenched stasis in the Liver collaterals. The treatment principle was changed to enriching the Liver, unblocking the collaterals, moderating tension, and relieving pain. Trichosanthes Fruit Powder *(guā lóu sǎn)* continued to be prescribed along with modifications of Linking Decoction *(yī guàn jiān)* and Peony and Licorice Decoction *(sháo yào gān cǎo tāng)* as follows:

Trichosanthis Semen *(guā lóu rén)* [stir-fried] 30g
Trichosanthis Pericarpium *(guā lóu pí)* 10g
Carthami Flos *(hóng huā)* 5g
Glehniae Radix *(běi shā shēn)* 30g
Ophiopogonis Radix *(mài mén dōng)* 30g
Rehmanniae Radix *(shēng dì huáng)* 30g
Paeoniae Radix alba *(bái sháo)* 40g
Glycyrrhizae Radix *(gān cǎo)* 15g
Tribuli Fructus *(cì jí lí)* 10g
Bombyx batryticatus *(bái jiāng cán)* [thoroughly stir-fried, finely crushed,
   and taken mixed into the hot decoction with 3g each dose] 10g
Notoginseng Radix *(sān qī)* [powdered then taken mixed into the
   hot decoction with 3g each dose] 10g

OUTCOME

After six packets of herbs the patient noticed a gradual reduction in the stabbing pain in her ribs, and by the time she had taken twelve packets, the pain had completely subsided.

Disease	Main Symptoms	Differential Diagnosis	Treatment Method	Formula
Herpes zoster	The skin over the ribs is red and surrounds groups of vesicles.	Injury of the Liver yin by fire toxin	Drain fire, resolve toxicity, enrich the Liver, and moisten dryness	Trichosanthes Fruit Powder *(guā lóu sǎn)* with Rhinoceros Horn and Rehmannia Decoction *(xī jiǎo dì huáng tāng)*, Linking Decoction *(yī guàn jiān)* Special herb: Trichosanthis Fructus *(guā lóu)*

Reflections and Clarifications

PHYSICIAN D   It seems to me that the mechanism for post-herpetic neuralgia is very similar to that for the initial stage of the disorder and thus a modified version of Trichosanthes Fruit Powder *(guā lóu sǎn)* should be appropriate. Is this correct, and if so, what modifications are indicated?

DR. YU   While this formula can be useful for later stage herpes zoster with pain, I don't think that this would be appropriate for post-herpetic neuralgia without any vesicles. In that situation, I usually use either Peony and Licorice Decoction *(sháo yào gān cǎo tāng)* with 30-60g of Paeoniae Radix alba *(bái sháo)* and 15-30g of Glycyrrhizae Radix *(gān cǎo)* or a version of that formula with normal dosages of those two ingredients in combination with Dredge the Liver Decoction *(shū gān tāng)*. The treatment is different because the pathodynamic is different. Post-herpetic neuralgia is attributable to a lack of nourishment, as the fire toxin has caused the yin and blood to be insufficient, and the result is a lack of flow through the collateral vessels. The pain comes from this, so the combination of sour and sweet flavors that is Peony and Licorice Decoction *(sháo yào gān cǎo tāng)* can transform the yin and stop the pain.

PHYSICIAN C   Dr. Yu, you have examined your past missteps and have made the proper adjustments. You use Trichosanthes Fruit Powder *(guā lóu sǎn)*, Rhinoceros Horn and Rehmannia Decoction *(xī jiǎo dì huáng tāng)*, and Linking Decoction *(yī guàn jiān)*. I understand that in this treatment Rhinoceros Horn and Rehmannia Decoction *(xī jiǎo dì huáng tāng)* clears heat and resolves toxicity, cools the blood, and disperses stasis, while Linking Decoction *(yī guàn jiān)* enriches and nourishes Liver yin and dredges the Liver and regulates qi. This is easy to understand. However, Trichosanthes Fruit Powder *(guā lóu sǎn)* is not in modern formula textbooks and so we do not know the formula's construction and functions.

DR. YU   Trichosanthes Fruit Powder *(guā lóu sǎn)* originates from the famous Qing-dynasty physician Cheng Guo-Peng's book *Awakening of the Mind in Medical Studies (Yī xué xīn wù)*. A passage in that book states:

> Trichosanthes Fruit Powder *(guā lóu sǎn)* treats dry and tense Liver qi with rib pain or development of vesicles.
>
> Large Trichosanthis Fructus *(guā lóu)*
>   [including the peel, mash thoroughly] .... 1 fruit
> Glycyrrhizae Radix *(gān cǎo)* .... 2 *qián* [6g]
> Carthami Flos *(hóng huā)* .... 7 *fēn* [2g]
>
> Decoct and administer.

PHYSICIAN C   The source text does not say this formula treats herpes zoster.

DR. YU   The original text does not specifically mention using this formula to treat snake cluster sores (aka herpes zoster). I came up with the idea of applying the formula specifically to the treatment of snake cluster sores.

The case we are discussing today serves the purpose of providing an explanation of the treatment of herpes zoster. It is important to grasp information from the four examinations, determine the cause from investigating the evidence, and examine the cause to determine the treatment. By no means should one, upon seeing herpes zoster, simply conclude that it is damp-heat in the Liver or Gallbladder and blindly and mechanically prescribe Gentian Decoction to Drain the Liver *(lóng dǎn xiè gān tāng)*. That is the first point. Second, the formula we used in this case, Cheng Guo-Peng's Trichosanthes Fruit Powder *(guā lóu sǎn)*, can absolutely be used as a special formula for herpes zoster. I ask you all to try it in the clinic from today on.

PHYSICIAN C   Modern materia medica textbooks clearly state that Trichosanthis Fructus *(guā lóu)* enters the Lung, Stomach, and Large Intestine channels. The peel, Trichosanthis Pericarpium *(guā lóu pí)*, clears heat, transforms phlegm, moves qi, and loosens the chest. The seed, Trichosanthis Semen *(guā lóu rén)*, moistens the Lung, transforms phlegm, lubricates the Intestines, and unblocks the stool. The whole fruit, Trichosanthis Fructus *(guā lóu)*, thus has these same functions, and nowhere do the books say that it enters the Liver channel and treats the Liver.

Classical materia medica also record Trichosanthis Fructus *(guā lóu)* as entering the Lung, Stomach, and Large Intestine channels with no mention of the Liver channel. How can it treat the Liver?

DR. YU It is likely that Cheng Guo-Peng derived this usage from his observations in the clinic. I suspect that in those years, Cheng used large dosages of Trichosanthis Fructus *(guā lóu)* to treat Liver disorders and found that he got outstanding results. Long searching through classical materia medica and other medical texts will not yield any references to Trichosanthis Fructus *(guā lóu)* treating the Liver. Clinical practice gives rise to new knowledge; this is called getting rid of old doctrines while creating new ones.

PHYSICIAN A I feel that Cheng Guo-Peng's expression "Trichosanthis Fructus *(guā lóu)* treats the Liver" does not depart from the theoretical framework of China's traditional medicine. For example, we could posit that, first, Trichosanthis Fructus *(guā lóu)* enters the Lung (a metal channel). It clears the Lung and transforms phlegm, promotes the movement of qi, and loosens the chest. It also enters the Large Intestine (another metal channel) and moistens the Lung and transforms phlegm as it lubricates the Intestines and unblocks the stool. It clears metal and restrains wood, allowing wood qi to flow unimpeded and also calming wood-fire. Second, Trichosanthis Fructus *(guā lóu)* also enters the Stomach channel and eliminates that which is jammed up, unblocking plugs and thus unclogging earth qi. As a result, wood qi can perform its function of dredging, discharging, and thrusting outward. Third, the *Comprehensive Outline of the Materia Medica (Běn cǎo gāng mù)* records that Trichosanthis Fructus *(guā lóu)* "clears the toxin from abscesses, swellings and sores." Chapter 74 of the *Basic Questions (Sù wèn)* says, "Pain, sores, and itching all pertain to the Heart." Thus, Trichosanthis Fructus *(guā lóu)* can drain Heart fire. Chapter 69 of the *Classic of Difficulties (Nàn jīng)* says, "For excess, drain the child." Thus, draining Heart fire (the child) is draining Liver fire. From this we can see that, although Trichosanthis Fructus *(guā lóu)* does not directly enter the Liver, it can treat Liver illnesses. Since it treats the Lung, Large Intestine, Stomach, and Heart it also indirectly treats the Liver. This is the wonder of the generating and controlling cycles of five-phase theory: one can travel a winding path to a deep place. Do you have any thoughts about this?

DR. YU Now that does seem deep, doesn't it! Full of twists and turns, not unlike what is called "treatments once or twice removed" (隔二隔三之治 *gé èr gé sān zhī zhì*) that push the cycles of the five phases this way and that, so that anything at all can be explained. The explanation is complete, clear, and logical. Nowadays, there are some medical papers like this, lacking a single new idea. If everyone follows set ideologies in this fashion, writing in endless clichés in a subtle and skillful manner, yet unwilling to progress with the times and use new experiences to make new theories, to the extent that they dare not take a step out of predefined limits, then it is difficult to hope that we can make major breakthroughs and surpass our worthy predecessors.

PHYSICIAN C Pain in the costal region with vesicles that are distributed in belt-like clusters is diagnostic for herpes zoster. The pattern that Cheng Guo-Peng discusses, however, is one in which vesicles may or may not accompany the costal pain. If there is costal pain with no vesicles, can it still be herpes zoster?

DR. YU   In the clinic we have absolutely seen herpes zoster patients who, for the duration of the disorder, experience no vesicles (this is known as zoster sine herpete). This can easily lead to misdiagnosis. The question is, how do we avoid misdiagnosis and treatment in this situation?

Simply stated, a physician should follow the instructions found in Chapter 74 of the *Basic Questions (Sù wèn)*, which follows a description of the types of pathogens associated with specific groups of symptoms (e.g., "The various cases of a sudden onset of rigid stiffness are all due to wind"):

> Carefully observe the dynamics of disease and in each case control what is associated with them. If [the signs] are there, look for [the pathodynamic]. If [the signs] are missing, [also] look for it.

There are instances where pain, itching or both occur along the nerve path and no sores appear and there are also instances when pain, itching or both persist for several days before sores manifest. In these cases, one should not be deceived but should consider the possibility of herpes zoster. Generally speaking, if the weather is dry and the patient meets the following conditions, one should consider a diagnosis of herpes zoster:

- The patient complains of pain in the chest and costal region.
- Hepatic and gallbladder disease can be ruled out as the cause of the pain.
- The patient has not previously suffered from herpes zoster and has had chicken pox.

Years ago I mistakenly thought that herpes zoster only occurred in the spring and autumn and that it only affected those of a strong, yang constitution. Later, I saw several patients who displayed the above symptoms in winter or summer and who were not of robust constitution. Accordingly, I did not promptly give these patients Trichosanthes Fruit Powder *(guā lóu sǎn)* and this resulted in less than effective treatment. Nowadays, when I see the signs listed above I prescribe an appropriately modified version of this formula without delay.

Examine carefully the essential nature of the disorder, follow the trail, carefully survey the situation, and, without acting rashly, prescribe a formula.

Herb Index

Formula Index

General Index

Translators

Andrew Ellis first studied Chinese medicine with Dr. James Tin Yau So at the New England School of Acupuncture. He left New England in 1983 to study Chinese language in Taiwan where he apprenticed with Chinese herbalist Xu Fu-Su for several years. Later he studied internal medicine and gynecology at the Xiamen Hospital of Chinese Medicine. While there, he also specialized in the study of acupuncture with Dr. Shi Neng-Yun and dermatology with Dr. Zhang Guang-Cai. Andrew is the founding owner of Spring Wind Herbs in Berkeley, California and has authored, translated, or co-translated several books on Chinese medicine including *Grasping the Wind, The Clinical Experience of Dr. Shi Neng-Yun, Notes from South Mountain, Fundamentals of Chinese Medicine, Chinese Herbal Medicine: Formulas & Strategies,* and *Handbook of Formulas in Chinese Medicine.*

Craig Mitchell, M.S., PH.D., EAMP, is a graduate of the American College of Traditional Chinese Medicine in San Francisco. He studied Chinese language and medicine in Taiwan for several years, and has written numerous articles and translated several Chinese medical texts including the *Shang Han Lun (On Cold Damage).* He completed his doctoral degree at the China Academy of Chinese Medical Sciences in 2006. He is now President of the Seattle Institute of Oriental Medicine, where he sees patients, supervises in the clinic, and teaches classes on Chinese herbal medicine and medical Chinese. Craig also maintains a private practice in Seattle.

Michael FitzGerald is a graduate of the bilingual program in Traditional Chinese Medicine at the American College of Traditional Chinese Medicine in San Francisco. He spent several years in Taiwan and Beijing furthering his studies, with a focus on fertility, gastroenterology, cardiac illnesses, and dermatology. He is owner of Stone Mountain Medicine Acupuncture and Herbal Pharmacy in Berkeley, California.